Functional Medicine

Editor

ELIZABETH BRADLEY

PHYSICAL MEDICINE AND REHABILITATION CLINICS OF NORTH AMERICA

www.pmr.theclinics.com

Consulting Editor
SANTOS F. MARTINEZ

August 2022 • Volume 33 • Number 3

ELSEVIER

1600 John F. Kennedy Boulevard • Suite 1800 • Philadelphia, Pennsylvania, 19103-2899

http://www.theclinics.com

PHYSICAL MEDICINE AND REHABILITATION CLINICS OF NORTH AMERICA Volume 33, Number 3
August 2022 ISSN 1047-9651, 978-0-323-89702-0

Editor: Megan Ashdown
Developmental Editor: Diana Grace Ang

Reprints. For copies of 100 or more of articles in this publication, please contact the Commercial Reprints
Department, Elsevier Inc., 360 Park Avenue South, New York, NY 10010-1710. Tel.: 212-633-3874; Fax:
212-633-3820; E-mail: reprints@elsevier.com.

Physical Medicine and Rehabilitation Clinics of North America (ISSN 1047-9651) is published quarterly by
Elsevier Inc., 360 Park Avenue South, New York, NY 10010-1710. Months of issue are February, May,
August, and November. Business and Editorial Offices: 1600 John F. Kennedy Blvd., Suite 1800, Philadelphia,
PA 19103-2899. Customer Service Office: 3251 Riverport Lane, Maryland Heights, MO 63043. Periodicals post-
age paid at New York, NY and additional mailing offices. Subscription price per year is $332.00 (US individuals),
$905.00 (US institutions), $100.00 (US students), $377.00 (Canadian individuals), $932.00 (Canadian institutions), $100.00 (Canadian students), $477.00 (foreign individuals), $932.00 (foreign institutions), and $210.00
(foreign students). Foreign air speed delivery is included in all *Clinics* subscription prices. All prices are subject
to change without notice. **POSTMASTER:** Send address changes to *Physical Medicine and Rehabilitation
Clinics of North America*, Customer Service Office: Elsevier Health Sciences Division, Subscription Customer
Service, 3251 Riverport Lane, Maryland Heights, MO 63043. **Customer Service: 1-800-654-2452 (US).
From outside of the United States, call 314-447-8871. Fax: 314-447-8029. E-mail: JournalsCustomer
Service-usa@elsevier.com (for print support); JournalsOnlineSupport-usa@elsevier.com (for online
support).**

Physical Medicine and Rehabilitation Clinics of North America is indexed in *Excerpta Medica, MEDLINE/
PubMed (Index Medicus), Cinahl,* and *Cumulative Index to Nursing and Allied Health Literature.*

Contributors

CONSULTING EDITOR

SANTOS F. MARTINEZ, MD, MS
Physical Medicine and Rehabilitation, Assistant Professor, Department of Orthopaedic Surgery and Biomedical Engineering, University of Tennessee College of Medicine, Campbell Clinic Orthopaedics, Memphis, Tennessee, USA

EDITOR

ELIZABETH BRADLEY, MD, MS
Medical Director, Center for Functional Medicine, Cleveland Clinic, Cleveland, Ohio, USA

AUTHORS

MICHELLE BEIDELSCHIES, PhD
Research and Education Director, Center for Functional Medicine, Assistant Professor of Medicine, Cleveland Clinic Lerner College of Medicine, Cleveland Clinic, Cleveland, Ohio, USA

NAZLEEN BHARMAL, MD, PhD, MPP
Associate Chief of Community Health and Partnerships, Cleveland Clinic Community Care, Cleveland, Ohio, USA

ELIZABETH BRADLEY, MD, MS
Medical Director, Center for Functional Medicine, Cleveland Clinic, Cleveland, Ohio, USA

DAVID CELLA, PhD
Professor and Chair, Department of Medical Social Sciences, Northwestern University Feinberg School of Medicine, Chicago, Illinois, USA

CHRISTOPHER R. D'ADAMO, PhD
Senior Research Advisor, Institute for Functional Medicine, Federal Way, Washington, USA; Assistant Professor, Department of Family and Community Medicine, Director, Center for Integrative Medicine, Department of Epidemiology and Public Health, University of Maryland School of Medicine, East Hall, Baltimore, Maryland, USA

ANNE MARIE FINE, NMD, FAAEM
Medical Director, Environmental Medicine Education International, LLC, Mancos, Colorado, USA

SARA GOTTFRIED, MD
Director of Precision Medicine, Marcus Institute of Integrative Health, Clinical Assistant Professor, Department of Integrative Medicine and Nutritional Sciences, Sidney Kimmel Medical College, Thomas Jefferson University, Philadelphia, Pennsylvania, USA

MARK HYMAN, MD
Pritzker Foundation Chair in Functional Medicine, Cleveland Clinic Lerner College of
Medicine, Founder and Senior Advisor, Cleveland Clinic Center for Functional Medicine,
Lenox, Massachusetts, USA

IRENE KATZAN, MD, MS
Medical Director, Patient-Entered Data, Director, Center for Outcomes Research and
Evaluation, Neurological Institute, Cleveland Clinic, Cleveland, Ohio, USA

DATIS KHARRAZIAN, PhD, DHSc, DC, MMSc
Department of Neurology, Harvard Medical School, Boston, Massachusetts, USA;
Department of Neurology, Massachusetts General Hospital, Charlestown,
Massachusetts, USA; Department of Preventive Medicine, Loma Linda University School
of Medicine, Loma Linda, California, USA

VALTER D. LONGO, PhD
Longevity Institute and Davis School of Gerontology, University of Southern California,
Los Angeles, California, USA; IFOM, FIRC Institute of Molecular Oncology, Milano, Italy

AMRENDRA MISHRA, PhD
Longevity Institute and Davis School of Gerontology, University of Southern California,
Los Angeles, California, USA

SEEMA M. PATEL, MD, MPH
Staff, Center for Functional Medicine, Cleveland Clinic, Center for Functional Medicine
Q-21, Cleveland, Ohio, USA

LYN PATRICK, ND
Educational Director, Environmental Medicine Education International, LLC, Mancos,
Colorado, USA

ALICE PRESCOTT SULLIVAN, DO
Staff Physician, Center for Functional Medicine, Cleveland Clinic, Cleveland, Ohio, USA

TERRY L. WAHLS, MD, IFMCP
Clinical Professor of Medicine, Departments of Internal Medicine, Neurology, and
Epidemiology, University of Iowa, Carver College of Medicine, Iowa City, Iowa, USA

MELISSA C. YOUNG, MD
Staff, Center for Functional Medicine, Cleveland Clinic, Cleveland Ohio, USA Center for
Functional Medicine, Chagrin Falls, Ohio, USA

Contents

Food is not just calories; food is information. Food is a complex array of macronutrients, vitamins, minerals, and phytochemicals that upgrade or downgrade our biological software with every bite. The standard American diet lacks essential nutrients and is rich in refined flour, sugar, and inflammatory oils that drive dysbiosis, metabolic dysfunction, and chronic disease. Modern medicine focuses on diagnosing and treating disease with drugs, not creating health. Functional medicine organizes the body into a network of interconnected systems. It focuses on correcting the underlying functional imbalances that drive disease while restoring health using personalized diet, lifestyle, and nutrition interventions.

The food we eat becomes the basic building blocks of our biology. A poor diet creates poor-functioning cells, tissues, organs, and biological systems and leads to disease. A nutrient-rich whole foods diet does the opposite. Inflammation is a common denominator in most chronic diseases, and our modern-day lifestyle is primarily to blame. An overload of processed foods, sugar, starch, and exposure to toxic chemicals damages our mitochondria, overwhelms our detox organs, creates oxidative stress, hormonal and mood imbalances, cognitive decline, and so much more. Functional Medicine treats disease by removing what is causing damage and providing the body with what it needs to repair itself to regain proper functionality.

Small intestinal bacterial overgrowth (SIBO) can exist in common conditions such as irritable bowel syndrome, obesity, cirrhosis, and Parkinson. Using the functional medicine matrix broadens the lens of how to evaluate SIBO. Assessing the predisposing factors, triggers, and contributors of SIBO enables the provider to better understand possible management strategies. Applying the functional medicine 5R program, remove, replenish, repair, reinoculate, and rebalance includes conventional treatment of SIBO and expands the provider's toolbox on different modalities to restore gut function

Although there is no dietary pattern than has been proven to be effective for reducing the number of relapses or enhancing lesions in patients with multiple sclerosis (MS), several pilot studies have demonstrated the efficacy of dietary plans to reduce MS-related symptoms. Low saturated fat (Swank), low fat vegan (McDougall), modified Paleolithic (Wahls), gluten free, Mediterranean, intermittent fasting, calorie restriction, and intermittent calorie restriction (fasting mimicking diet) all have been associated with reduction of MS-related symptoms such as reduced fatigue, improved mood, and improved quality of life. Mediterranean diet has proven effectiveness for prevention and reduction of comorbid disease severity.

Cardiovascular disease was previously considered a problem for men, despite more women dying annually from cardiovascular causes. As a result of flawed assumptions, clinical research relied on men, leading to biased guidelines and treatment protocols. Emerging evidence demonstrates that women have unique sex and gender differences that must be considered, particularly their cardiometabolic health, in a systems biology framework that can be organized into a functional medicine model of care. Our aim is to help clinicians recognize the value added by functional medicine in the assessment of women vis-à-vis cardiometabolic pathways, phenotypes, and differences in risk compared with men.

Mold toxin exposure by inhalation and ingestion has significant health consequences for humans. In this article, we discuss the sources of these everyday toxins and their relevance to patient health. The effects of mycotoxins can present across all body systems, and the resulting symptoms can be acute, cumulative, and chronic. These effects can occur discretely, but they can also present alongside other clinical entities. It is important for the clinician to recognize the phenomenon of mycotoxin illness, because as a primary cause, it does not resolve with current standards of care for conditions secondary to it.

The functional medicine matrix provides us with an opportunity to understand how social determinants of health (SDOH) and health related social needs may be root causes and contributors to current health and illness among patients. The matrix also allows us to map and recognize the intersectionality of SDOH on exposures and behaviors that influence antecedents, triggers, mediators, lifestyle factors, and clinical imbalances. Incorporating SDOH into clinical evaluations helps uncover and address the complex factors that lead to health disparities in order to provide more optimal patient-centered care.

Michelle Beidelschies, David Cella, Irene Katzan, and Christopher R. D'Adamo

The functional medicine model of care is focused on patient-centered rather than disease-centered care. Patient-centered care incorporates the patient's voice or experience of their condition alongside conventional biological factors to provide a "more complete" account of health. PROMIS Global, an NIH-validated patient-reported outcome (PRO) measure that evaluates the health-related quality of life, can be incorporated within the functional medicine model of care to evaluate self-reported physical, mental and social well-being across various conditions and guide personalized management strategies. Proper incorporation of PROMIS Global into clinical care and research is warranted to expand the available evidence base.

Amrendra Mishra and Valter D. Longo

Worldwide obesity has risen to record levels generating a major risk factor for metabolic syndrome, diabetes, hypertension, and cardiovascular disease as well as cancer and neurodegenerative diseases. Herein, the authors discuss the impact of obesity on life span and cardiometabolic disease in mice and humans and how different types of fasting can help prevent and treat them. The authors argue that specific types of fasting regimens, which are associated with low burden, high long-term compliance, and safety, can reduce obesity and other disease risk factors, lower morbidity, and extend health span.

Anne Marie Fine and Lyn Patrick

Environmental toxicant exposure, according to many researchers in the field, is the leading cause of chronic disease and premature death globally. For the purposes of this review, we will use obesity and type 2 diabetes as examples of toxicant-induced chronic diseases. Endocrine Disrupting chemicals (EDCs) such as phthalates and bisphenols, per- and polyfluoroalkyl substances (PFAS), and persistent organic pollutants (POPs) have been linked to increased risk for obesity and type 2 diabetes in both animal and large epidemiologic studies. These two conditions are well-documented examples of evidence for mechanisms of both adipose metabolism disruption and pancreatic cell dysfunction. The implications for health care directives to both identify, prevent, and treat these exposures are reviewed.

Datis Kharrazian

Neurodegenerative diseases impact more than 6 million Americans, and current predictions estimate the rates of neurodegenerative diseases will double in the next 30 years. These diseases are progressive with increasing loss of brain function throughout their course. Overtime, those suffering from neurodegenerative diseases will lose their ability to work and function efficiently in society. Families and society are burdened with skyrocketing costs to provide care for those who are unable to perform activities of daily living. There is an urgent need to develop treatment strategies to both reduce the incidence of neurodegenerative diseases and to delay the progression of the disease.

PHYSICAL MEDICINE AND REHABILITATION CLINICS OF NORTH AMERICA

SERIES OF RELATED INTEREST

Orthopedic Clinics
https://www.orthopedic.theclinics.com/
Neurologic Clinics
https://www.neurologic.theclinics.com/
Clinics in Sports Medicine
https://www.sportsmed.theclinics.com/

VISIT THE CLINICS ONLINE!
Access your subscription at:
www.theclinics.com

Foreword

Contrarian or Mainstream

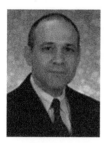

Santos F. Martinez, MD, MS
Consulting Editor

Incorporating Functional Medicine into our *Physical Medicine and Rehabilitation Clinics of North America* series was not a difficult decision. Functional Medicine probably has a different connotation to the Physical Medicine and Rehabilitation (PMR) specialist, as we pride ourselves as experts providing strategies for a wide range of functionally limiting disorders. I would ask the PMR specialist to keep an open mind and allow our fine guests to present useful information that reveals itself as they peel back some of the layers in patient care that we may have lost along the way. Although some may consider this evolving field somewhat of a nonconformist or eccentric anomaly in an RVU-dependent existence, its focus is inherent to all fields of medicine. The use of teamwork to obtain one's optimal potential utilizing a systematic approach to wellness, nutrition, and when appropriate, pharmacologic support seems obvious, but sadly has frequently been forfeited to a more compartmentalized approach for expediency. It is a disappointing observation that with medical expenses reaching 20% of our gross domestic product, many fields, including ours, still do not incorporate some basic care considerations, as everyone thinks the obligation belongs to another subspecialty. A large number of rehabilitation cases (eg, strokes, cardiac disease, vascular- and metabolic-related amputation, some cancers) may be the direct end product and pathologic expression of a number of conditions that Functional Medicine addresses directly.

I could not be more delighted that Dr Bradley took on this task, providing a fresh series of articles written by a lineup of world-class authorities. I am truly indebted to her

Phys Med Rehabil Clin N Am 33 (2022) xi–xii
https://doi.org/10.1016/j.pmr.2022.05.002
1047-9651/22/© 2022 Published by Elsevier Inc.

team for sharing information with what may be a new PMR audience and even more so for our patients who will benefit from this information.

Santos F. Martinez, MD, MS
Physical Medicine and Rehabilitation
Department of Orthopaedic Surgery and
Biomedical Engineering
University of Tennessee College of Medicine
Campbell Clinic Orthopaedics
Memphis, TN 38104, USA

E-mail address:
smartinez@campbellclinic.com

Preface

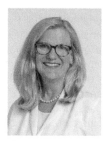

Elizabeth Bradley, MD, MS
Editor

I am honored to dedicate this issue of *Physical Medicine and Rehabilitation Clinics of North America* to Functional Medicine. Nutrition and medicine have been my passion for the past 30 years, and using food as medicine to address chronic disease and individually treat patients is part of the foundational approach of functional medicine.

Chronic disease is crippling our health care system, as it contributes to 1.5 million deaths annually. Recently, the *GAO* (U.S. Government Accountability Office)[1] presented a national strategy to address nutritionally many chronic diseases that are diet related,specifically cardiovascular diseases, cancer, and diabetes. Functional medicine is positioned to use our model to prevent and treat these diseases.

Functional medicine is the science of addressing complex chronic diseases through the functional medicine lens of systems-based biology. Functional medicine looks at each individual to determine the underlying root causes of their unique genomics, nutrition, lifestyle, and environmental influences. Functional medicine starts with a patient's story to develop a timeline while including individual mediators and triggers. Their complete medical history and evaluation are organized in a matrix-like format that involves the following clinical nodes of the matrix: Assimilation, Defense and Repair, Energy, Biotransformation and Elimination, Transport, Communication, and Structural Integrity. The matrix nodes are reviewed in more detail throughout this issue.

Experts in functional medicine address the nodes of the matrix in order to help all professionals use a different lens when evaluating chronic disease. Dr Mark Hyman provides an extensive overview of food as medicine and functional medicine concepts. The gut microbiome and digestive disorders are core to the functional medicine approach, and Dr Seema Patel's review of small intestinal bacterial overgrowth outlines this in detail. Further discussions related to the immune system (defense/repair) with specific dietary interventions are reviewed by Dr Terry Walhs.

Diving deeper into the matrix, this issue also focuses on hormones, inflammation, and mitochondrial health, as in Dr Sara Gottfried's article on Women: Diet, Cardiometabolic Health, and Functional Medicine, Dr Valter Longo's extensive review of intermittent fasting, and Dr Datis Kharrazian's Functional Medicine Approach to Neurodegeneration.

Phys Med Rehabil Clin N Am 33 (2022) xiii–xiv
https://doi.org/10.1016/j.pmr.2022.05.001
1047-9651/22/© 2022 Published by Elsevier Inc.

Environmental toxins influencing chronic disease is a hot topic these days; Dr Alice Prescott's detailed article explores mycotoxins, and Drs Anne Marie Fine and Lyn Patrick give an overview of toxicants and environmental medicine.

Functional medicine provides patient-centered care in both clinical and community settings. Beidelschies et al[2–4] recently demonstrated that functional medicine delivered by way of shared medical appointments (or group appointments) in a clinical setting significantly improved key patient-reported and biometric outcomes beyond those achieved in individual appointments and was less costly to deliver.[4] Dr Nazleen Bharmal reviews the positive health benefits of this care delivery model in a local, community setting. Then, Dr Michelle Beidelschies discusses the value of collecting patient-reported outcomes for clinical and research purposes, and why these outcomes are integral components to delivering functional medicine care.

I would like to thank all the contributing authors, the Institute for Functional Medicine, and my colleagues at the Center for Functional Medicine for advancing functional medicine in clinical, research, and educational settings. I foresee functional medicine being incorporated into every aspect of medical care and easing the burden of chronic diseases in our society.

Elizabeth Bradley, MD, MS
Center for Functional Medicine
Cleveland Clinic
9500 Euclid Avenue, Q-2
Cleveland, OH 44195, USA

E-mail address:
lizbradleymd@gmail.com

REFERENCES

1. United States Government Accountability Office, GAO 100. Highlights of GAO-21-593. Chronic health conditions, https://www.gao.gov/assets/gao-21-593.pdf, 2021, United States Government Accountability Office.
2. Engel G. The need for a new medical model: a challenge for biomedicine. Science 1977;196(4286):129–36.
3. Beidelschies M, Alejandro-Rodriquez M, Xinge J, et al. Association of the functional medicine model of care with patient-reported health quality-of-life outcomes. JAMA Netw Open 2019;2(10):e1914017.
4. Beidelschies M, Alejandro-Rodriquez M, Ning G, et al. Patient outcomes and costs associated with functional medicine-based care in a shared versus individual setting for patients with chronic conditions: a retrospective cohort study. BMJ Open 2021;11:e048294.

Food, Medicine, and Function: Food Is Medicine Part 1

Mark Hyman, MD[a], Elizabeth Bradley, MD[b],*

KEYWORDS

- Functional medicine • Obesity • Diabetes • Chronic disease • Inflammation
- Gut microbiome • Phytochemicals

KEY POINTS

- Food interacts with our genes to promote health or create disease.
- The standard American diet consists of disease-causing foods and lacks protective foods, driving the diabesity and chronic disease epidemic.
- Chronic disease can be reversed by correcting the underlying functional imbalances.
- Functional medicine identifies and treats the root cause of disease using personalized nutrition and lifestyle interventions to give the body what it needs to repair and thrive.
- The gut microbiome can promote health or disease; optimizing the gut flora is critical for preventing, treating, and reversing chronic disease.

What is food? Food is a source of pleasure and sustenance, a cause for gathering with family and community: something associated with happy memories, childhood pleasures, smells, and tastes that connect us to our past and bring joy in the moment. It is all that and more. Eating is the most important, connected act we perform every day: an act that connects us to nature, ecological cycles, our own biological functions and, of course, to each other. We are part of a great web of nature that provides the raw materials for creating a vibrant, alive, healthy life.

We evolved in an intimate relationship to our diet: consuming thousands of species of wild foods, both animals and plants, all interacting with our biology to regulate nearly every function of our bodies.[1] Although food is energy or calories, science has revealed it is far more than that. Food is information. Food is medicine. Food is the most powerful regulator of the biological response modifier in our body. In fact, the most important part of food may not be calories, protein, fat, carbohydrates, fiber, vitamins, or minerals, but the tens of thousands of medicinal compounds embedded in plants and even animal foods.[2] These medicinal compounds are called *phytonutrients*, and they regulate, modulate, and influence nearly every single one of the 37 billion, billion chemical reactions that occur inside our bodies every second.[3]

[a] Cleveland Clinic Lerner College of Medicine, Cleveland Clinic Center for Functional Medicine, 55 Pittsfield Road Suite 9, Lenox, MA 01240, USA; [b] Cleveland Clinic Center for Functional Medicine, 9500 Euclid Avenue, Cleveland, OH 44195, USA
* Corresponding author.
E-mail address: lizbradleymd@gmail.com

Phys Med Rehabil Clin N Am 33 (2022) 553–570
https://doi.org/10.1016/j.pmr.2022.04.001
1047-9651/22/© 2022 Elsevier Inc. All rights reserved.

This process of coevolution could be described as *symbiotic-phytoadaptation*. Our biology has adapted to use the phytochemicals found in food to beneficially influence our biological systems.[4] Through evolution, we have borrowed molecular signaling embedded in foods to optimize our biology.[1] For example, humans cannot synthesize vitamin C or manufacture omega-3 fats.[5,6] Our biology is lazy. We only synthesize what we must make to survive. The rest we get from nature—not just essential fatty acids like omega-3 fats from fish, or essential amino acids from protein, or vitamins and minerals, but what might be called the dark matter of food. The hidden conductor of the symphony of our biology, the 25,000 phytochemicals in the plant kingdom, that to date, have not been deemed essential are now recognized as critical for creating health.[2] Surprisingly, they are also found in animals, such as grass-fed beef, consuming a wide array of nutrient-dense plant foods.[7] Although the deficiency of these components may not result in acute deficiency diseases like scurvy, rickets, and protein malnutrition, they do produce long-latency deficiency diseases, what we call chronic illness—heart disease, diabetes, hypertension, obesity, dementia, depression, and more.[4,8,9]

In plant and animal foods exist a wide array of molecules that influence every aspect of our biology: protein, fats, carbohydrates, vitamins, minerals, soluble, insoluble, and resistant fibers, prebiotics, probiotics, vitamins and minerals, antioxidants, phytochemicals, and even microRNA, and the genetic material of plants, which we absorb and which communicate with our own DNA.[1] Foods are not made of ingredients but of complex array of compounds all dynamically influencing our biology with every bite.[1,4,7–9]

OUR STANDARD AMERICAN DIET

The standard American diet (SAD) is over 60% ultra-processed food,[10] mostly from commodity crops—wheat,[11] corn,[12] and soy.[13] These three crops are turned into hundreds of thousands of food-like products, which bear little resemblance to our evolutionary diet. Those who eat the most of these addictive foods are the most obese and sick.[14] This nutrient depleted diet not only makes us obese and sick but also drives us to consume more and more "food-like substances" looking for the missing nutrients, such as iron-deficient children with pica who eat dirt.[15] Only 11% of our diet is nuts, seeds, fruits, vegetables, whole grains, and beans.[16] Only 3% of our cropland is used to grow fruits, vegetables, and nuts.[17] Destructive agricultural techniques have destroyed our soil where plants get their nutrients.[18–20] Certain fruits and vegetables, such as broccoli, have over 40% less nutrients than they did over 50 years ago.[21,22] Today, our vegetables have been bred for yield, starch content, disease resistance, drought, shape, shelf stability, and hardiness for transport,[18–22] not for flavor, nutrient density, or phytochemical richness. Consider the difference in taste between a store-bought cardboard like perfect looking tomato in the middle of winter, then try an organic, heirloom tomato picked from the vine in late August.

Our SAD diet is nutritionally limited, and the abundance of disease-causing foods and lack of protective foods drives obesity and disease.[8–16] Globally, more than half of our calories come from three crops—wheat, corn, and rice.[23] There are about 6000 cultivated edible plant species, yet nearly all crop production comes from just nine species (sugar cane, maize, rice, wheat, potatoes, soybeans, oil-palm fruit, sugar beet, and cassava).[24] Most of those foods are the raw materials for the food industry to produce highly processed, disease-promoting foods and are not eaten in their original form.

WHY QUALITY MATTERS

The most important factor to consider when choosing what to eat is quality, which also brings along flavor, nutrient density, and phytochemical richness.[4,7–9] Meat is so much more than protein. Does feedlot beef affect our biology in the same way as wild elk? Do wild dandelion greens differ from iceberg lettuce? Is highly refined hybrid gluten rich white bread the same as heirloom whole kernel German rye bread? Is shortening different from fats found in sardines? All are meat, vegetables, grains, or fats. Calorie for calorie, gram for gram of protein, and carbs or fat they are the same. However, each has profoundly different effects on human biology.

There are major differences within the categories of protein, fat, and carbohydrate. Protein from plants is limited in key amino acids and requires combining different plants (grains, beans, nuts, seeds) to have adequate protein to build muscle.[25,26] It also requires us to consume much more volume (which comes with more calories and starch).[27] Animal protein is more nutrient dense, bioavailable, and better able to build muscle.[28] Plant proteins have "antinutritional factors" like tannins which may inhibit absorption of nutrients and amino acids, reducing the availability of amino acids needed for building new protein in the body.[29] Dietary fats are infinitely more complex—monounsaturated, polyunsaturated omega-3 and omega-6 fats, and saturated fats (and there are 10 types of saturated fats each with different effects on our biology). Carbohydrates are clearly very different across the board. Asparagus is a carbohydrate and so is a bowl of sugar. Are they the same when we eat them? Obviously not. Even fibers are different, some are simply inert indigestible roughage like cellulose and others preferentially feed the good microbes in our gut, which benefit our overall health. So, simply focusing on ratios or percentages of protein, fat, carbohydrate, and fiber in the diet is not helpful.

What is the quality of the food? What other compounds are included with that food or removed from it? How was it grown, in what soil, in what environment, when was it picked? For example, some areas of China have low selenium levels in the soil, whereas other areas high levels.[30] In the regions with high selenium, the cure rate for COVID-19 was three times higher than the areas with the lowest levels of selenium.[31] The death rate in the low-selenium areas was five times higher.[31] Tibetan doctors go to medical school for 11 years and spend summers high in the Himalayas studying plant medicine. The same plants grow in different environments or picked at different seasons can have profoundly different medical benefits.

THE MEDICINAL MAGIC OF PLANTS (AND ANIMALS)

But why do plants have these compounds in the first place? How does it benefit them? They likely don't make them for our benefit, despite the fact that we hijack them for our own purposes. The 25,000 + phytochemicals found in the edible plant kingdom are the plants messaging system, a means of protection, defense, and survival.[2,29] These compounds deter pests, prevent them being eaten,[32] and even communicate messages to other plants, animals, and even the trillions of microbes and fungi within the soil.[33] These compounds proclaiming themselves through their bright colors are antioxidants, anti-inflammatory, detoxifying, anticancer, and disease fighting (**Table 1**).[4]

We should all eat the rainbow of colors on a regular basis including a multitude of spices—concentrated sources of beneficial phytonutrients.[4] We have bred these protective chemicals out of most of our foods. A wild strawberry is an explosion of flavor and phytochemicals. A store bought, large, starchy, conventional strawberry is mealy, tasteless and limited in phytochemicals.[34] It is the phytochemical richness of plants that drives flavor. The total flavonoid content of purple corn is 25% greater than our modern yellow-hued corn on the cob,[35] purple potatoes have 1200% more than white potatoes,[36] and red oak leaf lettuce has 10 times more total flavonoids than iceberg lettuce.[37]

Table 1
Color of fruits and vegetables, select phytochemicals, and physiologic effects

Color	Fruits	Vegetables	Select Phytochemicals	Physiologic Effects
Red	Apples; blood oranges; cherries; cranberries; lingonberries; nectarines; pink grapefruit; pomegranate; raspberries; redcurrants; red pears; red plums; strawberries; watermelon	Radicchio; radishes; red beets; red bell peppers; red cabbage; red chard; red jalapeño pepper; red onion; red potatoes; tomatoes	Anthocyanins; carotenoids; ellagic acid; elagitannins; fisetin; flavones; lycopene; phloretin; quercetin	1. Anti-inflammatory 2. General antioxidant activity 3. Immune modulation
Orange	Apricots; blood oranges; cantaloupe; kumquat; mandarins; mangoes; nectarines; oranges; papaya; passion fruit; peaches; persimmons; tangerines	Carrots; orange bell peppers; pumpkin; sweet potatoes; turmeric yams	Alpha-carotene; beta-carotene; beta-cryptoxanthin; bioflavonoids; carotenoids; curcuminoids	1. Antioxidant for fat-soluble tissues; 2. endocrine modulation; and 3. role in ovulation and fertility processes
Yellow	Apples (golden delicious); Asian pears; bananas; lemon; pineapple; star fruit	Corn; ginger; potatoes (Yukon); squash (acorn, buttercup, butternut, summer, winter); yellow bell peppers; yellow onions	Bioflavonoids; bromelain; Gingerol; lutein; nobiletin; prebiotic fibers; rutin; zeaxanthin	1. Antioxidant; 2. enzymatic activity; 3. gastric motility and regulation; 4. reduce glycemic impact; and 5. role in fostering a healthy gut microbiome
Green	Avocado; Brussels sprouts; green tea; green apples; limes; olives; pears	Artichokes; asparagus; bamboo sprouts; bean sprouts; bell peppers; bitter melon; bok choy; broccoli; broccolini; cabbage; celery; cucumbers; edamame; green beans; green peas; greens (beet, chard, collards, dandelion, kale, lettuce, mustard, spinach, turnip); okra; rosemary and other herbs; snow peas; watercress	Catechins; chlorogenic acid; chlorophyll; epigallocatechin gallate; flavonoids; folates; glucosinolates; isoflavones; isothiocyanates; L-theanine; nitrates; oleocanthal; oleuropein; phytosterols; silymarin; sulforaphane; tannins; theaflavins; tyrosol; vitexin	1. Antioxidant; 2. blood vessel support; 3. role in healthy circulation and methylation
Blue-purple	Blackberries; blueberries; boysenberries; figs; huckleberries; prunes; purple grapes; raisins	Eggplant; plums; purple bell peppers; purple cabbage; purple carrots; purple cauliflower; purple kale; purple potatoes	Anthocyanidins; flavonoids, Phenolic acids, Proanthocyanidins, Pterostilbene, Resveratrol, Stilbenes	1. Antioxidant; 2. Cognitive support; 3. Healthy mood balance; 4. Role in neuronal health

From Minich DM. A review of the science of colorful, plant-based food and practical strategies for "eating the rainbow". J Nutr Metab 2019;19; with permission.

Even animal foods can contain phytonutrients. Animals, when given the freedom to self-select their diet, seek out a wide variety of plants for their nutrient value and medicinal compounds. These compounds end up in the meat.[38] Some plants may have more selenium, others contain more anti-inflammatory phytochemicals, and some even contain compounds that reduce methane production.[39] Grass fed or regeneratively raised cows grow much faster (as fast as a feed lot cow) when given the chance to graze on diverse tannin-containing legumes than when just grazing on one type of grass.[40,41] Remarkable research has found a wide array of medicinal plant compounds in the flesh of grass fed and wild animals that improve human health.[7,38] For example, goat's milk from goats allowed to forage on wild shrubs contains more catechins (the anti-inflammatory, detoxifying, anticancer compounds found in green tea) per 100 mL[42] than the same exact volume as brewed green tea.[43]

It is not only what we eat that matters. It is whatever we are eating ate. If plants are grown in soil rich in microbial life necessary to extract nutrients from soil for the plant, if they are grown without agrochemicals, if they are from seeds designed for flavor (which always is driven by the phytochemical richness of the plant), and if they are picked ripe and eaten soon after harvest and not transported over long distances we will be eating a cornucopia of nutrients and plant medicines.[44–48] When seeds are bred for flavor, not size or starch or the ability to be stacked neatly in a box for shipping, the side effect is extraordinary tasting medicinal foods. If we eat industrial food, even vegetables, our diet will be depleted.[49] If we are eating a factory-farmed cow fed a simplified diet of low-quality grains,[50] chicken excrement,[51] and candy,[52] ground-up animal parts the meat will be inflammatory and disease producing[50] but not if we eat a wild elk or regeneratively raised beef foraging on dozens of medical plants.

The consequences for our health have been disastrous. Our focus on the production of abundant calories to feed a hungry world with industrial agriculture had led to far too many starchy, sugary calories with almost no nutrients, and even less phytonutrients.[53] The result—2.1 billion overweight in the world[54] and chronic diseases, mostly caused by poor diet, now accounting for 71% of all global deaths.[55] Eleven million people die every year from poor diet—an overabundance of ultra-processed foods and lack of protective foods, making diet the number one cause of global deaths, exceeding smoking.[56] It also accounts for depression,[57] disability,[58] and economic stress for hundreds of millions (maybe billions) worldwide.[59] The greatest discovery of the last 50 years is that food is medicine with the power to prevent, treat, and even reverse most chronic disease and quickly.[60,61] A discovery mostly ignored by medicine.[62] We are literally upgrading or downgrading our biological software with every bite. The question is how does it work? Functional medicine is an approach for disease treatment and health creation that incorporates this new understanding of food as medicine. What we put at the end of our fork is more powerful than almost anything we will ever find in a prescription bottle. It works faster, better, and cheaper, and all the side effects are good ones.

FUNCTIONAL MEDICINE: THE SCIENCE OF CREATING HEALTH

What is functional medicine? It is the science of creating health. It is the application of the latest advances in science redefining health and disease—the science of systems medicine or network medicine.[63,64] The body is a biological ecosystem, a network of dynamically interacting, interconnected biological systems, not the usual ones we think of such as the cardiovascular, respiratory or neurologic system. The paradigm shift is from a reductionist to a systems view of health and disease. Rather than the 155,000 diseases in the ICD-10, there are seven core physiologic systems that underlie nearly all disease which results from imbalances in those systems.[65,66] Functional medicine focuses on restoring health in the system, not just treating the symptoms. Functional medicine is also the best expression of personalized medicine and nutrition, precision medicine and nutrition.[60–66]

Modern medicine is focused on diagnosis and treatment of disease. The goal is to diagnose diseases based on symptoms and geography. If a patient presents with pain and inflammation in certain joints, a positive rheumatoid factor, anti-CCP antibodies, an elevated sedimentation rate laboratory tests, and articular erosions or deformity on radiograph, we give a diagnosis of rheumatoid arthritis (RA). That is the end of thinking. We name the disease and the patient is told that RA is the cause of their joint pain. It is not the cause, but simply the name. The causes could be anything that causes inflammation—Lyme disease, gluten, increased intestinal permeability, *Entamoeba histolytica*, environmental toxins, or mercury; for example, naming the disease tells us nothing about the cause. We typically treat the downstream symptoms instead of the upstream causes. We know RA is an inflammatory disease. The solution? Powerful drugs including steroids, chemotherapy drugs, and biologics that suppress inflammation all with significant side effects.

A better approach is to diagnose and address the cause. If gluten is the cause stop eating it. If a leaky gut is the cause, fix it. If Lyme disease is the cause, treat it. No two patients are the same, even if they have the same diagnosis. All may cause RA, and each requires a very different treatment. The roadmap we have for disease is wrong. We need a new map. Functional medicine is that map.

The best example of a discovery that completely disrupts our old notion of disease is the microbiome. Something that was not even discussed or even named as factor in medicine until 20 years ago.[67] The microbiome breaks the old notion of single cause, single disease, and single drug model inherited from Louis Pasteur—pneumococcal bacteria cause pneumonia and is cured with penicillin.

However, how can that model explain how changes in our microbiome are linked to cancer,[68] heart disease,[69] obesity,[70] diabetes,[71] autism,[72] depression,[73] dementia,[74] asthma,[75] fibromyalgia,[76] autoimmune disease,[77] allergies,[78] skin disorders,[79] and much more? How does it explain the fact that transplanting the stool from a healthy child into autistic kids improves their autism?[80] Or that transplanting stool from a thin person to a person with metabolic syndrome reverses insulin resistance?[81] It cannot. We need a different model to explain these new discoveries. Just as Einstein turned physics upside and challenged Newton's paradigm, so too functional medicine overturns our outdated understanding of biology, human health, and disease.

Functional medicine focuses on the root cause. The approach to restoring health is simple. Remove and address the triggers and root cause of disease and add the ingredients for health. The body's natural intelligence and healing mechanisms do the rest. We start with removing the cause (or causes), and then replacing what the body needs to thrive. There are only a few causes that result in almost all diseases (other than dominant inherited genetic diseases like Down's syndrome); toxins (both internal and external such as pesticides, herbicides, plastics, heavy metals, and more); allergens (environmental and food); microbes (bacteria, viruses, parasites, worms, ticks, including imbalances in the microbiome); and poor diet and stress (physical or psychological).[82] These triggers of disease interact with our genes and all seven basic biological networks.[83] In addition to the triggers of disease, there are necessary ingredients for health—real food, nutrients, hormones, light, water, air, rest, rhythm, sleep, movement, love, connection, meaning and purpose. These are the raw materials, each needed in proper balance, different for each individual, to create a healthy human. Disease occurs when we have too many triggers and not enough of the right ingredients. Creating health is simply a matter of identifying and removing the triggers and replacing the necessary ingredients for health.

So, what does food have to do with any of this? Food, it turns out is the biggest driver of imbalances in our biological networks, and the biggest lever for rapid change, reversal of disease and creation of health. Dramatic improvements in health outcomes result from applying the latest advances in understanding systems and network medicine. Autoimmune diseases remit,[84,85] depression and anxiety subside,[86] migraines end,[87] children with autism improve speech and function,[88] psoriasis and eczema improve,[89,90] Alzheimer's patients improve their memory,[91,92] and type 2 diabetics often go into remission.[93] These are not anomalies or spontaneous remissions, but reproducible results based on applying food as medicine with the model of functional medicine.

How does food work to change disease, to create health? There is no other activity that has more power to change our biology than diet. We ingest pounds of foreign material into our body daily. If all calories were the same, it would not matter what we eat, but they are not. Food carries information molecules, instructions, and code that programs our biology with every bite for better or worse. Industrial food drives inflammation,[94] imbalances in hormones,[95] brain chemistry changes,[96] damages our microbiome,[97] and changes our gene expression to turn on disease causing genes.[95] Real whole nutrient and phytonutrient rich food does the opposite. It turns off inflammation, increases antioxidant systems,[4-9] balances hormones and brain chemistry,[83-93,95,96] optimizes the microbiome,[98] and turns on disease preventing, health-promoting genes.[95]

HOW IS THE BODY ORGANIZED?

Sadly, it is not organized by medical specialties, despite our medical training. What drives all disease imbalances in the fundamental networks underlying disease, networks that are all dynamically interacting every moment with our lifestyle, disease triggers, and genes.[99]

Nearly everyone one of the 155,000 diseases listed in the disease classification system known as ICD-10 is caused by imbalances in seven interconnected systems. Fix those systems and we do not have to treat the actual disease directly.[63-66]

What are those systems? (**Fig. 1**)

1. Assimilation (digestion, absorption, microbiome, digestive system, respiration)
2. Defense and repair (immune, inflammation, infections, microbiota)
3. Energy (energy regulation, mitochondrial function)
4. Biotransformation and elimination (toxicity, detoxification)
5. Transport (cardiovascular, lymphatic system)
6. Communication (endocrine, neurotransmitters, immune messengers)
7. Structural integrity (from subcellular membranes to musculoskeletal structure)

Although all of the triggers of disease noted above (toxins, allergens, microbes, poor diet, and stress) and all the ingredients for health (food, nutrients, hormones, air, water, light, rest, rhythm, movement, sleep, love, connection, meaning, and purpose) impact these networks to create balance or imbalance, by far the biggest regulator of all these networks is food. Common links between many seemingly separate diseases are now clear—inflammation, oxidative stress and loss of cellular energy and mitochondrial dysfunction, toxic overload and impaired detoxification, imbalances in the microbiome, hormonal, and cell-signaling imbalances and structural imbalances (such as sarcopenia)—changes in our cells, tissues, muscles, and bones that promote disease. What do Alzheimer's, autism, cancer, diabetes, depression, autoimmune disease,

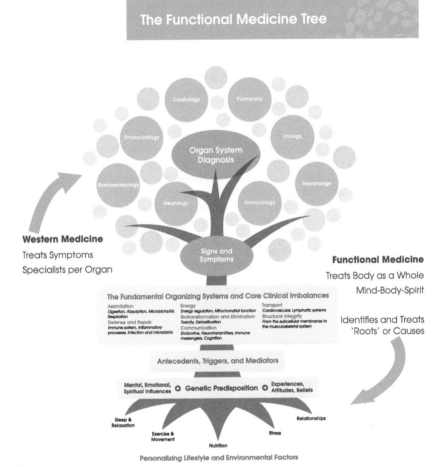

Fig. 1. The Institute for Functional Medicine (IFM) Functional Medicine Tree. Imbalances in the seven biological systems (trunk) lead to symptoms and diseases (branches and leaves). Western Medicine addresses the symptoms. Functional medicine addresses the root cause (diet, environment, genetics, and lifestyle factors) that predisposes an individual to disease. (*Used with permission from* The Institute for Functional Medicine (IFM), the global leader in Functional Medicine)

heart disease, allergies, asthma, skin conditions, and obesity have in common—inflammation, oxidative stress, imbalances in the microbiome, and often toxic overload and imbalances in cell messengers.[68–79] Rather than treating all these diseases as distinct entities, the focus is on uncovering the root causes for each person. Ten kids with autism, or 10 patients with RA, or 10 patients with heart disease may each have different causes and need different treatments. Today, we prescribe treatments based on the diagnosis not usually the cause. Once we get a diagnosis thinking often stops and standard of care is applied for any specific condition. Most chronic disease is at best managed but not cured and the treatments often have serious side effects. Food and its myriad components from amino acids, fatty acids, carbohydrates, fibers, vitamins, minerals, and phytochemicals are the natural ligands for cell receptors that are the targets of pharmaceuticals, but without adverse side effects. By focusing on restoring balance in the basic biological networks of our body, diseases often improve or resolve.[64]

Food is the biggest lever to impact all these systems. The wrong food harms each system and the right food helps optimize each system. The right food regulates the health of our microbiome, our immune system, reduces levels of inflammation, oxidative stress, and improves our mitochondrial function.[100] Food balances our hormones and brain chemistry, supports detoxification, and improves the function and health of our circulatory systems, and even provides the raw materials for every cell, muscle, tissue, organ, and bone in our body.[101–103]

We will explore how food influences each of these networks, this network of networks.

FOOD THROUGH THE LENS OF FUNCTIONAL MEDICINE

Food interacts with each of our biological networks, the seven systems at the root of all health and disease. How actually does food interact with our biology specifically?

FOOD AND OUR GUT

The microbiome, the extraordinary kingdom of microbes living in us, may be the most important organ in the body orchestrating every function of our biology. Bacteria in our microbiome outnumber our own cells 10 to one.[104] Bacterial genes outnumber our own genes 100 to one.[105] Genes make proteins and metabolites. There may be more metabolites from microbes in our bloodstream than our own human metabolites. Every metabolic and chemical reaction in our body is called the metabolome, but there is also a metabolome of the microbiome.[106] Much of its function is yet to be discovered. An unhealthy microbiome can cause heart disease, cancer, diabetes, obesity, autism, autoimmunity, dementia, allergies, asthma, fibromyalgia, Parkinson's, skin disorders like acne, asthma, eczema, and psoriasis,[68–79,107] not to mention all the digestive disorders including irritable bowel, reflux, or colitis.[108] And, it can also heal those conditions. They key is learning to optimize the microbiome.

FOOD IS MEDICINE: HOW THE GUT IS HARMED

Just as right foods keep our inner garden healthy, the wrong foods create havoc, often feeding the unwanted potentially pathogenic bacteria. These pathogenic bacteria drive inflammation and contribute to intestinal permeability.[109] A great example is breast milk versus formula. Breast milk contains oligosaccharides that are indigestible for humans. Their role is simply to feed the baby's microbiome, particularly *Bifidobacterium infantis*.[110] It is food for the microbiome that produces the critical short-chain fatty acid, butyrate, the main source of energy for the intestinal epithelium and regulates immunity and inhibits oncogenes.[111] Formula does not contain oligosaccharides, and the sugars in formula fertilize bacteria that produce propionic acid.[112] This compound causes brain inflammation, oxidative stress, impairs detoxification systems, and damages the mitochondria all which are found in autism.[113] Autism can be induced in rat models simply by giving intrathecal propionic acid. Omega-3 fats and vitamin B12 help reduce the effects of propionic acid on the brain and autism.[114]

Dysbiotic bacteria grow for two reasons: first, not eating enough of the foods that feed the beneficial flora and eating too many foods that feed pathogenic bacteria. Gluten and dysbiosis are the most significant cause of increased intestinal permeability. Wheat contains inflammatory proteins called gliadin that increases zonulin, which in turn increases intestinal permeability.[115,116] Even in those who are not gluten-sensitive, eating a lot of gluten tends to disrupt gut function, not to mention that most wheat today is sprayed with the weed killer, glyphosate, at harvest to dry it out.[117,118] Our morning Cheerios has more glyphosate than vitamins B12 and D which are actually added to the cereal.[119] Why is that bad? Aside from being a known carcinogen, glyphosate destroys our microbiome.[120] Starch and sugar promote overgrowth of toxic bacteria and yeast and often lead to SIBO or small intestinal bacterial overgrowth and SIFO, small intestinal fungal overgrowth.[121,122] Different fats also have different impacts on the gut. Soybean oil, a refined omega-6 seed oil that runs rampant in the SAD, has increased 1000-fold over the past 100 years.[123] Soybean oil, among other industrialized vegetable seed oils, triggers metabolic endotoxemia.[124] Our metabolism is affected by toxic byproducts of certain bacteria, endotoxins known as lipopolysaccharides, triggering tumor necrosis factor alpha and cytokine production worsening insulin resistance, leading to obesity and type 2 diabetes.[125] Omega-3 fats do the opposite.[6]

Additives, thickeners, and emulsifiers in most processed food including carrageenan and gums also adversely affect the microbiome and intestinal permeability and have been linked to autoimmune diseases.[126] Medications are another driver of dysbiosis especially proton pump inhibitors to treat reflux. These medications not only prevent the absorption of calcium, vitamin B12, iron, zinc, and magnesium but also lead to overgrowth of bugs in our small intestine and irritable bowel.[127–129] Other drugs either trigger overgrowth of dysbiotic bacteria, and yeast or increase intestinal permeability including antibiotics, steroids, hormones, birth control, NSAIDS, and aspirin.[130]

FOOD IS MEDICINE: GUT-HEALING FOODS

With every bite we are feeding our microbiome. Fertilizing either symbiotic or dysbiotic flora. The gut is responsible for digesting and absorbing the raw materials from food (amino acids, sugars, fats, vitamins, mineral, phytochemicals, and even beneficial microbial metabolites). It is also the main location of 70% of our immune system.[131] It is the first line of defense forming a barrier between the inside of our gut (basically a tube that is outside of us filled with bacteria and foreign food proteins). It can break down for many of the reasons noted above resulting in increased intestinal permeability. Food and bacterial toxins are absorbed driving inflammation throughout the body. All those diseases noted above are inflammatory diseases. The right flora and the right food help keep that barrier intact, and the wrong flora and foods break it down.[132]

How do we feed the good flora? Fiber is critical. Certain foods have high levels of prebiotic fiber-artichokes, asparagus, Jerusalem artichokes, plantains, seaweed, and more. Any fiber-rich foods help keep the flora healthy—vegetables, fruits, nuts, seeds, whole grains, and beans. Probiotic-rich foods also help support a healthy gut, traditional fermented foods such as sauerkraut, pickles, tempeh, miso, natto, and kimchi. Polish women eat 30 pounds of sauerkraut a year in Poland. When they move to the United States, they stop eating it. Polish women in the United States have dramatically higher rates of breast cancer than their cousins in Poland consuming kraut.[133] Some of the exciting discoveries around the microbiome involve the role of polyphenols, the colorful phytonutrients found in plants. The good flora feed on them and, in turn, those bugs protect us. For example, *Akkermansia mucinophilia* is fueled by cranberry, pomegranate, green tea, and other polyphenols.[134] When it is in abundance, it creates a protective layer in the gut preventing a leaky gut, autoimmune disease, and even heart disease and diabetes.[135–137] This bacterium is also necessary for certain cancer treatments to work, such as immunotherapy.[138]

Our gut also needs other nutrients to function well. Zinc from pumpkin seeds and oysters is necessary for digestive enzyme function. Omega-3 fats from fish such as sardines or herring are needed to regulate inflammation and heal a leaky gut. Vitamin D from small, cold-water fish, egg yolks, and the sun is also necessary for gut healing. Foods with L-glutamine such as bone broth, containing *glycosaminoglycans*, also help heal the gut.[139] Kudzu, a Japanese root, is a powerful gut-soothing food.[140]

Food is the most important regulator of our microbiome. Children in Africa eating traditional diets have a healthy microbiome. Kids in Europe have modern gut busting diets and unhealthy microbiomes resulting in more disease.[141] We do not just eat for our own health, but the health of our microbiome.

DISCLOSURE

This project received no funding. Dr Mark Hyman is the owner of Hyman Digital, a health information company. He is the author of numerous books on food and nutrition that receive royalties and the host of *The Doctor's Farmacy*, a podcast that earns income from advertising in the food and health space.

REFERENCES

1. Stover PJ, Caudill MA. Genetic and epigenetic contributions to human nutrition and health: managing genome-diet interactions. J Am Diet Assoc 2008;108(9): 1480–7.

2. Carlsen MH, Halvorsen BL, Holte K, et al. The total antioxidant content of more than 3100 foods, beverages, spices, herbs and supplements used worldwide. BMC Nutr 2010;9:3.

3. Rodriguez A. The encounter. In: Wall street international. 2021. Available at: https://wsimag.com/feature/65608-the-encounter. Accessed November 13, 2021.

4. Minich DM. A review of the science of colorful, plant-based food and practical strategies for "eating the rainbow". J Nutr Metab 2019;19:1–19.

5. National Institute of Health Office of Dietary Supplements. Vitamin C. In: NIH ODS. 2021. Available at: https://ods.od.nih.gov/factsheets/VitaminC-Health Professional/. Accessed October 30, 2021.

6. National Institute of Health Office of Dietary Supplements. Omega-3 Fatty Acids. In: NIH ODS. 2021. Available at: https://ods.od.nih.gov/factsheets/Omega3 FattyAcids-HealthProfessional/. Accessed October 30, 2021.

7. Van Elswyk ME, McNeill SH. Impact of grass/forage feeding versus grain finishing on beef nutrients and sensory quality: the U.S. experience. Meat Sci 2014; 96(1):535–40.

8. Liu RH. Health-promoting components of fruits and vegetables in the diet. Adv Nutr 2013;4(3):384S-92S.

9. Liu RH. Dietary bioactive compounds and their health implications. J Food Sci 2013;78(1):A18–25.

10. Steele EM, Baraldi LG, Louzada ML, et al. Ultra-processed foods and added sugars in the US diet: evidence from a nationally representative cross-sectional study. BMJ Open 2016;6(3):1–8.

11. Economic Research Service U.S. Department of Agriculture. Wheat. In: ERS U.S. Department of agriculture. 2021. Available at: https://www.ers.usda.gov/topics/crops/wheat/. Accessed October 30, 2021.

12. Economic Research Service U.S. Department of Agriculture. Corn & other feed-grains. In: ERS USDA. 2021. Available at: https://www.ers.usda.gov/topics/crops/corn-and-other-feedgrains/. Accessed October 30, 2021.

13. Economic Research Service U.S. Department of Agriculture. Soybean & oil crops overview. In: ERS USDA. 2021. Available at: https://www.ers.usda.gov/topics/crops/soybeans-oil-crops/. Accessed October 30, 2021.

14. Elizabeth L, Machado P, Zinöcker M, et al. Ultra-processed foods and health outcomes: a narrative review. Nutrients 2020;12(7):1955.

15. Schulte EM, Avena NM, Gearhardt AN. Which foods may be addictive? The roles of processing, fat content, and glycemic load. PLoS One 2015;10(2):1–18.

16. Shan Z, Rehm CD, Rogers G, et al. Trends in dietary carbohydrate, protein, and fat intake and diet quality among US adults, 1999-2016. JAMA 2019;322(12):1178–87.

17. Mulik K, O'Hara JK. The healthy farmland diet. In: Union of concerned scientists reports & multimedia. 2013. Available at: https://www.ucsusa.org/resources/healthy-farmland-diet#ucs-report-downloads. Accessed November 8, 2021.

18. Jones DL, Cross P, Withers PA, et al. Review: nutrient stripping: the global disparity between food security and soil nutrient stocks. J Appl Ecol 2013;50:851–62.

19. Mayer AM. Historical changes in the mineral content of fruits and vegetables. Br Food J 1997;99(6):207–11.

20. Davis DR, Epp MD, Riordan HD. Changes in USDA food composition data for 43 garden crops, 1950 to 1999. J Am Coll Nutr 2004;23(6):669–82.

21. Farnham MW, Grusak MA, Wang M. Calcium and magnesium concentration of inbred and hybrid broccoli heads. J Amer Hort Sci 2000;125(3):344–9.

22. Davis DR. Declining fruit and vegetable nutrient composition: what is the evidence? J Am Soc Hortic Sci 2009;44(1):15–9.

23. Awika JM. Major cereal grains production and use around the world. In: Awika JM, Piironen V, Bean S, editors. Advances in cereal science: implications to food processing and health promotion1089. Washington, DC: American Chemical Society; 2011. p. 1–13.

24. Piling D, Bartley D, Baumung R, et al. The status and trends of biodiversity for food and agriculture. In: Bélanger J, Pilling D, editors. FAO Commission on genetic resources for food and agriculture. Rome: Food and Agriculture Organization; 2019. p. 113–87.

25. Berrazaga I, Micard V, Gueugneau M, et al. The role of the anabolic properties of plant- versus animal-based protein sources in supporting muscle mass maintenance: a critical review. Nutrients 2019;11(8):1825.

26. Mariotti F, Gardner CD. Dietary protein and amino acids in vegetarian diets-a review. Nutrients 2019;11(11):2661.

27. Gorissen SH, Horstman AM, Franssen R, et al. Ingestion of wheat protein increases in vivo muscle protein synthesis rates in healthy older men in a randomized trial. J Nutr 2016;146(9):1651–9.

28. Van Vliet S, Burd NA, Loon LJ. The skeletal muscle anabolic response to plant-versus animal-based protein consumption. J Nutr 2015;145(9):1981–91.

29. Sarwar G, Wu C, Cockell K. Impact of antinutritional factors in food proteins on the digestibility of protein and the bioavailability of amino acids and on protein quality. BJN 2012;108(2):315–32.

30. Sun GX, Meharg A, Li G, et al. Distribution of soil selenium in China is potentially controlled by deposition and volatilization? Sci Rep 2016;6:20953.

31. Zhang J, Taylor EW, Bennett K, et al. Association between regional selenium status and reported outcome of COVID-19 cases in China. Am J Clin Nutr 2020; 111(6):1297–9.
32. Stiller A, Garrison K, Gurdyumov K, et al. From fighting critters to saving lives: polyphenols in plant defense and human health. Intl J Mol Sci 2021;22(16):8995.
33. Witzany G. Plant communication from biosemiotic perspective. Plant Signal Behav 2006;1(4):169–78.
34. Najda A, Dyduch-Siemińska M, Dyduch J, et al. Comparative analysis of secondary metabolites contents in Fragaria vesca L. fruits. Ann Agric Environ Med 2014;21(2):339–43.
35. Lao F, Sigurdson GT, Giusti MM. Health benefits of purple corn (*Zea mays* L.) phenolic compounds. Comp Rev Food Sci Food Saf 2017;16(2):234–46.
36. Park SY, Lee SY, Yang JW, et al. Comparative analysis of phytochemicals and polar metabolites from colored sweet potato (*Ipomoea batatas* L.) tubers. Food Sci Biotechnol 2016;25(1):283–91.
37. Gan YZ, Azrina A. Antioxidant properties of selected varieties of lettuce *(Lactuca sativa* L.) commercially available in Malaysia. Int Food Res 2016;23(6): 2357–62.
38. Van Vliet S, Provenza FD, Kronberg SL. Health-promoting phytonutrients are higher in grass-fed meat and milk. Front Sustain Food Syst 2021;4:299.
39. Ku-Vera JC, Jiménez-Ocampo R, Valencia-Salazar S, et al. Role of secondary plant metabolites on enteric methane mitigation in ruminants. Front Vet Sci 2020;7:584.
40. Lagrange SP, MacAdam JW, Villalba JJ. The use of temperate tannin containing forage legumes to improve sustainability in forage–livestock production. Agronomy 2021;11(11):2264.
41. MacAdam JW, Villalba JJ. Beneficial effects of temperate forage legumes that contain condensed tannins. Agriculture 2015;5(3):475–91.
42. Delgadillo-Puga C, Cuchillo-Hilario M, León-Ortiz L, et al. Goats' feeding supplementation with *Acacia farnesiana* pods and their relationship with milk composition: fatty Acids, polyphenols, and antioxidant activity. Animals 2019; 9(8):515.
43. Rains TM, Agarwal S, Maki KC. Antiobesity effects of green tea catechins: a mechanistic review. J Nutr Biochem 2011;22(1):1–7.
44. Montgomery DR, Biklé A. Soil health and nutrient density: beyond organic vs. conventional farming. Front Sustain Food Syst 2021.
45. Managa MG, Tinyani PP, Senyolo GM, et al. Impact of transportation, storage, and retail shelf conditions on lettuce quality and phytonutrients losses in the supply chain. Food Sci Nutr 2018;6:1527–36.
46. Arah IK, Amaglo H, Kumah E, et al. Preharvest and postharvest factors affecting the quality and shelf life of harvested tomatoes: a mini review. Int J Agron 2015; 2015:6.
47. Kiura IN, Gichimu BM, Rotich F. Proximate and nutritional composition of stored bulb onions as affected by harvest and postharvest treatments. Int J Agron 2021;2021:9.
48. Turner E, Luo Y, Buchanan R. Microgreen nutrition, food safety, and shelf life: a review. J Food Sci 2020;85(4):870–82.
49. Pikosky M, Cifelli C, Agarwal S, et al. Do Americans get enough nutrients from food? Assessing nutrient adequacy with NHANES 2013-2016. CDN 2019;3(1): 18–40.

50. Provenza FD, Kronberg SL, Gregorini P. Is grassfed meat and dairy better for human and environmental health? Front Nutr 2019;6:26.

51. Rankins DL Jr, Poore MH, Capucille DJ, et al. Recycled poultry bedding as cattle feed. Vet Clin North Am Food Anim Pract 2002;18(2):253–66.

52. Goldberg E. Skittles highway spill reveals awful trend in the food industry. In: The huffington post. 2017. Available at: https://www.huffpost.com/entry/skittles-highway-spill-cattle-feed-candy_n_5886270de4b070d8cad3d74e. Accessed: November 20, 2021.

53. KC KB, Dias GM, Veeramani A, et al. When too much isn't enough: Does current food production meet global nutritional needs? PLoS One 2018;13(10):1–16.

54. Ng M, Fleming T, Robinson M, et al. Global, regional, and national prevalence of overweight and obesity in children and adults during 1980-2013: a systematic analysis for the Global Burden of Disease Study 2013. Lancet 2014; 384(9945):766–81.

55. World Health Organization. Noncommunicable diseases. WHO; 2021. Available at: https://www.who.int/news-room/fact-sheets/detail/noncommunicable-diseases. Accessed November 7, 2021.

56. Global Burden Disease 2017 Diet Collaborators. Health effects of dietary risks in 195 countries, 1990-2017: a systematic analysis for the Global Burden of Disease Study 2017. Lancet 2019;393(10184):1958–72.

57. Luppino FS, de Wit LM, Bouvy PF, et al. Overweight, obesity, and depression: a systematic review and meta-analysis of longitudinal studies. Arch Gen Psychiatry 2010;67(3):220–9.

58. Tremmel M, Gerdtham UG, Nilsson PM, et al. Economic burden of obesity: a systematic literature review. Int J Environ Res Public Health 2017;14(4):435.

59. Specchia ML, Veneziano MA, Cadeddu C, et al. Economic impact of adult obesity on health systems: a systematic review. Eur J Public Health 2015; 25(2):255–62.

60. Smith R. Let food be thy medicine. BMJ 2004;328(7433):0.

61. Abuajah CI, Ogbonna AC, Osuji CM. Functional components and medicinal properties of food: a review. J Food Sci Technol 2015;52(5):2522–9.

62. Downer S, Berkowitz SA, Harlan TS, et al. Food is medicine: actions to integrate food and nutrition into healthcare. BMJ 2020;369:m2482.

63. Bland J. Defining *function* in the functional medicine model. IMCJ 2017; 16(1):22–5.

64. Hanaway P. Form follows function: a functional medicine overview. Perm J 2016; 20(4):16–109.

65. Bland JS. Systems biology meets functional medicine. IMCJ 2019;18(5):14–8.

66. Bland JS, Minich DM, Eck BM. A systems medicine approach: translating emerging science into individualized wellness. Adv Med 2017;2017:1–5.

67. Prescott SL. History of medicine: origin of the term microbiome and why it matters. Hum 2017;4:24–5.

68. Jain T, Sharma P, Are A, et al. New insights into cancer-microbiome-immune axis: decrypting a decade of discoveries. Front Immunol 2021;12:102.

69. Trøseid M, Andersen GØ, Broch K, et al. The gut microbiome in coronary artery disease and heart failure: Current knowledge and future directions. EBioMedicine 2020;52:102649.

70. Tseng C, Wu C. The gut microbiome in obesity. J Fla Med Assoc 2019;118:S3–9.

71. Li WZ, Stirling K, Yang JJ, et al. Gut microbiota and diabetes: From correlation to causality and mechanism. World J Diabetes 2020;11(7):293–308.

72. Fouquier J, Moreno Huizar N, Donnelly J, et al. The gut microbiome in autism: study-site effects and longitudinal analysis of behavior change. ASM 2021; 6(2):e00848-20.
73. Barandouzi ZA, Starkweather AR, Henderson WA, et al. Altered composition of gut microbiota in depression: a systematic review. Front Psychiatry 2020; 11:541.
74. Saji N, Murotani K, Hisada T, et al. Relationship between dementia and gut microbiome-associated metabolites: a cross-sectional study in Japan. Sci Rep 2020;10(1):8088.
75. Frati F, Salvatori C, Incorvaia C, et al. The role of the microbiome in asthma: the gut-lung axis. Int J Mol Sci 2018;20(1):123.
76. Erdrich S, Hawrelak JA, Myers SP, et al. Determining the association between fibromyalgia, the gut microbiome and its biomarkers: a systematic review. BMC Musculoskelet Disord 2020;21(1):181.
77. Xu H, Liu M, Cao J, et al. The dynamic interplay between the gut microbiota and autoimmune diseases. J Immunol Res 2019;2019:1–14.
78. Pascal M, Perez-Gordo M, Caballero T, et al. Microbiome and allergic diseases. Front Immunol 2018;9:1584.
79. De Pessemier B, Grine L, Debaere M, et al. Gut-skin axis: current knowledge of the interrelationship between microbial dysbiosis and skin conditions. Microorganisms 2021;9(2):353.
80. Kang DW, Adams JB, Coleman DM, et al. Long-term benefit of microbiota transfer therapy on autism symptoms and gut microbiota. Sci Rep 2019;9(1):58271.
81. Kootte R, Levin E, Salojarvi J, et al. Improvement of insulin sensitivity after lean donor feces in metabolic syndrome is driven by baseline intestinal microbiota composition. Cell Met 2017;26(4):611–9.
82. The Institute for Functional Medicine.. Functional medicine: a clinical model to address chronic disease and promote well-being. In: Ifm. 2021. Available at: https://functionalmedicine.widen.net/s/pkcvf2wzlj/ifm_functional_medicine_descriptive_paper. Accessed November 13. 2021.
83. Beidelschies M, Alejandro-Rodriguez M, Ji X, et al. Association of the functional medicine model of care with patient-reported health-related quality-of-life outcomes. JAMA Netw Open 2019;2(10):e1914017.
84. Alwarith J, Kahleova H, Rembert E, et al. Nutrition interventions in rheumatoid arthritis: the potential use of plant-based diets. A review. Front Nutr 2019;6:141.
85. Bagur MJ, Murcia MA, Jiménez-Monreal AM, et al. Influence of diet in multiple sclerosis: a systematic review. Adv Nutr 2017;8(3):463–72.
86. Firth J, Marx W, Dash S, et al. The effects of dietary improvement on symptoms of depression and anxiety: a meta-analysis of randomized controlled trials. Psychosom Med 2019;81(3):265–80.
87. Hindiyeh NA, Zhang N, Farrar M, et al. The role of diet and nutrition in migraine triggers and treatment: a systematic literature review. Headache 2020;60(7): 1300–16.
88. Doreswamy S, Bashir A, Guarecuco JE, et al. Effects of diet, nutrition, and exercise in children with autism and autism spectrum disorder: a literature review. Cureus 2020;12(12).
89. Katsimbri P, Korakas E, Kountouri A, et al. The effect of antioxidant and anti-inflammatory capacity of diet on psoriasis and psoriatic arthritis phenotype: nutrition as therapeutic tool? Antioxidants 2021;10(2):157.
90. Kanda N, Hoashi T, Saeki H. Nutrition and atopic dermatitis. J Nippon Med Sch 2021;88(3):171–7.

91. Bredesen DE. Reversal of cognitive decline: a novel therapeutic program. Aging 2014;6(9):707–17.

92. Bredesen DE. Inhalational Alzheimer's disease: an unrecognized - and treatable - epidemic. Aging 2016;8(2):304–13.

93. Taheri S, Zaghloul H, Chagoury O, et al. Effect of intensive lifestyle intervention on bodyweight and glycaemia in early type 2 diabetes (DIADEM-I): an open-label, parallel-group, randomized controlled trial. Lancet Diabetes Endocrinol 2020;8(6):477–89.

94. Christ A, Lauterbach M, Latz E. Western diet and the immune system: an inflammatory connection. Immunity 2019;51(5):794–811.

95. Ryan KK, Seeley RJ. Physiology. Food as a hormone. Science 2013;339(6122): 918–9.

96. Selhub E. Nutritional psychiatry: your brain on food. Harvard Health Blog; 2020. Available at: https://www.health.harvard.edu/blog/nutritional-psychiatry-your-brain-on-food-201511168626. Accessed November 13, 2021.

97. Zinöcker MK, Lindseth IA. The Western diet-microbiome-host interaction and Its role in metabolic disease. Nutrients 2018;10(3):365.

98. Dahl WJ, Rivero Mendoza D, Lambert JM. Diet, nutrients and the microbiome. Prog Mol Biol Transl Sci 2020;171:237–63.

99. Guarneri E. Identifying Root Cause for Better Treatment Outcome. Institute for Functional Medicine. Available at: https://www.ifm.org/news-insights/identifying-root-cause-better-treatment-outcome/. Accessed December 19, 2021.

100. Haß U, Herpich C, Norman K. Anti-Inflammatory diets and fatigue. Nutrients 2019;11(10):2315.

101. Hodges RE, Minich DM. Modulation of metabolic detoxification pathways using foods and food-derived components: a scientific review with clinical application. J Nutr Metab 2015;2015:760689.

102. Medina-Remón A, Casas R, Tressserra-Rimbau A, et al. Polyphenol intake from a Mediterranean diet decreases inflammatory biomarkers related to atherosclerosis: a substudy of the PREDIMED trial. Br J Clin Pharmacol 2017;83:114–28.

103. Institute of Medicine (US). Committee on Diet and Health. In: Woteki CE, Thomas PR, editors. Eat for life: the food and nutrition board's guide to reducing your risk of chronic disease. Washington DC: National Academies Press; 1992. Available at: https://www.ncbi.nlm.nih.gov/books/NBK235023/?report=classic.

104. National Institute of Health. NIH Human microbiome project defines normal bacteria makeup of the body. U.S. Department of Health and Human Services; 2012. Available at: https://www.nih.gov/news-events/news-releases/nih-human-microbiome-project-defines-normal-bacterial-makeup-body. Accessed November 13, 2021.

105. Qin J, Li R, Raes J, et al. A human gut microbial gene catalogue established by metagenomic sequencing. Nature 2010;464:59–65.

106. Van Treuren W, Dodd D. Microbial contribution to the human metabolome: implications for health and disease. Annu Rev Pathol 2020;15:345–69.

107. Jackson A, Forsyth CB, Shaikh M, et al. Diet in Parkinson's Disease: Critical Role for the Microbiome. Front Neurol 2019;10:1245. https://doi.org/10.3389/fneur.2019.01245.

108. Weiss GA, Hennet T. Mechanisms and consequences of intestinal dysbiosis. Cell Mol Life Sci 2017;74(16):2959–77.

109. Ferreira R, Mendonça L, Ribeiro C, et al. Relationship between intestinal microbiota, diet and biological systems: an integrated view. Crit Rev Food Sci Nutr 2020;1–21.

110. Chichlowski M, Shah N, Wampler JL, et al. *Bifidobacterium longum* subspecies *infantis* (*B. infantis*) in pediatric nutrition: current state of knowledge. Nutrients 2020;12(6):1581.

111. Li Z, Zhu H, Ma B, et al. Inhibitory effect of *Bifidobacterium infantis*-mediated sKDR prokaryotic expression system on angiogenesis and growth of Lewis lung cancer in mice. BMC Cancer 2012;12:155.

112. Edwards CA, Parrett AM, Balmer SE, et al. Faecal short chain fatty acids in breast-fed and formula-fed babies. Acta Paediatr 1994;83(5):459–62.

113. Frye RE, Rose S, Chacko J, et al. Modulation of mitochondrial function by the microbiome metabolite propionic acid in autism and control cell lines. Transl Psychiatry 2016;6(10):e927.

114. Alfawaz H, Al-Onazi M, Bukhari SI, et al. The independent and combined effects of omega-3 and vitamin B12 in ameliorating propionic acid induced biochemical features in juvenile rats as rodent model of autism. J Mol Neurosci 2018;66(3):403–13.

115. Drago S, El Asmar R, Di Pierro M, et al. Gliadin, zonulin and gut permeability: effects on celiac and non-celiac intestinal mucosa and intestinal cell lines. Scand J Gastroenterol 2006;41(4):408–19.

116. El Asmar R, Panigrahi P, Bamford P, et al. Host-dependent zonulin secretion causes the impairment of the small intestine barrier function after bacterial exposure. Gastroenterology 2003;124(1):275.

117. Caio G, Lungaro L, Segata N, et al. Effect of gluten-free diet on gut microbiota composition in patients with celiac disease and non-celiac gluten/wheat sensitivity. Nutrients 2020;12(6):1832.

118. Roseboro K. Why is glyphosate sprayed on crops right before harvest? Eco-Watch. 2016. Available at: https://www.ecowatch.com/roundup-cancer-1882187755.html. Accessed November 13, 2021.

119. Naidenko O, Temkin A. In new round of tests, Monsanto's weedkiller still contaminates food marketed to children. Environmental Working Group; 2019. Available at: https://www.ewg.org/childrenshealth/monsanto-weedkiller-still-contaminates-foods-marketed-to-children. Accessed November 13, 2021.

120. Leino L, Tall T, Helander M, et al. Classification of the glyphosate target enzyme (5-enolpyruvylshikimate-3-phosphate synthase) for assessing sensitivity of organisms to the herbicide. J Hazard Mater 2021;408:124556.

121. Hoffmann C, Dollive S, Grunberg S, et al. Archaea and fungi of the human gut microbiome: correlations with diet and bacterial residents. PLoS One 2013;8(6):e66019.

122. Saffouri GB, Shields-Cutler RR, Chen J, et al. Small intestinal microbial dysbiosis underlies symptoms associated with functional gastrointestinal disorders. Nat Commun 2019;10(1):2012.

123. Blasbalg TL, Hibbeln JR, Ramsden CE, et al. Changes in consumption of omega-3 and omega-6 fatty acids in the United States during the 20th century. Am J Clin Nutr 2011;93(5):950–62.

124. Yan JK, Zhu J, Gu BL, et al. Soybean oil-based lipid emulsion increases intestinal permeability of lipopolysaccharide in caco-2 cells by downregulation of p-glycoprotein via ERK-FOXO 3a Pathway. Cell Physiol Biochem 2016;39(4):1581–94.

125. Singer-Englar T, Barlow G, Mathur R. Obesity, diabetes, and the gut microbiome: an updated review. Expert Rev Gastroenterol Hepatol 2019;13(1):3–15.

126. Lerner A, Matthias T. Changes in intestinal tight junction permeability associated with industrial food additives explain the rising incidence of autoimmune disease. Autoimmun Rev 2015;14(6):479–89.

127. Ito T, Jensen RT. Association of long-term proton pump inhibitor therapy with bone fractures and effects on absorption of calcium, vitamin B12, iron, and magnesium. Curr Gastroenterol Rep 2010;12(6):448–57.

128. Farrell CP, Morgan M, Rudolph DS, et al. Proton pump inhibitors interfere with zinc absorption and zinc body stores. Gastroenterol Res 2011;4(6):243–51.

129. Spiegel BM, Chey WD, Chang L. Bacterial overgrowth and irritable bowel syndrome: unifying hypothesis or a spurious consequence of proton pump inhibitors? Am J Gastroenterol 2008;103(12):2972–6.

130. McGettigan M, Menias C, Gao Z. Imaging of drug-induced complications in the gastrointestinal system. Radiographics 2016;36(1):71–87.

131. Vighi G, Marcucci F, Sensi L, et al. Allergy and the gastrointestinal system. Clin Exp Immunol 2008;153(Suppl 1):3–6.

132. Valdes AM, Walter J, Segal E, et al. Role of the gut microbiota in nutrition and health. BMJ 2018;361:k2179.

133. Pathak DR, Stein AD, He JP, et al. Cabbage and sauerkraut consumption in adolescence and adulthood and breast cancer risk among US-resident polish migrant women. Int J Environ Res Public Health 2021;18(20):10795.

134. Zhou K. Strategies to promote abundance of *Akkermansia muciniphila*, an emerging probiotics in the gut, evidence from dietary intervention studies. J Funct Foods 2017;33:194–201.

135. Naito Y, Uchiyama K, Takagi T. A next-generation beneficial microbe: *Akkermansia muciniphila*. J Clin Biochem Nutr 2018;63(1):33–5.

136. Bian X, Wu W, Yang L, et al. Administration of *Akkermansia muciniphila* Ameliorates Dextran Sulfate Sodium-Induced Ulcerative Colitis in Mice. Front Microbiol 2019;10:2259.

137. Zhang L, Qin Q, Liu M, et al. Akkermansia muciniphila can reduce the damage of gluco/lipotoxicity, oxidative stress and inflammation, and normalize intestine microbiota in streptozotocin-induced diabetic rats. Pathog Dis 2018;76(4):1–15.

138. Routy B, Le Chatelier E, Derosa L, et al. Gut microbiome influences efficacy of PD-1-based immunotherapy against epithelial tumors. Science 2018; 359(6371):91–7.

139. Camilleri M. Leaky gut: mechanisms, measurement and clinical implications in humans. Gut 2019;68(8):1516–26.

140. Song X, Dong H, Zang Z, et al. Kudzu resistant starch: an effective regulator of type 2 diabetes mellitus. Oxid Med Cell Longev 2021;2021:4448048.

141. De Filippo C, Cavalieri D, Di Paola M, et al. Impact of diet in shaping gut microbiota revealed by a comparative study in children from Europe and rural Africa. Proc Natl Acad Sci U S A 2010;107(33):14691–6.

Food, Medicine, and Function: Food is Medicine Part 2

Mark Hyman, MD[a], Elizabeth Bradley, MD[b],*

KEYWORDS

- *Functional medicine* • *Chronic disease* • *Inflammation* • *Microbiome* • *Mitochondria*
- *Detoxification* • *Insulin* • *Neurotransmitters*

KEY POINTS

- Chronic, inflammatory diseases are driven by poor diet and lifestyle.
- Removing inflammatory triggers (food, environmental toxins) and adding in therapeutic foods can correct underlying functional imbalances.
- Optimizing our mitochondrial health can prevent, treat, and reverse chronic disease and promote healthy aging and longevity.
- Hormones and neurotransmitters are controlled mainly by our diet and require key vitamins and minerals to function optimally.
- What we eat determines the structure and function of our cells and tissues.

FOOD AND INFLAMMATION AND IMMUNITY

What do nearly all modern diseases have in common? Inflammation. Depression, autism, cancer, heart disease, obesity, diabetes, dementia, allergies, asthma, chronic fatigue, and autoimmune disease are all inflammatory diseases. That begs the question, what is causing all this rampant inflammation? It is mostly our food. Too many inflammatory foods and not enough anti-inflammatory foods. Our immune system attempts to keep a perfect balance, on surveillance for danger. Appropriate immune activation is good, overactivation is not. The severe illness and death caused by COVID-19 is the result of our own immune system overreacting causing a "cytokine storm".[1] It mostly affects those whose immune systems are both suppressed and inflamed at the same time. Poor diet accounted for 63% of COVID-19 hospitalization.[2] Studies show that the risk factors for COVID-19 infection, severity, and death are

[a] Cleveland Clinic Lerner College of Medicine, Cleveland Clinic Center for Functional Medicine, 55 Pittsfield Road Suite 9, Lenox, MA 01240, USA; [b] Cleveland Clinic Center for Functional Medicine, 9500 Euclid Avenue, Cleveland, OH 44195, USA
* Corresponding author. The UltraWellness Center, 55 Pittsfield Road, Suite 9, Lenox Commons, Lenox, MA 01240.
E-mail address: lizbradleymd@gmail.com

Phys Med Rehabil Clin N Am 33 (2022) 571–586
https://doi.org/10.1016/j.pmr.2022.04.002
1047-9651/22/© 2022 Elsevier Inc. All rights reserved.

Abbreviations	
mTOR	The mammalian target of rapamycin
FOXO	Forkhead family of transcription factors
DAF	Abnormal dauer formation protein
DDT	Dichlorodiphenyltrichloroethane
PCB	Polychlorinated biphenyls
BPA	Bisphenol A
dL	Deciliter
DMSA	Dimercaptosuccinic acid
EDTA	Ethylenediaminetetraacetic acid
NO	Nitric oxide
ADHD	Attention-deficit/hyperactivity disorder
PMS	Premenstrual syndrome
GMO	Genetically modified organism
EEG	Electroencephalogram
ATP	Adenosine triphosphate
MIT	Massachusetts Institute of Technology
SAD	Standard American diet

modifiable.[3] Although there are other causes of inflammation—toxins, allergen, infections, and stress, food plays the largest role.

How does food trigger inflammation? Often it starts in the gut. Moreover, high levels of sugar and refined starch in the diet are the main drivers of inflammation. Sugar and refined starch spike blood glucose, which in turn spikes insulin. Insulin drives sugar, starch, and free fatty acids to be stored in visceral *adipocytes*. These adipocytes produce *adipocytokines* that drive metabolic and hormonal dysfunction. As we ingest more and more sugar and starch (the main calories in our modern diet), we need more and more insulin to overcome the resistance to its effects. More insulin, more fat storage, more inflammation.[4,5] Although sugar drives inflammation, it also suppresses our immune response to infections.[6] It also fuels dysbiotic flora resulting in leaky gut and further inflammation.[7,8]

Fats may be another trigger of inflammation. Although still debated in the science, the sheer volume of processed food has increased our intake of refined oils that contain large amounts of omega 6 fats. They are essential for cellular health but excess may cause adverse health consequences. As hunter gathers, we consumed omega 6 fats from nuts and seeds and other plants, not from gallons of industrially produced, solvent extracted, heat-treated oxidized oils.[9] We have eliminated most foods containing omega 3 fats except for some seafood. The balance is key, too many omega 6 fats can inhibit the anti-inflammatory effects of omega 3 fats resulting in inflammation.[10] Ideally, omega 6 fats should come from whole foods such as nuts and seeds or unrefined plant oils. Adequate omega 3 fats from small wild fish are also critical to maintain the balance between omega 3 and omega 6 fatty acids.

The other main trigger of inflammation in our diet are food sensitivities and food reactions, not true allergies type 1 hypersensitivity IgE-mediated reactions such as a peanut allergy but low-grade type IV delayed hypersensitivity IgG-mediated response that can result in chronic inflammation from gluten, dairy, soy, or other common foods. In addition food additives, chemicals, and emulsifiers drive changes in the microbiome resulting in increased intestinal permeability.[11,12] Food sensitivities affect up to 20% of the population and have increased significantly during the past couple of decades.[13] True celiac has increased 400% during the last 50 years.[14] Increased intestinal permeability is caused by our modern lifestyle and Westernized diet—low fiber, high starch and sugar diet, processed foods, chronic stress, toxins, and changes in food genetics.[15,16] When partially digested food proteins leak across the intestinal barrier and encounter the immune system, it triggers an inflammatory response to the food antigens, bacterial antigens, or lipopolysaccharides.[16] The inflammation can attack any organ or system in our body, including our brain.[17] The most common foods that create reactions are gluten, dairy, grains, beans, soy, nuts and seeds, and night-shades.[15,18,19,20] Often healing the gut and repairing the increased intestinal perme-ability will reduce or eliminate these delayed hypersensitivity reactions. An elimination diet may be a powerful tool for anyone with an inflammatory condition.

Although many ways foods can trigger inflammation, food is also the most powerful source of anti-inflammatory compounds. Many of the 25,000 + phytochemicals in plants are powerful anti-inflammatories. The polyphenols in plant foods are among na-ture's best inflammation fighting compounds and found in colorful plant foods—red, green, yellow, orange, purple.[21] Extra virgin olive oil contains oleocanthal, for example, which actives the same anti-inflammatory receptors as ibuprofen without the side effects.[22]

Spices are anti-inflammatory powerhouses including turmeric, ginger, and rose-mary.[23] Meat cooked with spices neutralizes any potential inflammation.[24] Omega 3 fats found in wild foods, fish, seafood, and some nuts and seeds are also powerful anti-inflammatories. Mushrooms including Shitake, Maitake, Reishi, Chaga, Turkey tail, and Cordyceps contain powerful immune regulating and anticancer compounds called polysaccharides.[25,26] Moreover, foods rich in vitamins and minerals boost im-munity and reduce inflammation including vitamin C, zinc, selenium, and vitamin D. Vitamin D alone regulates hundreds of genes that affect inflammation and immunity.[27] A meal of guavas and parsley (vitamin C), pumpkin seeds and oysters (zinc), Brazil nuts and sardines (selenium), and porcini mushrooms and herring (vitamin D) is an im-mune boosting, anti-inflammatory super meal.

FOOD AND ENERGY

The energy stored in food in the form of fat, protein, and carbohydrates is metabolized with oxygen in the *mitochondria*. The food and oxygen then produce ATP, the main fuel source for our biology. Some foods are easily metabolized, and create limited free radicals, others create a significant amount of oxidative stress that damages our tissues and cells. Endogenous antioxidant systems including catalase, superoxide dismutase, and glutathione peroxidase mitigate the harm from free radicals produced by oxidative phosphorylation. However, our endogenous antioxidant systems are insufficient to address the oxidative stress when we eat too much sugar, starch, and processed foods and too few nutrients or are exposed to environmental toxins.

The key to longevity and health is optimizing mitochondria. Poorly functioning mito-chondria are found in most chronic diseases including obesity, diabetes, heart dis-ease, dementia, Parkinson disease, chronic fatigue, fibromyalgia, and autism. It can also present as fatigue, brain fog, muscle pain, intolerance to exercise, and acceler-ated aging.[28]

How we feed our bodies affects the number and function of our mitochondria. Longevity research reflects that the key to longevity and healthy aging is optimizing the function of mitochondria.[29] Although environmental toxins, infections, food aller-gens, an unhealthy gut microbiome, nutrient deficiencies can all damage mitochon-dria, the biggest factor is food. What we eat but also when we eat. Aging researchers have identified key regulatory genes (sirtuins, mTOR, FOXO, DAF-2, and others) that control the aging process by affecting the health and function of our mitochondria.[30]

Leonard Guarente from MIT, who discovered *sirtuins*, found that sugar and refined starches damages the mitochondria and turns off the longevity genes. Americans eat nearly a cup of sugar a day, which may partly explain why life expectancy is going down for the first time in history.[31] The other problem is just too much food. We never give our metabolic engines a rest. Snacking, late-night eating and bingeing are American pastimes, much to our detriment. Since 1961, the average American consumes an extra 720 calories a day,[32] calories that have to be stored or burned, overwhelming mitochondria producing more free radicals overwhelming our endogenous antioxidants driving more disease and rapid aging. It also explains why during the same time period obesity rates in America climbed from 13% to 40%, a more than 300% increase.[33]

Our mitochondria can function like a hybrid engine and can run on 2 fuel sources: fat or carbohydrates. The typical American diet is more than 42% low-quality, refined carbohydrates a dirty burning, inefficient fuel, instead of clean burning fats.[4] Harmful fats damage the mitochondria including trans fats and oxidized oils (especially from deep frying).[34,35] Certain fats called ketones are the preferred fuel for mitochondria and help them repair, renew, and rebuild optimizing their function.[36] Turns out human biology is exquisitely adapted to starvation. Time restricted eating, intermittent fasting, fasting mimicking diets, calorie restriction all activate protective endogenous protective and regenerative biological systems.[37] However, our modern culture rarely provides those periods of scarcity, even an overnight fast of 12 to 16 hours can have a profound impact on health and the mitochondria. When there is a lack of food, we switch to fat burning. We have weeks' worth of fat stored on our bodies. When we burn the fat on our bodies (or in the case of a ketogenic diet, the fat in our diet), it results in multiple downstream benefits. Our cells clean up waste and debris, recycle old parts to make new cells, through autophagy and mitophagy, activate our antioxidant and anti-inflammatory systems, reduce visceral fat, increase muscle and bone, heighten brain function (so we can find the next meal!). The process inhibits the rate of aging and reverses many chronic diseases.[36,37]

New science on longevity has identified key mechanisms that get turned on with starvation or anything that mimics starvation including calorie restricted diets, time restricted eating (eating in an 8-hour, 10-hour, or 12-hour window), intermittent fasting (skipping a day of eating a week or 2 days of very low-calorie intake a week), ketogenic diets, and fasting mimicking diets (5 days of calorie restriction).[37] They all have similar biological effects. When we eat turns out to be just as important as how much or what we eat. Combining high-quality nutrient dense foods, with the optimal timing will enhance mitochondrial function and repair.

Muscle is where we have the most mitochondria. Therefore, diets that cause muscle loss—high starch and sugar and low protein diets—also leave us with less and poorer functioning mitochondria. Especially as we age, we need more protein, and higher quality protein.[38] Animal protein is the most bioavailable and the most effective way to build muscle but vegan proteins can help build muscle if supplemented with certain amino acids that are lower in plant foods such as leucine and other branched chain amino acids (BCAAs).[39,40]

In addition to calories and oxygen, ATP production requires specific vitamins and minerals and other nutrients: B vitamins, coenzyme Q10, carnitine, zinc, magnesium, selenium, omega 3 fats, lipoic acid, n-acetylcysteine, vitamin E, vitamin K, sulfur, and others.[41] Our modern nutrient depleted diet provides very few of these mitochondrial boosters. Food is a great source of these and other phytonutrients that supercharge our mitochondria including blueberries, pomegranate seeds, grass fed beef and butter, broccoli, sardines, extra virgin olive oil, avocados, and almonds. One of the best fuel sources for the mitochondria is medium-chain triglyceride oil found in unrefined coconut oil but may also be bought separately. It is the cleanest burning preferred fuel for our mitochondria and an excellent performance enhancer before exercise.[42]

Properly fueling mitochondria, consuming clean burning fuels, avoiding sugar and starch, increasing good fats and ensuring optimal levels of key nutrients can provide a metabolic tune up at little cost and no risk.[43,44] The use of time restricted, intermittent fasting and ketogenic diets can be regenerative.[36,37]

FOOD AND DETOXIFICATION

When we hear "detox" most of us think of drug or alcohol rehab or fad "cleansing" diets. However, we have an endogenous detoxification system designed to handle internal metabolic waste and environmental toxins. The process of detoxification can be hindered by an overload of toxic processed food, sugar, starch, and an overload of environmental toxins. It also requires a host of foods, phytochemicals, protein, vitamins and minerals, fiber, and water to function optimally.

The problem occurs when we get overloaded, overwhelming our detoxification system. Although most physicians are not trained adequately in this part of our physiology, it turns out it is linked to so many of the diseases we see today. Sadly, both the diagnosis and treatment of impaired detoxification are almost never made. Many of our common diseases are linked to an overload of toxins including heart disease, diabetes, cancer, autism, and Alzheimer disease.[45] Environmental toxins have even been dubbed *obesogens*, which cause weight gain,[46] and *autogens*, which cause autoimmune disease.[47]

Eighty thousand chemicals have been introduced into the environment since the Industrial Revolution—most have never been tested for safety. They cause inflammation, oxidative stress, damage the mitochondria, disrupt our gut function, create hormonal imbalances, and overload our detoxification systems.[45] A study of 10 newborns done by the Environmental Working Group, found 270 known toxins in the umbilical cord blood, before they even took their first breath. Pesticides, DDT, PCBs, phthalates, parabens, flame retardants, BPA, mercury, lead, and more.[48] We are born prepolluted. A lifetime of ongoing exposures compounds our toxic load.

Even though the medical literature confirms the link between toxins and most of our chronic diseases, most doctors do not address this clinically. For example, lead levels more than 2 µg/dL (normal is less than 10), had dramatically higher risks for heart attack, stroke and death because high cholesterol and blood pressure are directly linked to high blood lead levels.[49,50] In fact lead levels more than 2 µg/dL, increase the risk of cardiovascular disease more than dyslipidemia. Yet, it is not often addressed. Lead overload is straightforward to treat with the right foods, nutrients, and sometimes chelators such as DMSA or EDTA. Parkinson disease has a well-recognized link to environmental toxins. Farmers have the highest rates from exposure to pesticides.[51] Children exposed to pesticides, in one study, lost 27 million Intelligence quotient (IQ)points during a span of 15 years, which seems small compared with flame-retardants that resulted in a loss of 162 million IQ points in children.[52] Toxins are also linked to autism and even type 2 diabetes. Arsenic, pesticides, and bisphenol A cause diabetes.[53]

Our detoxification systems were not designed for such an overwhelming load of toxins. In addition to air and water pollution, many toxins lurk in our food. Fatty liver is the number one cause of liver transplants. What causes fatty liver? Sugar and starch.[54] Ducks are force-fed corn to make foie gras (which is French for fatty liver). The biggest causes of kidney failure—high blood pressure and diabetes, again are caused mostly by sugar and starch in our diet. Add to that load of sugar and refined carbs the 5 lb of food additives we eat every year,[55] the pesticides and weed killers in our food, the mercury in our fish, and the arsenic and toxins in our water, and our endogenous detoxification systems are overwhelmed. Alcohol, acetaminophen, and other prescription medicines often add to the toxic overload.

Food contains nearly all the ingredients our bodies need to eliminate waste. Adequate intake of water helps remove waste through the kidneys and digestive system. Fiber is essential for helping waste products get through our colon quickly. Hepatic detoxification is more complicated, energy and nutrient intensive. Phase 1 detoxification, our cytochrome P450 system metabolizes toxins, often producing highly reactive intermediates that then must be processed through phase 2 detoxification—methylation, glucuronidation, acetylation, and glutathione conjugation. Each of these pathways requires both nutrients and phytonutrients for optimal function. The food group that best boosts these pathways are the cruciferous vegetable family (broccoli, collards, kale, cabbage, Brussel sprouts) that contains compounds with sulfur that enhance the production of glutathione, the body's master antioxidant—glucosinolates, sulforaphane.[56] Garlic and onions also provide the sulfur needed for detoxification. Adequate amino acids from protein are also essential to fuel these pathways. Green tea chelates (binds) to heavy metals and is a super detoxifier, which may be why Japanese are able to handle the mercury overload from too much tuna sushi.[57] The liver also needs adequate levels of B1, B2, B3, B6, B12 and folate, manganese, magnesium, zinc, and selenium as cofactors for detoxification enzymes. These are found in animal protein, seafood, nuts, seeds, and green vegetables. It also needs a rich array of phytochemicals including flavonoids, and compounds found it herbs and spices. Curcumin, found in the Indian spice turmeric, not only reduces inflammation and oxidative stress but also is powerful in aiding detoxification.[58] Rosemary, ginger, cilantro, dandelion greens, parsley, lemon peel, watercress, burdock root, artichokes are all powerful detoxifying foods to add to our diet on a regular basis.[59]

Food is both the cause of overload of our detoxification systems—too much sugar, starch, processed foods, pesticides, and additives—and the solution. Adding high-quality protein, phytonutrients, vitamins, and mineral rich foods along with lots of fiber and fresh clean water keeps our detoxification functioning optimally and our toxic load low.

FOOD AND TRANSPORT (CIRCULATORY AND LYMPHATIC CIRCULATION)

How do cell-signaling molecules find their receptors? How do the nutrients and phytochemicals find the right receptors to act on? How does the body clear waste? It is our transportation systems—our circulatory system (all the blood vessels) and our lymphatic system, a parallel set of vessels that clear all the metabolic waste from our tissues and returns it to the heart to be cleansed by the liver and kidneys.

The biggest killer in the world today is cardiovascular disease, which in turn is mostly caused by insulin resistance, prediabetes, or type 2 diabetes.[60] Atherosclerosis is the biggest killer and causes heart attacks, strokes, amputations in diabetics, and even dementia. However, contrary to the popular understanding, this is not a plumbing problem that can be fixed by a bypass, angioplasty, or stents. It is not just cholesterol that is the problem. Atherosclerosis is triggered when inflammation and hormonal changes turn our cholesterol into fragile plaques that coat our arteries.[60,61] Heart disease is an inflammatory disease, a disease of hormonal imbalance. What causes the inflammation and hormonal dysregulation (insulin resistance)? Our diet. Although environmental toxins, stress, our microbiome and genetics all pay a role, our diet is the biggest driver of cardiovascular disease. Studies have shown that 90% of all heart disease can be prevented by changes in diet and lifestyle changes like regular exercise and not smoking.[62]

Our body contains about 60,000 miles of blood vessels, enough to go around the earth about 2.5 times.[63] However, these vessels are not just inert tubes that carry blood, they are also immune and hormonal organs and require the right diet to function optimally. When the *endothelium* is dysfunctional, it causes high blood pressure and lays down atherogenic cholesterol and plaque. What drives this dysfunction? Our modern industrial, processed, high starch, sugar, and refined fat inflammatory diet that is low in protective medicinal foods. Studies show that a single fast food meal harms blood vessels.[64] Much of the adverse effects can be offset by consuming phytonutrients and antioxidants.[64,65] It may be that absence of medicinal phytochemicals and antioxidants is an important driver of heart disease (and most other diseases). Eating a nutrient dense whole foods diet also rich in phytonutrients will prevent the damage in the first place.[65] Interestingly, any harmful effects of eating meat are neutralized when consumed with lots of spices and phytonutrients.[18]

The other important foods for vascular health are foods that increase nitric oxide, or NO, a molecule that helps increase blood flow. The amino acid arginine is the precursor for NO, and the best food sources are pumpkin seeds, sesame seeds, walnuts, almonds, turkey breast, soybeans, and seaweed. Omega 3 fat from wild fish also helps improve endothelial function, blood vessel health, and prevents clotting.[66] The heart healthy benefits of olive oil are likely due to the effect of polyphenols on endothelial function and reducing blood vessel inflammation.[67]

High blood pressure leads to heart attacks, heart failure, strokes, and kidney failure. However, what leads to high blood pressure? Although genetics play a role, and a few people are salt sensitive, and environmental pollution and heavy metals such as lead and mercury are a factor but for most, it is driven by insulin resistance—which in turn is driven by our high starch and sugar diet, low in nutrients. Hyperinsulinemia and visceral fat and the resultant inflammation and oxidative stress cause high blood pressure. In addition, 75% of Americans are consuming a magnesium-deficient diet.[68] Low magnesium contributes to high blood pressure. Magnesium relaxes blood vessels. Stress, alcohol, caffeine, and sugar all deplete magnesium. It is found in foods we eat too little of—nuts, seeds, and greens.

What we eat and what we do not eat regulates the health of our cardiovascular system.

THE OTHER VASCULAR SYSTEM: OUR LYMPHATICS

A much-neglected aspect of our health is our lymphatic system. We cannot see it, we cannot touch it, it does not show up on an X-ray but it is working all the time to clear the metabolic waste from our tissues. Our lymphatic system also absorbs fats from our gut and transports it into our general circulation and brings white blood cells to and from lymph nodes to help us fight infection. It can be out of balance when we have a high intake of processed foods, low levels of nutrients, and a lack of physical activity and can contribute to arthritis, headaches, digestive and skin disorders, excess weight, and fatigue.

The heart pumps the blood around our blood vessels but our lymphatic vessels need our movement, muscle activity, and breathing to pump the waste fluid back into our heart. There are several ways to improve lymphatic circulation including exercise, lymphatic massage, hot and cold showers, steam and saunas followed by cold dips, dry brushing, lots of hydration, and deep breathing, which facilitates lymphatic flow return to the heart.[69–73] However, what we eat matters too. Foods that tend to impair lymphatic function are the common culprits—processed foods, dairy, sugar, sweeteners, and too much salt. Moreover, there are many foods that help improve lymphatic function including green leafy vegetables, ground flaxseeds, chia seeds, avocados, garlic, nuts, seaweed, citrus fruits, and cranberries. Phytochemically rich herbs such as echinacea, astragalus, cilantro, and parsley can also help.

As for each of our biological systems, the major regulator is food. Bad foods cause imbalance, dysfunction, and disease and good foods optimize their function.

FOOD AND COMMUNICATION

Neurotransmitters, hormones, and cytokines are cell-signaling molecules that regulate much of our biology. Many things influence their function. Diet, nutrient deficiencies, stress, toxins, the microbiome, and more but the greatest influence is our diet with powerful measurable effects.

When these messengers, such as instruments in a symphony orchestra, play out of tune, diseases such as depression, anxiety, violent behavior, ADHD, impaired learning and cognitive dysfunction, premenstrual syndrome, polycystic ovarian syndrome, sexual dysfunction, breast, cervical, and uterine cancer, low libido and erectile dysfunction, inflammation, allergy, and autoimmune disease develop.

HORMONES AND DIET

The single biggest hormonal disorder we face is insulin resistance. One in 2 Americans has prediabetes or type 2 diabetes.[74] A whopping 75% of Americans are overweight,[27] and 88% are metabolically unhealthy[75]—all suffering from one thing in common. Too much insulin, the result of the mountains of sugar and flour we consume. That insulin in turn creates a domino effect. It drives all those excess calories into visceral fat cells that produce messengers that increase hunger, slow metabolism, prevent fat burning, and increase inflammation. In women, too much insulin turns estrogen into testosterone.[76] The result is something misleadingly called polycystic ovarian syndrome. It is not an ovarian problem. It is dietary problem. The excess testosterone in women causes hair loss, facial hair, acne, and infertility. In men, the testosterone is converted to estrogen, which is why men with large amounts of visceral fat often have gynecomastia, low testosterone, erectile dysfunction, and loss of hair on their bodies. The same high sugar and starch diet also spikes cortisol. When we eat a sugar-laden diet, our body literally perceives it as a stress, just like being chased by a tiger. Adrenalin and cortisol increase, worsening insulin resistance and increasing cravings for sugar and starch.[77] The cure: essentially a whole food, good fat, plant rich, fiber rich, low glycemic, phytonutrient rich diet.

Many hormonal problems also result from imbalances in sex hormone metabolism—menopause, PMS, cancers in women. We live in a culture that drives excess estrogen, and increases toxic estrogens in the body. Too much sugar, low fiber diets, nutritional deficiencies, alcohol, xenoestrogens (pesticides, plastics, environmental chemicals that mimic estrogen), stress, lack of exercise all drive hormonal imbalances.

Estrogen metabolized and excreted through the liver and bile. Constipation or an unhealthy gut microbiome (mostly caused by our low fiber, processed diet) result in increased enterohepatic circulation estrogens increasing the risk for breast and uterine cancer and worsening PMS and menopause.[78] Certain fibers, for example, in flaxseeds, contain lignans, which help detoxify and improve estrogen metabolism reducing cancer risk.[79] The multiple forms of estrogen can all have different effects on the body. Some are anticancer, and some promote cancer. For example, 2-OH estrogen is protective, and 16-OH estrogen is carcinogenic. Eating a diet high in sugar and starch increases the 16-OH, whereas eating a diet high in flaxseeds, isoflavones from whole non-GMO soy and high in cruciferous vegetables such as broccoli increases the 2-OH estrogen.[80] These metabolites can be measured in the urine. Studies show that activating the 2-OH pathway with extracts of cruciferous vegetables called *diindolemethane* can reverse cervical dysplasia.[81]

For men, testosterone levels are inversely related to their insulin levels. Reducing sugar and increasing fat raises testosterone levels.[82] Our sex hormones are made from cholesterol. The best treatment of sexual dysfunction is to stop the SAD diet and eat foods that help blood flow (see Food and Flow) and increasing good fats.

Thyroid function is also affected by what we eat, and low thyroid function is extremely prevalent condition that affects more than 1 in 5 women and 1 in 10 men. Low thyroid function can be triggered by gluten, too many raw kale smoothies (raw cruciferous veggies can be goitrogens at high doses), and diets low in zinc, selenium, vitamin D, and iodine.[83] Environmental toxins often found in our food such as pesticides and mercury also damage our thyroid.[84] Adding foods rich in zinc (pumpkin seeds and oysters), selenium (sardines and Brazil nuts), vitamin D (herring and porcini mushrooms), and iodine (seaweed and fish) can help optimize thyroid function.

FOOD, MIND, MOOD, AND BEHAVIOR

The association between diet and our brain health is profound. Depression, anxiety, ADHD, autism, dementia, behavior problems, violence, and mild cognitive dysfunction can all be linked to poor food choices. The fastest way to address these problems is to start with diet.

Whole new fields of research such as nutritional psychiatry and metabolic psychiatry have emerged in the last decade. Studies show that simply swapping out processed, sugary starchy foods for whole foods is effective in treating depression; in fact, 400% better than the control group on a typical Western diet.[85] One study of violent juveniles found that children simply giving them a vitamin and mineral supplement reduced violent acts by 39% compared with a control group.[86] Why were they violent? Their brains were starving for nutrients that regulate mood and behavior including iron, magnesium, B12, and folate. Giving these children vitamins for 3 months fixed their abnormal brain waves on EEG.

Children with poor diets, who do not eat fruits and vegetables and have vitamin and mineral deficiencies, have worse academic performance, including lower test scores, lower grades, poor cognitive function with less alertness, attention, memory, processing of visual information, problem-solving, and increased absenteeism.[87] The result is that kids are inattentive, disruptive, late, or absent.[88]

Although they are not eating enough brain food, they are also eating too many chemicals, including about 5 lb of dyes, preservatives, and additives that are linked to hyperactivity and worse.[89] Calcium propionate, a preservative found in all flour and bread products, is linked to severe behavior changes and even autism.[90]

Medical practice is slow to catch up to all the research and use food as medicine, not in an abstract way, but very specific, science-based ways to treat disease and optimize function.

FOOD: WHAT WE ARE MADE FROM?

Every cell in our body turns over every 7 years. Some turn over daily, some weekly, some take longer. We make new cell, organs, tissues, skin, muscles, bone, and even brain cells every day. The raw materials all come from what we eat. Do we want to be made of Doritos or grass-fed steak? Coca cola or wild blueberries? Our structure, which determines our function, depends on what we eat for the building blocks—the proteins, fats, and minerals that make up who we are. Carbohydrates are not considered an essential nutrient. The problem is that our processed diet is about 50% to 60% carbohydrate, mostly low-quality refined starches and sugars that are the raw materials for processed food. If those carbohydrates do not become our structure, where do they go? We burn some but most are turned into dangerous disease-causing visceral fat.

Our structure matters. Every part of our body has a structure but also a function. If we are made from poor-quality parts, we will create a poorly functioning body. Muscle loss and bone loss are very significant factors in aging and age-related diseases. Muscle is the main location of our metabolism—low muscle mass results in insulin resistance, inflammation, hormonal dysregulation (lower growth hormone and testosterone and increased cortisol).[91] The effect of poor-quality muscles, marbled fat in the muscles, is an increase in diabetes, inflammation, and aging.[92]

What do cells do? They are the units of a very large coordinated network of cells, and those cells make up organs, tissues, muscles, and bones. What are cells made of? The raw materials from our diet that are synthesized into the appropriate molecule or tissue. Every cell membrane is the docking station for all the thousands of cell signaling molecules. Every cell membrane is made of fat. If it is made of hydrogenated fats, it is stiff, hard, and dysfunctional. If it is made of omega 3 fats, it is soft, pliable, and able to receive cellular messengers.

Imagine building a house out of rotten wood, disintegrating bricks. Why build the body from defective ingredients? High-quality fats are essential in our diet—our brain is 60% fat, our nerve coverings are all made from fat, every one of our 10 trillion cells is wrapped in a little fatty membrane.[93] Do we really want to make them from oxidized damaged refined oils in French fries or Kentucky Fried Chicken (KFC)? We also need the best quality protein. The body makes most of its important molecules from protein including muscles, cells, and immune molecules. Not all protein is the same. The best type of protein to build muscle is other muscle—animal protein. Protein also is found in plant foods but the quality is lower, and it has lower levels of essential amino acids needed to synthesize new muscle, especially the BCAAs, leucine, isoleucine, and valine and also lysine and sulfur-based amino acids.[39] There compounds such as phytates in plant proteins such as beans and nuts that impair protein absorption. Rather than being turned into muscle, plant proteins are often just burned as calories. Vegans, especially as they age, need to increase overall volume of protein-rich plant foods, adding protein powders and supplementing with BCAA.[40] Combining small amounts of meat and including more plant proteins helps the body use the plant protein from beans.

In addition, vitamins and minerals are needed to build tissues, muscles, and bones including vitamin D, vitamin K, calcium, magnesium, and more. If food is information, then it is critical to consume the right instructions to upgrade our biological software.

SUMMARY

Food is so essential to the proper functioning of our biology, to creating health, and living a long vibrant life. Food is medicine and plays a role in our network of biological networks, our systems of systems that are the true foundation of health. The wrong foods create imbalances in those systems that lead to disease and accelerated aging. A few examples for each of the systems hopefully provided a quick glimpse into the complexity of how everything connects and how everything is connected to what we eat (or do not eat). There are thousands more examples. The most important choice we make every day for our health is the food we eat, and how in turn the choice of what we eat not only affects us but our human community, the environment, and the climate and connects us to the things that matter most.

DISCLOSURE

This project received no funding. Dr Mark Hyman is the owner of Hyman Digital, a health information company. He is the author of numerous books on food and nutrition that receive royalties and the host of *The Doctor's Farmacy*, a podcast that earns income from advertising in the food and health space.

REFERENCES

1. Ragab D, Salah Eldin H, Taeimah M, et al. The COVID-19 cytokine storm; what we know so far. Front Immunol 2020;11:1446.
2. O'Hea rn M, Liu J, Cudhea F. Coronavirus disease 2019 hospitalizations attributable to the cardiometabolic conditions in the United States: a comparative risk assessment analysis. J Am Heart Assoc 2021;10(5):e019259.
3. Simon M, Pizzorno J, Katzinger J. Modifiable risk factors for SARS-CoV-2. Integr Med (Encinitas) 2021;20(5):8–14.
4. Ludwig DS, Hu FB, Tappy L, et al. Dietary carbohydrates: role of quality and quantity in chronic disease. BMJ 2018;361:k2340.
5. Ludwig DS, Ebbeling CB. The carbohydrate-insulin model of obesity: beyond "calories in, calories out. JAMA Intern Med 2018;178(8):1098–103.
6. Shomali N, Mahmoudi J, Mahmoodpoor A, et al. Harmful effects of high amounts of glucose on the immune system: An updated review. Biotechnol Appl Biochem 2021;68(2):404–10.
7. Christ A, Lauterbach M, Latz E. Western diet and the immune system: an inflammatory connection. Immunity 2019;51(5):794–811.
8. Zinöcker MK, Lindseth IA. The Western diet-microbiome-host interaction and Its role in metabolic disease. Nutrients 2018;10(3):365.
9. Blasbalg TL, Hibbeln JR, Ramsden CE, et al. Changes in consumption of omega-3 and omega-6 fatty acids in the United States during the 20th century. Am J Clin Nutr 2011;93(5):950–62.
10. Innes JK, Calder PC. Omega-6 fatty acids and inflammation. Prostaglandins Leukot Essent Fatty Acids 2018;132:41–8.
11. Lerner A, Matthias T. Changes in intestinal tight junction permeability associated with industrial food additives explain the rising incidence of autoimmune disease. Autoimmun Rev 2015;14(6):479–89.
12. Tuck CJ, Biesiekierski JR, Schmid-Grendelmeier P, et al. Food intolerances. Nutrients 2019;11(7):1684.
13. Lomer MC. Review article: the aetiology, diagnosis, mechanisms and clinical evidence for food intolerance. Aliment Pharmacol Ther 2015;41(3):262–75.
14. Rubio-Tapia A, Kyle RA, Kaplan EL, et al. Increased prevalence and mortality in undiagnosed celiac disease. Gastroenterology 2009;137(1):88–93.
15. Camilleri M. Leaky gut: mechanisms, measurement and clinical implications in humans. Gut 2019;68(8):1516–26.

16. Bischoff SC, Barbara G, Buurman W, et al. Intestinal permeability–a new target for disease prevention and therapy. BMC Gastroenterol 2014;14:189.

17. Riccio P, Rossano R. Undigested food and gut microbiota may cooperate in the pathogenesis of neuroinflammatory diseases: a matter of barriers and a proposal on the origin of organ specificity. Nutrients 2019;11(11):2714.

18. Vojdani A, Afar D, Vojdani E. Reaction of lectin-specific antibody with human tissue: possible contributions to autoimmunity. J Immunol Res 2020;2020:1438957.

19. Brennan D. What foods should you avoid if you have leaky gut syndrome? MedicineNet. 2021. Available at: https://www.medicinenet.com/foods_to_avoid_if_you_have_leaky_gut_syndrome/article. Accessed November 17, 2021.

20. Luo EK. What to know about nightshade allergies. Brighton, East Sussex (UK). MedicalNewsToday; 2018. Available at: https://www.medicalnewstoday.com/articles/321883. Accessed November 17, 2021.

21. Minich DM. A review of the science of colorful, plant-based food and practical strategies for "eating the rainbow". J Nutr Metab 2019;19:1–19.

22. Beauchamp GK, Keast RS, Morel D, et al. Phytochemistry: ibuprofen-like activity in extra-virgin olive oil. Nature 2005;437(7055):45–6.

23. Yashin A, Yashin Y, Xia X, et al. Antioxidant activity of spices and their impact on human health: a review. Antioxidants (Basel) 2017;6(3):70.

24. Li Z, Henning SM, Zhang Y, et al. Antioxidant-rich spice added to hamburger meat during cooking results in reduced meat, plasma, and urine malondialdehyde concentrations. Am J Clin Nutr 2010;91(5):1180–4.

25. Guggenheim AG, Wright KM, Zwickey HL. Immune modulation from five major mushrooms: application to integrative oncology. Integr Med (Encinitas) 2014; 13(1):32–44.

26. Zhang Y, Zhang M, Jiang Y, et al. Lentinan as an immunotherapeutic for treating lung cancer: a review of 12 years clinical studies in China. J Cancer Res Clin Oncol 2018;144(11):2177–86.

27. Ramagopalan SV, Heger A, Berlanga AJ, et al. A ChIP-seq defined genome-wide map of vitamin D receptor binding: associations with disease and evolution. Genome Res 2010;20:1352–60.

28. Nicolson GL. Mitochondrial dysfunction and chronic disease: treatment with natural supplements. Integr Med (Encinitas) 2014;13(4):35–43.

29. Habiballa L, Salmonowicz H, Passos JF. Mitochondria and cellular senescence: Implications for musculoskeletal ageing. Free Radic Biol Med 2019;132:3–10.

30. Pan H, Finkel T. Key proteins and pathways that regulate lifespan. J Biol Chem 2017;292(16):6452–60.

31. New Hampshire Department of Health and Human Services Department of Public Health Services. How much sugar do you eat? You might be surprised! NH DHHS-DPHS-Health promotion in motion. Available at: https://www.dhhs.nh.gov/dphs/nhp/documents/sugar.pdf. Accessed December 11, 2021.

32. Gould S. 6 charts that show how much more Americans eat that they used to. Insider. 2017. Available at: https://www.businessinsider.com/daily-calories-americans-eat-increase-2016-07. Accessed: December 11, 2021.

33. Fryar CD, Carroll MD, Afful J. Prevalence of overweight, obesity, and severe obesity among adults aged 20 and over: United States, 1960–1962 through 2017–2018. NCHS Health E-Stats; 2020.

34. Longhi R, Almeida RF, Pettenuzzo LF, et al. Effect of a trans fatty acid-enriched diet on mitochondrial, inflammatory, and oxidative stress parameters in the cortex and hippocampus of Wistar rats. Eur J Nutr 2018;57(5):1913–24.

35. Dhibi M, Brahmi F, Mnari A, et al. The intake of high fat diet with different trans fatty acid levels differentially induces oxidative stress and non alcoholic fatty liver disease (NAFLD) in rats. Nutr Metab 2011;8:65.

36. Miller VJ, Villamena FA, Volek JS. Nutritional ketosis and mitohormesis: potential implications for mitochondrial function and human health. J Nutr Metab 2018; 2018:5157645.

37. Longo VD, Panda S. Fasting, circadian rhythms, and time-restricted feeding in healthy lifespan. Cell Metab 2016;23(6):1048–59.

38. Baum JI, Kim IY, Wolfe RR. Protein consumption and the elderly: what is the optimal level of intake? Nutrients 2016;8(6):359.

39. Berrazaga I, Micard V, Gueugneau M, et al. The role of the anabolic properties of plant- versus animal-based protein sources in supporting muscle mass maintenance: a critical review. Nutrients 2019;11(8):1825.

40. Van Vliet S, Burd NA, Loon LJ. The skeletal muscle anabolic response to plant-versus animal-based protein consumption. J Nutr 2015;145(9):1981–91.

41. Wesselink E, Koekkoek WAC, Grefte S, et al. Feeding mitochondria: potential role of nutritional components to improve critical illness convalescence. Clin Nutr 2019;38(3):982–95.

42. Wang Y, Liu Z, Han Y, et al. Medium Chain Triglycerides enhances exercise endurance through the increased mitochondrial biogenesis and metabolism. PLoS One 2018;13(2):e0191182.

43. Ames BN. A role for supplements in optimizing health: the metabolic tune-up. Arch Biochem Biophys 2004;423(1):227–34.

44. Ames BN. The metabolic tune-up: metabolic harmony and disease prevention. J Nutr 2003;133(5 Suppl 1):1544S-8S.

45. Sears MR, Genuis SJ. Environmental determinants of chronic disease and medical approaches: recognition, avoidance, supportive therapy, and detoxification. J Environ Public Health 2012;2012:356798.

46. Holtcamp W. Obesogens: an environmental link to obesity. Environ Health Perspect 2012;120(2):a62–8.

47. Kieber-Emmons T, Kohler H. Evolutionary origin of autoreactive determinants (autogens). Proc Natl Acad Sci U S A 1986;83(8):2521–5.

48. Environmental Working Group. Body burden: the pollution in newborns. Washington, DC: Environmental Working Group; 2005. Available at: https://www.ewg.org/research/body-burden-pollution-newborns. Accessed December 11, 2021.

49. Menke A, Muntner P, Batuman V, et al. Blood lead below 0.48 micromol/L (10 microg/dL) and mortality among US adults. Circulation 2006;114(13):1388–94.

50. Navas-Acien A, Guallar E, Silbergeld EK, et al. Lead exposure and cardiovascular disease–a systematic review. Environ Health Perspect 2007;115(3):472–82.

51. Gorell JM, Johnson CC, Rybicki BA, et al. The risk of Parkinson's disease with exposure to pesticides, farming, well water, and rural living. Neurology 1998; 50(5):1346–50.

52. Gaylord A, Osborne G, Ghassabian A, et al. Trends in neurodevelopmental disability burden due to early life chemical exposure in the USA from 2001 to 2016: A population-based disease burden and cost analysis. Mol Cell Endocrinol 2020;502:110666.

53. Evangelou E, Ntritsos G, Chondrogiorgi M, et al. Exposure to pesticides and diabetes: A systematic review and meta-analysis. Environ Int 2016;91:60–8.

54. Jensen T, Abdelmalek MF, Sullivan S, et al. Fructose and sugar: A major mediator of non-alcoholic fatty liver disease. J Hepatol 2018;68(5):1063–75.

55. Mancini F. The truth about food additives: how they threaten your health. London (UK): Ecologist; 2012. Available at: https://theecologist.org/2012/jan/18/truth-about-food-additives-how-they-threaten-your-health. Accessed December 11, 2021.

56. Minich DM, Brown BI. A review of dietary (phyto)nutrients for glutathione support. Nutrients 2019;11(9):2073.

57. Anacleto P, Barbosa V, Alves RN, et al. Green tea infusion reduces mercury bio-accessibility and dietary exposure from raw and cooked fish. Food Chem Toxicol 2020;145:111717.

58. Joe B, Vijaykumar M, Lokesh BR. Biological properties of curcumin-cellular and molecular mechanisms of action. Crit Rev Food Sci Nutr 2004;44(2):97–111.

59. Hodges RE, Minich DM. Modulation of metabolic detoxification pathways using foods and food-derived components: a scientific review with clinical application. J Nutr Metab 2015;2015:760689.

60. Ormazabal V, Nair S, Elfeky O, et al. Association between insulin resistance and the development of cardiovascular disease. Cardiovasc Diabetol 2018;17:122.

61. Laakso M, Kuusisto J. Insulin resistance and hyperglycaemia in cardiovascular disease development. Nat Rev Endocrinol 2014;10:293–302.

62. Cleveland Clinic. 90 percent of heart disease is preventable through healthier diet, regular exercise, and not smoking. Cleveland (OH): Cleveland Clinic Newsroom; 2021. Available at: https://newsroom.clevelandclinic.org/2021/09/29/90-percent-of-heart-disease-is-preventable-through-healthier-diet-regular-exercise-and-not-smoking/. Accessed: November 18, 2021.

63. Bautch VL, Caron KM. Blood and lymphatic vessel formation. Cold Spring Harb Perspect Biol 2015;7(3):a008268.

64. Barringer TA, Hacher L, Sasser HC. Potential benefits on impairment of endothelial function after a high-fat meal of 4 weeks of flavonoid supplementation. Evid Based Complement Alternat Med 2011;2011:796958.

65. van Bussel BC, Henry RM, Ferreira I, et al. A healthy diet is associated with less endothelial dysfunction and less low-grade inflammation over a 7-year period in adults at risk of cardiovascular disease. J Nutr 2015;145(3):532–40.

66. Zehr KR, Walker MK. Omega-3 polyunsaturated fatty acids improve endothelial function in humans at risk for atherosclerosis: A review. Prostaglandins Other Lipid Mediat 2018;134:131–40.

67. Schwingshackl L, Christoph M, Hoffmann G. Effects of olive oil on markers of inflammation and endothelial function-a systematic review and meta-analysis. Nutrients 2015;7(9):7651–75.

68. Uwitonze AM, Razzaque MS. Role of magnesium in vitamin D activation and function. J Am Osteopath Assoc 2018;118(3):181–9.

69. Hespe GE, Kataru RP, Savetsky IL, et al. Exercise training improves obesity-related lymphatic dysfunction. J Physiol 2016;594(15):4267–82.

70. Vairo GL, Miller SJ, McBrier NM, et al. Systematic review of efficacy for manual lymphatic drainage techniques in sports medicine and rehabilitation: an evidence-based practice approach. J Man Manip Ther 2009;17(3):e80-9.

71. Mooventhan A, Nivethitha L. Scientific evidence-based effects of hydrotherapy on various systems of the body. N Am J Med Sci 2014;6(5):199–209.

72. Moseley AL, Piller NB, Carati CJ. The effect of gentle arm exercise and deep breathing on secondary arm lymphedema. Lymphology 2005;38(3):136–45.

73. Nagashio S, Ajima K, Maejima D, et al. Water intake increases mesenteric lymph flow and the total flux of albumin, long-chain fatty acids, and IL-22 in rats: new

concept of absorption in jejunum. Am J Physiol Gastrointest Liver Physiol 2019; 316(1):G155–65.

74. Menke A, Casagrande S, Geiss L, et al. Prevalence of and trends in diabetes among adults in the United States, 1988-2012. JAMA 2015;314(10):1021–9.

75. Araújo J, Cai J, Stevens J. Prevalence of optimal metabolic health in American adults: National Health and Nutrition Examination Survey 2009-2016. Metab Syndr Relat Disord 2019;17(1):46–52.

76. Unluhizarci K, Karaca Z, Kelestimur F. Role of insulin and insulin resistance in androgen excess disorders. World J Diabetes 2021;12(5):616–29.

77. Chao AM, Jastreboff AM, White MA, et al. Stress, cortisol, and other appetite-related hormones: Prospective prediction of 6-month changes in food cravings and weight. Obesity (Silver Spring) 2017;25(4):713–20.

78. Alizadehmohajer N, Shojaeifar S, Nedaeinia R, et al. Association between the microbiota and women's cancers - cause or consequences? Biomed Pharmacother 2020;127:110203.

79. Kajla P, Sharma A, Sood DR. Flaxseed-a potential functional food source. J Food Sci Technol 2015;52(4):1857–71.

80. Minich D. The best foods for supporting estrogen metabolism. Dr. Deanna Minich 2020. Available at: https://deannaminich.com/the-best-foods-to-eat-for-supporting-estrogen-metabolism/. Accessed: November 18, 2021.

81. Sepkovic DW, Stein J, Carlisle AD, et al. Diindolylmethane inhibits cervical dysplasia, alters estrogen metabolism, and enhances immune response in the K14-HPV16 transgenic mouse model. Cancer Epidemiol Biomarkers Prev 2010; 19(2):628.

82. Fantus RJ, Halpern JA, Chang C, et al. The association between popular diets and serum testosterone among men in the United States. J Urol 2020;203(2): 398–404.

83. Liontiris MI, Mazokopakis EE. A concise review of Hashimoto thyroiditis (HT) and the importance of iodine, selenium, vitamin D and gluten on the autoimmunity and dietary management of HT patients. Points that need more investigation. Hell J Nucl Med 2017;20(1):51–6.

84. Fiore M, Oliveri Conti G, Caltabiano R, et al. Role of Emerging Environmental Risk Factors in Thyroid Cancer: A Brief Review. Int J Environ Res Public Health 2019; 16(7):1185.

85. Jacka FN, O'Neil A, Opie R, et al. A randomised controlled trial of dietary improvement for adults with major depression (the 'SMILES' trial). BMC Med 2017;15:23.

86. Schoenthaler S, Amos S, Doraz W, et al. The effect of randomized vitamin-mineral supplementation on violent and non-violent antisocial behavior among incarcerated juveniles. J Nutr Environ Med 1997;7(4):343–52.

87. Centers for Disease Control and Prevention. Health and academic achievement. 2014. Available at: https://www.cdc.gov/healthyyouth/health_and_academics/pdf/health-academic-achievement.pdf. Accessed: November 18, 2021.

88. Basch CE. Breakfast and the achievement gap among urban minority youth. J Sch Health 2011;81(10):635–40.

89. McCann D, Barrett A, Cooper A, et al. Food additives and hyperactive behaviour in 3-year-old and 8/9-year-old children in the community: a randomised, double-blinded, placebo-controlled trial. Lancet 2007;370(9598):1542.

90. Dengate S, Ruben A. Controlled trial of cumulative behavioural effects of a common bread preservative. J Paediatr Child Health 2002;38(4):373–6.

91. Suyoto PST, Aulia B. Low muscle mass and inflammation among patients with type 2 diabetes mellitus in Indonesia. Diabetol Int 2018;10(3):219–24.
92. Ibarguren M, López DJ, Escribá PV. The effect of natural and synthetic fatty acids on membrane structure, microdomain organization, cellular functions and human health. Biochim Biophys Acta 2014;1838(6):1518–28.
93. Chang CY, Ke DS, Chen JY. Essential fatty acids and human brain. Acta Neurol Taiwan 2009;18(4):231–41.

The Identification and Management of Small Intestinal Bacterial Overgrowth
A Functional Medicine Approach

Seema M. Patel, MD, MPH[a], Melissa C. Young, MD[b],*

KEYWORDS

- Small intestinal bacterial overgrowth
- Small intestinal bacterial overgrowth and treatment
- Small intestinal bacterial overgrowth and diet
- Small intestinal bacterial overgrowth and functional medicine • Functional medicine

KEY POINTS

- SIBO may coexist with many other conditions including irritable bowel syndrome, cirrhosis, scleroderma, Parkinson, obesity, and inflammatory bowel disease.
- A functional medicine approach may reveal pertinent antecedents, triggers, and mediators (ATMs) contributing to SIBO symptoms including low gastric acid, impaired motility, gut epithelial inflammation, use of certain medications, and other systemic inflammatory diseases such as diabetes, scleroderma, and Parkinson.
- Organization of ATMs within the functional medicine matrix may support a management strategy that extends beyond treating the bacterial overgrowth by way of antibiotic or herbal antimicrobial therapies to include possible root causes.

INTRODUCTION

Small intestinal bacterial overgrowth (SIBO) is a common yet underrecognized condition characterized by an excessive amount of bacteria in the small intestine. The true prevalence of SIBO is unknown, but it is more common in women and the elderly.[1–4] SIBO can exist in many common conditions such as irritable bowel syndrome (IBS), obesity, and cirrhosis.[1,2,4,5] Historically, SIBO was defined as an excess of bacteria exceeding 10^5 colony-forming units (CFU) per milliliter, which is seen more commonly with stagnant loop conditions.[1,6,7] Recently, the American College of Gastroenterology guidelines recommend the threshold of 10^3 CFU/mL by jejunal aspirate and

[a] Cleveland Clinic Functional Medicine, 9500 Euclid Avenue, Q-2 Cleveland, OH 44159, USA;
[b] Center for Functional Medicine, 551 Washington Street, Chagrin Falls, OH 44022, USA
* Corresponding author.
E-mail addresses: patels2@ccf.org (S.M.P.); pyoungm9@ccf.org (M.C.Y.)

Phys Med Rehabil Clin N Am 33 (2022) 587–603
https://doi.org/10.1016/j.pmr.2022.04.003
1047-9651/22/© 2022 Elsevier Inc. All rights reserved.

culture as diagnostic for SIBO.[7–10] In complex patients, systemic symptoms that extend beyond the gut often coincide with a SIBO diagnosis. Using a functional medicine-based approach focused on a root-cause analysis may help providers broaden the lens of how to identify and manage SIBO as well as guide the provider to recognize underlying dysfunctions that need to be balanced.

IDENTIFICATION OF SMALL INTESTINAL BACTERIAL OVERGROWTH
Common Symptoms

Patients with SIBO present with various gastrointestinal symptoms including abdominal pain, bloating, nausea, constipation, diarrhea, and/or flatulence.[5,7,8,11] More severe patients present with weight loss, malnutrition, and malabsorption of iron, calcium, magnesium, and vitamins A, B_{12}, D, and E.[5,7,11–13] Because SIBO is associated with intestinal permeability, or "leaky gut," patients may also present with systemic symptoms such as rosacea, migraines, joint pain, as well as neurologic complaints like brain fog, memory loss, anxiety, and depressive symptoms.[5,11,14]

Owing to the variety of symptoms and complexity of patients with SIBO, using a functional medicine approach may help identify underlying dysfunctions. Functional medicine providers first create a timeline of antecedents, triggers, and mediators (or ATMs). Antecedents are predisposing factors. Triggers are events that occur before disease onset or provoke the onset of the disease. Last, mediators are factors that perpetuate continual symptoms and/or disease.

The patient's symptoms are then organized into a matrix. The functional medicine matrix is a "whole person" approach that helps clinicians appreciate the interconnectedness of different organ systems from a biochemical and physiologic process.[15] This organizing system may aid in the development of a personalized management strategy for SIBO.

ORGANIZING SMALL INTESTINAL BACTERIAL OVERGROWTH ANTECEDENTS, TRIGGERS, AND MEDIATORS IN THE FUNCTIONAL MEDICINE MATRIX

Table 1 overviews how ATMs are organized within the functional medicine matrix.

Impaired Digestion Leading to Mucosal Inflammation

Matrix node: assimilation and digestion

Impaired digestion can result from a reduction in levels of gastric acid, bile salts, and pancreatic enzymes as well as malabsorption syndromes. A reduction in levels of digestive enzymes, bile acids, and/or gastric acid diminish their antibacterial effect[3,5,8,11] decreasing the protection of the small intestine. Furthermore, a low level of bile salts and/or exocrine pancreatic insufficiency can result in mucosal inflammation, increase endotoxemia, and impair absorption of critical vitamins.[5,6,8,9,16]

There are various ATMs associated with impaired digestion. Antecedents include congenital pancreatic insufficiency and/or celiac disease. Triggers/mediators are conditions that negatively affect the production and secretion of various digestive supports. Triggers can be surgery and/or radiation. Mediators may include the following: lowered gastric acid can be from chronic proton pump inhibitor (PPI) use, age-related achlorhydria, autoimmune gastritis, *Helicobacter pylori* infection, and/or postsurgical achlorhydria.[5,6,8,9,16] Patients presenting with chronic pancreatitis have a propensity for SIBO due to diminished level of gastric acid, intestinal dysmotility, and disturbance in gut immune defense.[17] SIBO evaluation should be considered for patients with refractory celiac disease. The exact mechanism relating these

Table 1
Antecedents, triggers, and mediators for small intestinal bacterial overgrowth using the functional medicine matrix

	Matrix Node			
ATMs	Assimilation and digestion Impaired digestion leading to mucosal inflammation	Structural integrity Impaired intestinal motility and structural changes	Defense and repair Chronic inflammation and immune deficiencies	Biotransformation and elimination Environmental toxicants
Antecedents	• Congenital pancreatic insufficiency • Celiac disease Celiac disease not treated or refractory can lead to intestinal mucosal inflammation and decrease in gut defense Pancreatic insufficiency can lead to malabsorption	• Congenital and acquired anatomic issues • EDS Anatomic alterations can change motility. EDS can have defective collagen, poor motility, and redundant bowel	• Selective IgA deficiency • Common variable immune deficiency Decreased IgA can increase intestinal permeability and risk for bacterial translocation	• Genetic variability in detoxification • Nutritional status Genetic defects can decrease ability to detoxify Nutritional status if depleted can decrease ability to detoxify
Triggers	• Surgery • Radiation Surgery and radiation can decrease digestive support and alter motility	• Radiation enteritis • Obstruction/pseudo-obstruction • Past abdominal/pelvic surgery with resulting adhesions Radiation alters gut epithelium and can alter motility Anatomic disease and surgical adhesions can result in narrowing and stasis leading to SIBO	• TBIs • Infection: acute, chronic, or stealth; viral, tick, fungal, bacterial, parasites • Food poisoning • TBI: exact mechanism unknown but disruption in gut-brain axis leads to dysbiosis, which can worsen neural inflammation • Infections: exact mechanism uncertain but possible dysbiosis • Food poisoning can trigger an autoimmune reaction against the MMC	• Environmental toxicants • Mold/mycotoxin • Heavy metals Toxicants can cause dysbiosis, a loss of diversity of microbiota, increased intestinal permeability, and inflammation

(continued on next page)

Table 1
(continued)

Matrix Node			
Mediators			

• Low gastric acid
• Low bile salts
• Exocrine pancreatic insufficiency
• Chronic pancreatitis
• Celiac disease
	• Blind loops/bypass surgery
	• Adhesions or disease
	• Strictures from inflammatory bowel disease or other
	• Small bowel diverticulosis
	• Volvulus
	• Intussusception
	• Tumor or abdominal and/or pelvis malignancy
	• Altered collagen/EDS
	• Scleroderma/amyloidosis
	• Radiation
	• Opioid medications
	• Antidiarrheal medicines
	• Anticholinergic medicines
	• Untreated/partially treated hypothyroid states
	• Ileocecal valve disorders
	• Damage to MMC
	• Gastroparesis
	• IBS
		• Immunodeficiency states
		  ○ HIV
		  ○ Congenital and/or acquired deficiency
		• Anti CDT-B or anti-vinculin antibody
		• Aging/obesity
		• Scleroderma/amyloidosis
		• CAD
		• NAFLD/cirrhosis
		• Parkinson
		• Diabetes, DM neuropathy
		• Stress
			• Environmental toxicants
			• Mold/mycotoxin
			• Heavy metals
			• Genetic variability in detoxification
			• Nutritional status

• Gastric acid, bile salts, and pancreatic enzymes have an antibacterial effect • With low gastric acid levels, incoming bacteria may not be destroyed and can increase risk for SIBO • Low levels of pancreatic enzymes and bile salts decrease absorption of	• Anatomic disease and surgical adhesions can result in narrowing & impaired motility • Epithelial alterations of the gut can cause dysmotility • Medications and hypothyroid states may impact motility	• Decreased IgA levels can increase intestinal permeability and risk for bacterial translocation • Food poisoning can lead to antibodies against predominant MMC • SCI may increase intestinal inflammation	Toxicants can cause dysbiosis, a loss of diversity of microbiota, increased intestinal permeability, and inflammation Genetic defects can decrease ability to detoxify Nutritional status if depleted can decrease ability to detoxify

critical vitamins and can increase endotoxemia and mucosal inflammation

- The ileocecal valve dysfunction can cause retrograde movement of colonic bacteria into the SI
- MMC damage can lead to stasis and inflammation
- IBS and gastroparesis are multifactorial in origin

- Stress decreases beneficial bacteria and decreases secretory IgA and protective mucins on the intestinal mucosa

The matrix was adapted for SIBO education and reflects the authors' viewpoints only.

Abbreviations: CAD, coronary artery disease; CDT-B, cytolethal distending toxin B; DM, diabetes mellitus; EDS, Ehlers-Danlos syndrome; HIV, immunodeficiency virus; IBS, irritable bowel syndrome; MMC, migrating motor complex; NAFLD, nonalcoholic fatty liver disease; TBI, traumatic brain injury; SI, small intestine; SCI, systemic chronic inflammation.

conditions is unclear but may result from possible intestinal mucosal damage and a decrease in immune defense.[13,18,19]

Impaired Intestinal Motility and Structural Changes

Matrix node: structural integrity

Impaired intestinal motility can result from a wide range of conditions. Impairments can be categorized as due to anatomic changes, alterations in the gut epithelium, medication-related hypomotility, ileocecal valve dysfunction, and/or damage to the migrating motor complex (MMC). MMC is a cyclical electromechanical activity in the gastrointestinal (GI) smooth muscle cells occurring in the fasting state. Diminished MMC activity can lead to stasis and risk for bacterial overgrowth.

Anatomic alterations can be antecedents, triggers, or mediators based on the patient's timeline. Anatomic alterations can be congenital and/or acquired resulting from surgical gastric bypass, adhesions or disease, strictures from inflammatory bowel disease (IBD) or other conditions, diverticulosis, volvulus, tumors, or abdominal/pelvic malignancies.[5,8,13,20]

Alterations in the gut epithelium can be antecedents or mediators. An antecedent is Ehlers-Danlos syndrome (EDS), which can be associated with disordered collagen, redundant bowel, and impaired motility, increasing their risk for SIBO.[21] Acquired alterations in the gut epithelium can be a trigger like radiation or mediators resulting from radiation, scleroderma, and/or amyloidosis.[7,8,14,22]

The remaining categories of impaired motility are mediators. Medications like opioids and anticholinergics[1,14,22] as well as an inadequately treated hypothyroid state can decrease motility. Ileocecal valve reflux may result from damage to the valve from surgery, inflammation, and/or intrinsic valve dysfunction. This reflux may cause retrograde transfer of colonic bacteria to the small intestine, increasing the risk of SIBO.[5,7,8,11,13,14] Damage to the MMC can be mediators such as opioid use, EDS, systemic diseases such as diabetes and Parkinson, and damage to nerves or muscles of the small intestine.[5,7] And the last group, IBS and gastroparesis may have dysmotility and are considered multifactorial in origin.[1,5]

Systemic Chronic Inflammation and Immune Deficiencies

Matrix node: defense and repair

A hyperactive or an underactive immune system can lead to systemic chronic inflammation (SCI). When the immune system is hyperactive, it is constantly overreacting, which may cause immune dysregulation and an increased inflammatory state possibly contributing to autoimmunity and chronic diseases such as heart disease, cancer, and dementia. When the immune system is underactive, it fails to protect the body against infections from different viruses, bacteria, fungi, ticks, and parasites. These infections can also contribute to SCI. Chronic inflammatory states may increase intestinal mucosal inflammation, which can impair motility and increase the risk of stasis.

There are many ATMs associated with immune deficiencies and/or infection related. Antecedents can be congenital immune conditions such as common variable immune deficiency and selective IgA deficiency.[5,7,8] Triggers may be acute, chronic, or stealth infections involving bacteria, viruses, fungi, ticks, and/or parasites. A trigger/mediator can be food poisoning causing an autoimmune reaction against proteins in the small intestine creating anti-CdT-B (cytolethal distending toxin B) and anti-vinculin antibodies, which damage predominant MMC leading to diarrhea-type SIBO.[23,24] Triggers and mediators can also be congenital and/or acquired immune deficiencies such as human immunodeficiency virus.[6,8]

Hyperinflammatory states are triggers and/or mediators. Traumatic brain injuries (TBIs) can be a trigger or mediator. The exact mechanism of how TBIs disrupt the gut-brain axis is unknown; however, the feedback loop initiated by the TBI leads to dysbiosis, and this pathogenic flora influences the gut-brain axis and increases neural inflammation.[25,26] The literature references Parkinson, scleroderma, amyloidosis, obesity, coronary artery disease, nonalcoholic fatty liver disease, cirrhosis, diabetes, diabetic neuropathy, and aging[4,8,14,27,28] as other chronic systemic inflammatory states associated with SIBO. However, because SCI exists in many other conditions, a SIBO diagnosis should be considered when the patient's condition worsens or is unresponsive to therapy. And last, stress can worsen any inflammatory state. Exposure to stress can reduce beneficial bacteria and encourage the growth of possible pathogens.[29] Chronic stress may also affect the production of secretory IgA and protective mucin on the mucosal surface.[29]

Environmental Toxicants

Matrix node: biotransformation and elimination

Humans are exposed to hundreds of environmental chemicals, which include, but are not limited to, air pollutants, heavy metals, pesticides, herbicides, persistent organic pollutants, polychlorinated biphenyls, perfluoroalkyl and polyfluoroalkyl substances phthalates, bisphenols, and mycotoxins from past exposure to water-damaged buildings.[30–33] These chemicals are ubiquitous, and humans have chronic exposure from food, water, air, plastic water bottles and food packaging, personal care products, cosmetics, and detergents.[30,31,34] An important antecedent is the wide spectrum of genetic variability in biotransformation and detoxification. These genetic polymorphisms can decrease detoxification ability and increase the risk of harm from these environmental toxicants.[35] The nutritional status of an individual can also influence the individual's ability to detoxify and can be an antecedent or mediator.[35] The environmental toxicants themselves can be triggers and/or mediators. With the explosion of research[30,36,37] on the gut microbiome, it is increasingly recognized that xenobiotics[30,36,37] alter the gut microbiome and this imbalance may contribute to systemic disease. The adverse impact of these environmental chemicals on the structure and function of gut microbiome includes dysbiosis,[36,37] intestinal permeability,[31,38] intestinal inflammation,[31] and loss of diversity.[39]

TESTING FOR SMALL INTESTINAL BACTERIAL OVERGROWTH
Breath Testing

Breath testing can be performed in a clinical or residential setting by way of commercially available home tests. Although the gold standard for SIBO testing is jejunal aspirates,[5,7,8] this is difficult to perform because of its invasive nature. Therefore, clinicians order a breath test to diagnose SIBO.[5,7,8,40]

In 2017, the North American Consensus statement was developed to streamline breath testing interpretation. An increase in hydrogen (H_2) of 20 ppm or more from baseline within 90 minutes and/or an increase in methane (CH_4) of 10 ppm or greater is considered positive[7,8,41,42]; they no longer recommend 2 peaks.[7,8,42] Methane overgrowth, called intestinal methanogen overgrowth (IMO) is produced by Archaea, which are not bacteria.[7] Methane is associated with chronic constipation and is likely to be colonized by *Methanobrevibacter smithii* in the small intestine.[2,43] The last gas is hydrogen sulfide. This gas is considered when the aforementioned gases give flat line on a traditional breath test.[42] There is currently only 1 test in the market, the Trio Test, that checks for all 3 gases.

There is a wide range in the sensitivity and specificity of the breath test. The glucose breath test sensitivity ranges from 20% to 100%, and the specificity can vary from 30% to 86%.[41,42,44] The lactulose breath test sensitivity varies from 31% to 68% and specificity ranges from 44% to 100%.[41,42,44] Owing to this wide spectrum in specificity and sensitivity for both these breath tests, there is concern for overdiagnosis of SIBO due to high false-positives.

There are many reasons for false-negatives and false-positives. False-negatives can occur if patients hyperventilate during the test, engage in exercise before or during the test, have recently used antibiotics, and/or have engaged in bowel purges. Conditions that delay the delivery of the carbohydrate or bypass the small intestine such as achalasia, partial gastric obstruction, and proximal enterocutaneous fistula can also lead to false-negatives.[41,45,46] False-positives can occur due to smoking, consumption of fermentable food/drinks before testing, failure to follow the preprocedure diet, and fasting, which allow for rapid fermentation. False-positives can occur in patients with a history of upper GI tract surgery and/or chronic constipation, which prolong the oral-cecal transit time.[41,45,46] To decrease false test results, strict adherence to test preparation and protocol is essential.

FUNCTIONAL MEDICINE MANAGEMENT OF SMALL INTESTINAL BACTERIAL OVERGROWTH

Functional medicine management of SIBO is a "whole person" approach; it expands to include treating the bacterial overgrowth, restoring gut and body function, as well as investigating and treating underlying dysfunctions.

Impaired Digestion Leading to Mucosal Inflammation

Matrix node: assimilation and digestion

The functional medicine diagnostic and treatment approach to SIBO focuses on improving the core functions of the digestive tract (digestion, absorption, regulated intestinal permeability, detoxification, and elimination) because disturbances in these functions may be attributed to symptoms. To address disturbances, functional medicine uses the 5R approach—an acronym for remove, replace, reinoculate, repair, and rebalance.[47] The first part involves removing triggers such as pathogenic bacteria or yeast in the GI tract as well as removing any food sensitivities and/or allergies. The second part involves replacing digestive factors such as digestive enzymes, if needed. The third part involves repopulating the intestinal tract with beneficial bacteria using prebiotics and/or probiotics. The fourth part involves repairing the gut lining by replenishing various nutrients needed to ameliorate mucosal inflammation and oxidation, and improve epithelial defense barrier. The fifth and last part involves rebalancing the lifestyle factors (meditation, exercise, and sleep) that affect the health of the digestive tract and calming sympathetic overactivity.

Remove

The first part of SIBO treatment is removing pathogenic agents. **Table 2** outlines standard antibiotic and herbal therapy for SIBO.

Standard therapeutic options: antibiotics

When using antibiotics, the goal is to *modify* the microbial community to improve symptoms, not to eradicate the entire bacterial flora.[5,7,48] For hydrogen-predominant SIBO, rifaximin is the antibiotic of choice because it exhibits local effects with the intestinal lining due to its poor absorption systemically. An additional benefit is its broad-spectrum activity against gram-positive and gram-negative microorganisms

Table 2
Small intestinal bacterial overgrowth treatment options based on (A) hydrogen (B) methane and (C) sulfur results

(A) If Hydrogen Result Is Positive, Consider One of the Following Antibiotic Options:

Name	Dosing	Duration
Rifaximin	400mg to550 mg 3×/d	Take for 2 wk.
Amoxicillin-clavulanic	500/125 mg 3×/d	If symptoms
Metronidazole	250 mg 3×/d	persist,
Ciprofloxacin	250 to 500mg mg 2×/d	take for an
Tetracycline	250 mg 4×/d	additional
Trimethoprim-sulfamethoxazole	1 double strength 2×/d	2 wk
Norfloxacin	800 mg daily or 400mg 2x/day	
Doxycycline	100 mg 2×/d	

If Hydrogen Result Is Positive, can Also Consider Following Herbal Options:
Recommend Using 2 Herbs to Treat Hydrogen SIBO

Name	Dosing	Duration
FC-Cidal	2 capsules 2–3×/d	Take for 2 mo
Dysbiocide	2 capsules 2–3×/d	
Candibactin-AR	1 capsule 3×/d	
Candibactin-BR	2 capsule 3×/d	
Berberine	1000 mg 3×/d	
Oil of oregano	100-200- mg 3×/d	
Neem	600 mg 3×/d	

(B) If Methane Result Is Positive, Combine the Following Antibiotic Options:

Name	Dosing	Duration
Rifaximin	550 mg 3×/d	Take for 2 wk
Neomycin	500 mg 2x/day	

If Methane Result Is Positive, Consider the Following Herbal Options:

Name	Dosing	Duration
Atrantil	2 caps 3×/d	Take for 2 mo
Allicin	600 mg 3×/d	
Combine one of the aforementioned with 2 hydrogen-treating herbs		

(C) If Sulfur Result Is Positive or There Is a Flat Line on the Breath Test, Consider the Following Antibiotic Option:

Name	Dosing	Duration
Rifaximin	550 mg 3×/d	Take for 2 wk

If Sulfur Result Is Positive or There Is a Flat Line on Breath Test, Consider One of the Following Herbal Options:

Name	Dosing	Duration
Oil of oregano	100-200 mg 2 caps 3×/d	Take for 1 mo
Molybdenum	100–150mcg 2×/d	
Combine the aforementioned 2 treatments with bismuth	500–540 mg 3×/d	
	20–40 mg daily	
Zinc acetate		

as well as aerobic and anaerobic bacteria.[7,8,11,49,50] The treatment dose can range from 400mg to 550 mg 3 times per day for 2 weeks. If symptoms recur, an additional 2-week course is recommended. Other antibiotics such as amoxicillin/clavulanate, metronidazole, ciprofloxacin, tetracycline, trimethoprim-sulfamethoxazole, and nor-floxacin[6,42,44] may be used when there are cost concerns, sensitivity to rifaximin, or previous failure with rifaximin. Rifaximin is also used to treat hydrogen sulfide gas, but there is minimal mention of hydrogen sulfide gas treatment in the literature.

Patients presenting with IMO may benefit from combination antibiotic therapy. Rifaximin monotherapy has a response rate of only 28% to 33% with IMO. However, combination therapy of neomycin and rifaximin for 2 weeks improves the response rate to 87%.[6,10,13,51]

Once antibiotic treatment is over and if patients have persistent symptoms, this may be due to small intestinal fungal overgrowth (SIFO). SIBO and SIFO can present with abdominal pain, bloating, gas, and diarrhea.[52,53] Using fluconazole 100 mg daily for 2 weeks after antibiotic therapy can help.[52,53]

Complications can occur with antibiotic treatment. Complications can include diarrhea, *Clostridium difficile* infection, yeast infections, allergic reactions, and/or financial strain.[6,13] It is not necessary to repeat SIBO testing after treatment if the patient improves.[6]

SIBO recurrences are common unfortunately. High-risk patients who have an underlying cause that cannot be changed (ie, surgical bypass, and so on) can be treated using 1 week of antibiotics per month, alternating norfloxacin with metronidazole monthly for 3 consecutive months.[6,14]

Emerging therapeutic options: herbal antimicrobials

Even though rifaximin is the treatment of choice, it can be cost prohibitive and prior authorizations are often denied. A study comparing rifaximin to herbal combination antimicrobial treatments showed that both treatments were efficacious and the herbal antimicrobial therapy cost was lower.[8,54] Based on their clinical expertise, some functional medicine providers may recommend single herbal treatments like berberine, oil of oregano, and/or neem with variable dosing and duration.[55]

For patients with IMO, combining 2 hydrogen-specific antimicrobials with either Atrantil, a combination herbal supplement, or allicin, medicinal garlic can be considered. Small studies demonstrate that Atrantil can improve constipation and bloating in subjects with IBS-C. Atrantil is prescribed as 2 capsules 3 times per day for 2 months.[56,57] Allicin is made by various nutraceutical companies and is prescribed as 900 to 950 mg 3 times per day for 2 months.[55]

For patients with hydrogen sulfide SIBO there are a few options, but evidence on their effectiveness is limited. Functional medicine providers will use high doses of oil of oregano 200 to 500 mg 3 times per day or molybdenum 100 to 150 µg 2 times per day combined with bismuth and zinc acetate for 1 month.[55,58,59]

Complications and recurrences of SIBO can occur with antimicrobial therapy as well. Complications can be allergic reactions, intolerance, and/or financial strain. For prevention of recurrences in high-risk patients, functional medicine providers are more likely to recommend daily low-dose herbal antimicrobials for 2 to 3 months. The most common nutraceuticals used are berberine, Atrantil, or a combination herbal supplement.

Removing offending foods

Removing certain foods may be beneficial for patients with SIBO. The most common dietary recommendation for hydrogen- and methane-predominant SIBO is the low FODMAP diet, which reduces or removes fermentable oligosaccharides, disaccharides, monosaccharide, and polyols. High-FODMAP foods are osmotically active and ferment in the small intestine increasing intestinal water volume and gas.[48,60,61] Although this diet has not undergone rigorous clinical study, it is commonly used clinically to reduce symptoms in patients with SIBO.[10,13] The low-FODMAP diet is prescribed for 6 to 8 weeks only because low-fiber diets for long term can decrease beneficial bacteria in the gut microbiome.[61]

Reintroduction of food is methodically done to identify foods that exacerbate symptoms. If the eliminated food on reintroduction does not worsen symptoms, it is incorporated back into the diet. However, if the patient feels worse, it is recommended to temporarily omit the food from the diet and attempt another reintroduction 6 to 8 weeks later. At the end, the patient creates a personalized modified FODMAP diet.

There are a few other dietary options to consider. The elemental diet may be beneficial especially in sensitive patients or those who have failed the low FODMAP diet. The elemental formula, a medical food, is readily absorbed in the small intestine and does not feed the bacteria. The elemental formula is used for 14 days, and if symptoms persist, it can be extended for 21 days.[8,48] There are also SIBO diets created by different providers that may be beneficial but have limited evidence. There is even less information on how to treat hydrogen sulfide SIBO with diet. Many functional medicine providers will recommend a low-sulfur diet for 1 month to reduce symptom burden.[58] The last dietary consideration is spacing meals out every 4 to 6 hours if there is concern about MMC dysfunction or impaired motility from other causes.

Replace

Because patients with SIBO may be deficient in gastric acid and digestive enzymes, replacing them may improve symptoms. If low gastric acid is a concern, replacing with betaine hydrochloric acid should be considered. Administration should be slowly started with 1 capsule with meals and increased as tolerated to 3 to 5 capsules if needed.[62] Weaning the patient off chronic PPIs should be considered *if appropriate* using functional medicine therapies. Stool studies can be performed to evaluate fecal pancreatic elastase and fecal fat. Pancreatic exocrine replacement therapy is indicated for pancreatic elastase levels less than 100 μg/g feces by fecal elastase test.[63] An insufficiency of pancreatic enzymes is considered by functional medicine providers when the pancreatic elastase level is between 100 and 200 μg/g and can be supported with a supplemental pancreatic enzyme. If there is an elevation of level of fecal fats, adding supplemental bile salts with meals may be beneficial. Many providers also use broad-spectrum digestive enzymes with meals to support the patient.

Repair

Repairing the intestinal mucosa is important because many patients with SIBO have a "leaky gut." Decreasing intestinal permeability can be accomplished using L-glutamine alone or in a combination formula or with a dairy-free immunoglobulin supplement during the bacterial treatment or following treatment depending on the patient's tolerance. In small studies, dairy-free immunoglobulin supplements improved patient symptoms due to refractory IBS with or without SIBO.[64,65] The repair formula is used for 2 to 4 months. Owing to intestinal mucosal inflammation, patients may have malabsorption of vitamins such as B_{12}, A, D, and E and iron, thus evaluating and replenishing is necessary if appropriate.[5,11,13]

Reinoculating

Reinoculating the gut microbiome is generally recommended after completing antimicrobial and antifungal treatments. Studies evaluating probiotics to manage SIBO have been mixed.[7,12,44,66] Functional medicine providers often start with soil-based probiotics, *Bacillus* species, free of prebiotics. One should consider slowly titrating upward, starting at a half capsule or 1 capsule 2 times per week and increase to daily. If the patient tolerates daily probiotics, increase to 2 capsules daily [67] If the patient is tolerating soil-based probiotics, probiotics rich in *Lactobacillus* and *Bifidobacterium* (free of prebiotics) should be considered. The probiotics should be slowly titrated upward starting with 1 capsule 2 times per week and increased to daily as tolerated. If yeast overgrowth is a concern, adding *Saccharomyces boulardii*, a probiotic yeast may be beneficial.[68] Soil-based probiotics are used for about 6 months and then weaned if able to use other probiotics but may vary by provider. The duration of other probiotics varies by patient condition and provider.

Because prebiotics propagate the growth of established gut bacteria, timing of their use in the management of SIBO is critical. If the pathogenic bacteria are not fully eradicated, the incorporation of prebiotics may contribute to a SIBO relapse. Conversely, if introduced at the appropriate time, prebiotics can strengthen the beneficial gut microbiome. Small studies demonstrate improvement using partially hydrolyzed guar gum for patients with SIBO as well as patients with IBS-D.[69,70] It is probably best to introduce prebiotics after the patient can tolerate all the aforementioned steps. Microdosing prebiotics twice weekly in small amounts and then slowly increasing the frequency seems better tolerated in clinical practice. The duration of prebiotic therapy can be months and is occurring simultaneously with the investigation of underlying causes.

Rebalance

Calming the body from a chronic sympathetic overdrive to a more balanced autonomic nervous system is critical. Regular engagement in calming practices like meditation, tapping, breath work, grounding, binaural beats, and advanced programs such as limbic or amygdala retraining for the severely ill may improve patient symptoms.[71] Important lifestyle modifications to enhance sleep and restorative movement practices are also recommended.

Impaired Intestinal Motility and Structural Changes

Matrix node: structural integrity

Impaired intestinal motility and structural changes are probably the most challenging underlying causes of SIBO to manage. Prokinetics both pharmacologic and herbal can improve intestinal motility.[8,14] Pharmacologic prokinetics include cisapride, tegaserod, low-dose erythromycin, and prucalopride.[8] Functional medicine providers also use compounded low-dose naltrexone 1 to 5 mg daily, which acts as an anti-inflammatory, improving motility and intestinal permeability.[72] Herbal prokinetics to consider are STW5[73] and nutraceuticals containing ginger and artichoke.[74] In clinical practice, combining herbal prokinetics with low-dose naltrexone seems effective, but no studies to date have examined this.

The remaining causes of impaired motility include medications, anatomic changes, and systemic diseases. Medications that reduce motility and their continued indication should be reviewed. It should be confirmed that the thyroid is properly functioning and replacement should be used if needed. Patients with anatomic causes such as strictures, adhesions, and or other abdominal pathologies of concern need appropriate referrals to surgery and/or gastroenterology for further diagnostic assessment and treatment.[14] Inflammatory conditions such as IBD, scleroderma, and amyloidosis can be mitigated applying functional medicine principles.

Other Functional Medicine Matrix Domains to Consider

Although patients may improve with the aforementioned treatments, some patients may continue to have persistent symptoms and may need a deeper dive into other root causes. Therefore, it may be valuable to pursue potential stealth infections or environmental toxicant exposures. However, there is a paucity of evidence supporting this.

Systemic Chronic Inflammation and Immune deficiencies

Matrix node: defense and repair

Systemic chronic inflammation and immune deficiencies can be ameliorated using functional medicine principles of an anti-inflammatory diet and lifestyle modifications. If stealth infections are a concern, investigating for chronic parasitic, tick-borne, viral, and bacterial infections may be indicated.

Environmental Toxicants

Matrix node: biotransformation and elimination

Environmental toxicants are ubiquitous and are often overlooked by conventional providers. When patients are not improving with the aforementioned therapies, have known genetic polymorphisms that affect detoxification and/or past and current exposures to environmental toxicants and water damaged buildings, evaluating for specific environmental toxicants and/or mycotoxins should be considered.

SUMMARY

SIBO is a common but underrecognized condition that is seen in many conditions including IBS, cirrhosis, scleroderma, Parkinson, obesity, and IBD. A functional medicine approach may uncover pertinent antecedents, triggers, and mediators contributing to SIBO such as low gastric acid states, impaired motility, gut epithelial inflammation, use of motility-affecting medications, and/or systemic inflammatory diseases such as diabetes, scleroderma, and immune deficiency syndromes. SIBO treatment using the functional medicine 5 R program may help reduce bacterial overgrowth and expand possible therapeutic options to manage the other underlying dysfunctions in SIBO. Organizing the ATMs within the functional medicine matrix may support a management strategy that extends beyond treating the bacterial overgrowth and uncovering underlying root causes that may need to be addressed.

DISCLOSURE

The authors have nothing to disclose.

REFERENCES

1. Shah A, Talley N, Jones M, et al. Small intestinal bacterial overgrowth in irritable bowel syndrome: a systematic review and meta analysis of case control studies. Am J Gastroenterol 2020;115(2):190–201.
2. Takakura W, Pimentel M. Small intestinal bacterial overgrowth and irritable bowel syndrome-an update. Front Psychiatry 2020;11:664.
3. Ghoshal UC, Shukla R, Ghoshal U. Small Intestinal Bacterial overgrowth and IBS: a bridge between Functional Organic Dichotomy. Gut Liver 2017;11(2):198–208.
4. Ghosh G, Jesudian AB. Small intestinal bacterial overgrowth in patients with cirrhosis. J Clin Exp Hepatol 2019;9(2):257–67.

5. Ghoshal UC, Ghoshal U. Small intestinal bacterial overgrowth and other intestinal disorders. Gastroenterol Clin North Am 2017;46(1):103–20.
6. Quigley EMM, Murray JA, Pimentel M. AGA clinical practice update on small intestinal bacterial overgrowth: expert review. Gastroentology 2020;159(4):1526–32.
7. Pimentel M, Saad R, Long M, et al. ACG clinical guideline: small intestinal bacterial overgrowth. Am J Gastroenterol 2020;115(2):165–78.
8. Rao SSC, Bhagatwala J. Small intestinal bacterial overgrowth: clinical features and therapeutic management. Clin Transl Gastroenterol 2019;10:10.
9. Jacobs C, Coss Adame E, Attaluri A, et al. Dysmotility and proton pump inhibitor use are independent risk factors for small intestinal bacterial overgrowth and/or fungal overgrowth. Aliment Pharmacol Ther 2013;37(11):1103–11.
10. Rezaie A, Buresi M, Lin H, et al. Hydrogen and Methane Based breath testing in gastrointestinal disorders: The North American Consensus statement. Am J Gastroenterol 2017;112(5):775–84.
11. Sachdev A, Pimentel M. Gastrointestinal Bacterial Overgrowth: Pathogenesis and Clinical Significance. Adv Chron Dis 2013;4(5):223–31.
12. Zhong C, Qu C, Wang B, et al. Probiotics for preventing and treating SIBO: A Meta-analysis and Systemic Review of Current Evidence. J Clin Gastroenterol 2017;51(4):300–11.
13. Adike A, DiBaise JK. Small intestinal bacterial overgrowth: nutritional implications, diagnosis, and management. Gastroenterol Clin North Am 2018;47(1):193–208.
14. Bures J, Cyrany J, Kohoutova D, et al. Small Intestinal Bacterial Overgrowth Syndrome. World J Gastroenterol 2010;28(16):2978–90.
15. Vasques A. Chapter 10: organ system function and underlying mechanisms: the interconnected web. In: *Textbook of functional medicine*, gig harbor. Institute for Functional Medicine; 2006. p. 99.
16. Bohm M, Shin A, Xu H, et al. Risk factors associated with upper aerodigestive tract or Coliform bacterial overgrowth of the small intestine in symptomatic patients. J Clin Gastroenterol 2020;54(1):150–7.
17. Ni Chonchubhair H, Bashir Y, Dobson M, et al. The prevalence of small intestinal bacterial overgrowth in non surgical patients with chronic pancreatitis and pancreatic exocrine insufficiency. Pancreatology 2018;18(4):379–85.
18. Losurdo G, Salvatore D'Abramo F, Indellicati G, et al. The influence of small intestinal bacterial overgrowth in digestive and extra-intestinal disorders. Int J Mol Sci 2020;21(10):3531.
19. Charlesworth R, Winter G. Small intestinal Bacterial Overgrowth and Celiac disease-coincidence or causation? Expert Rev Gastroenterol Hepatol 2020;14(5):305–6.
20. Mouillot T, Rhyman N, Gauthier C, et al. Study of small intestinal bacterial overgrowth in a cohort of patients with abdominal symptoms who underwent bariatric sugery. Obes Surg 2020;30(6):2331–7.
21. Xiong T, Baker J, Chey W, et al. Small intestinal bacterial overgrowth (SIBO) is common in patients with ehlers-danlos syndrome (EDS. Am J Gastroenterol 2019;114:S663–4.
22. Sakkas LI, Simopoulou T, Daoussis D, et al. Intestinal involvement in systemic sclerosis: a clinical review. Dig Dis Sci 2018;63(4):834–44.
23. Rezaie A, Park SC, Morales W, et al. Assessment of anti-viniculin and anti-cytolethal distending toxin b antibodies in subtypes of irritable bowel syndrome. Dig Dis Sci 2017;62(6):1480–5.

24. Pimentel M, Morales W, Pokkunuri V, et al. Autoimmunity links vinculin to the pathophysiology of chronic functional bowel changes following camplyobacter jejuni infection in a rat model. Dig Dis Sci 2015;60(5):1195–205.
25. Zhu CS, Grandhi R, Patterson Thomas T, et al. A review of traumatic brain injury and the gut microbiome: insights into novel mechanism of secondary brain injury and promising new targets for neuroprotection. Brain Sci 2018;8:113.
26. Zhang Y, Wang Z, Peng J, et al. Gut microbiota-brain interaction: an emerging immunotherapy for traumatic brain injury. Exp Neurol 2021;337:113585.
27. Augstyn M, Grys I, Kukla M. Small intestinal bacterial overgrowth and nonalcoholic fatty liver disease. Clin Exp Hepatol 2019;5(1):1–10.
28. Fialho A, Fialho A, Kochlar G, et al. Association between small intestinal bacterial overgrowth by glucose breath test and coronary artery disease. Dig Dis Sci 2018; 63(2):412–21.
29. James M. The gut liver axis: chapter 31 clinical approaches to detoxification and biotransformation. In: *The Textbook of functional medicine*, harbor gig. The Institute for Functional Medicine; 2006. p. 563.
30. Chiu K, Warner G, Nowak RA, et al. The impact of environmental chemicals on the gut microbiome. Toxicol Sci 2020;176(2):253–84.
31. Rosenfeld CS. Gut dysbiosis in animals due to environmental chemical exposures. Front Cell Infect Microbiol 2017;7:396.
32. Liew WP, Mohd-Redzwan S. Mycotoxin: its impact on gut health and microbiota. Front Cell Infect Microbiol 2018;8:60.
33. Shao M, Zhu Y. Long Term metal exposure changes gut microbioa of residents in surrounding a mining and smelt area. Sci Rep 2020;10:43–7.
34. Abdelsalam N, Ramadan AT, ElRakaiby MT, et al. Toxicomicrobiomics: the human microbiome vs pharmaceutical, dietary, and environmental xenobiotics. Front Pharmocol 2020;11:390.
35. Lyon M, Bland J, Jones DS. Chapter 31 clinical approaches to detoxification and biotransformation. In: *Textbook of functional medicine*, gig harbor. Institute for Functional Medicine; 2006. p. 543.
36. Lu K, Manbub R, Fox JG. Xenobiotics: interactions with the intestinal microflora. ILAR J 2015;56(2):218–27.
37. Giambo F,T,M, Costa C, Fenga C. Toxicology and microbiota: how do pesticides influence gut microbiota? a review. Int J Envir Res Public Health 2021;18:5510.
38. Choi YJ, Seelback MJ, Pu H, et al. Polychlorinated bisphenyls disrupt integrity via NADPH oxidase induced alterations of tight junction protein expression. Environ Health Perspect 2010;118(7):976–81.
39. Tu P, Chi L, Bodnar W, et al. Gut microbiome toxicity: connecting the environment and gut microbiome-associated diseases. Toxics 2020;8(1):19.
40. Andrei M, Nicolaie T, Stoicescu A, et al. Intestinal microbiome, SIBO and IBD: what are the connections? Curr Health Sci 2015;41:3.
41. Massey BT, Wald A. Small intestinal bacterial overgrowth syndrome: a guide for appropriate use of breath testing. Dig Dis Sci 2021;66(2):338–47.
42. Rezaie A, Buresi M, Lembo A, et al. Hydrogen and methane-based breath testing in gastrointestinal disorders: the North American Consensus statement. Am J Gasterol 2017;112(5):775–84.
43. Konstantinos T, Change C, Pimentel M. Methanogens: methane and gastrointestinal motility. J Neurogastroenterol Motil 2014;20(1):31–40.
44. Bushyhead D, Quigley E. Small intestinal bacterial overgrowth. Gastroenterol Clin North Am 2021;50(2):463–74.

45. Losordo G, Leandro G, Lerardi E, et al. Breath tests for the non invasive diagnosis of small intestinal bacterial overgrowth: a systemic review with meta-analysis. J Neurogasteroenterol Motil 2020;26(1):16–28.

46. Gasbarrini A, Corazza GR, Gabarrini G, et al. Ist rome H2 Breath testing Consensus Conference Working group. Methodology and Indications of H2-breath testing in gastrointestinal diseases: the Rome Consensus statment. Aliment Pharmcol Ther 2009;29:1–49supp.

47. The Institute for Functional Medicine. The institute for functional medicine toolbox. The Institute for Functional Medicine; 2016 [Online]. Available at:: https://functionalmedicine.widencollective.com/portals/o1ttcfkm/Toolkit_AllResourcesA-Z. Accessed December 2021.

48. Rezaie A, Pimentel M, Rao S. How to test and treat small intestinal bacterial overgrowth: an evidence-based approach. Curr Gastroenterol Rep 2016;18(2):8.

49. Pimentel M. Review article: potential mechanism of action of rifaximin in the management of irritable bowel syndrome with diarrhea. Aliment Pharmacol Ther 2016; 43(supplement 1):37–49.

50. Gatta L, Scarpignato C. Systemic Review with meta-analysis: rifaximin is effective and safe for the treatment of small intestinal bacterial overgrowth. Aliment Pharm Ther 2017;45(5):604–16.

51. Triantafyllou K, Chang C, Pimentel M. Methanogens, Methane and gastrointestinal motility. J Neurogastroenterol Motil 2014;20(1):31–40.

52. Erdogan A, Rao SS. Small Intestinal Fungal Overgrowth. Curr Gastroenterol Rep 2015;17(4):16.

53. Singh R, Mullin G. A wasting syndrome and malnutrition caused by small intestinal fungal overgrowth: a case report and review of the literature. Integr Med 2017; 16(3):48–51.

54. Chedid V, Dhalia S, Clarke JO, et al. Herbal therapy is equivalent to rifaximin for the treatment of small intestinal bacterial overgrowth. Glob Adv Health Med 2014; 3(3):16–24.

55. Siebecker, Allison, "siboinfo.com [Online]. Available at: https://www.siboinfo.com/herbal-antibiotics.html. Accessed 21 12 2021.

56. Brown K, Scott-Hoy B, Jennings LL. Repsonse of irritable bowel syndrome with constipation patients administered a combined quebracho/conker tree/M balsamea Willd extract. World J Gastroenterol 2016;7(3):463–8.

57. Brown K, Scott-Hoy B, Jennings L. Efficacy of a Quebracho, Conker Tree, and M Balsamea Wild Blended Extract in a Randomized Study in Patients with Irritable Bowel Syndrome with Constipation. J Gastro Hep Res 2015;4(9):1762–7.

58. Ruscio M. drruscio.com/hydrogen-sulfide-sibo/ [Online]. Available at:: https://drruscio.com/hydrogen-sulfide-sibo/. Accessed December 2021.

59. Minich, Deanna, "metagenics.com,". 2018 [Online]. Available at: https://www.metagenicsinstitute.com/pulse_patrol/plp-eps-5-sibo-sulfur/.   Accessed December 2021.

60. Staudacher HM, Whelan K. The low FODMAP diet: recent advances in understanding its mechanism and efficacy in IBS. Gut 2017;66(8):1517–27.

61. Altobelli E, Del Negro V, Angeletti PM, et al. Low FODMAP diet improves irritable bowel syndrome symptoms: A meta-analysis. Nutrients 2017;9(9):940.

62. Guilliam T, Drake L. Meal time supplementation with betaine HCL for functional hypochlorhydria: what is the evidence? Integratie Med A Clinician's J 2020; 19(1):32–6.

63. Struyvenberg MR, Martin CR, Freedman SD. Practical guide to exocrine insufficiency-Breaking the myths. BMC Med 2017;15(1):29.

64. Weinstock L, Jasion V. Serum derived immunoglobulin/protein isolate therapy for patients with refractory irritable bowel syndrome. Open J Gastroenterol 2014; 4(10):329–34.
65. Liaquat H, Ashat M, Stocker A, et al. Clinical efficacy of serum derived bovine immunoglobulin in patients with refractory inflammatory bowel disease. Am J Med Sci 2018;356(6):531–6.
66. Quigley E, Quera R. Small intestinal bacterial overgrowth: role of antibiotics, pre-biotics and probiotics. Gastroenterology 2006;130(2 suppl 1):S78–90.
67. Catinean A, Neag AM, Nita A, et al. Bacillus spp. Spores-A promising treatment option for patients with irritable bowel Syndrome. Nutrients 2019;11(9):1968.
68. Pais P, Almeida V, Yilmaz M, et al. Saccharomyces boulardii: What Makes It Tick as Successful Probiotic? J Fungi (Basel Switzerland) 2020;6(2):78.
69. Furnari M, Parodi L, Gemignani E, et al. Clinical Trial: the combination of rifaximin with partially hydrolyzed guar gum is more effective than rifaximin alone in erad-icating small intestinal bacterial overgrowth. Aliment Pharm Ther 2010;32(8): 1000–6.
70. Yasukawa Z, Inoue R, Ozeki M, et al. Effect of repeated consumption of partially hydrolyzed guar gum on fecal characteristics and gut microbiota: a randomized, doubl blind, placebo-controlled, and parallel group clinical trial. Nutrients 2019; 11:2170.
71. Sanabria-Mazo J, Montero-Marin J, Feliu-Soler A, et al. Mindfulness based pro-gram pluse amygdala and insula retraining (MAIR) for the treatment of women with fibromyalgia: a pilot randomized controlled trial. J Clin Med 2020;9(10):1–16.
72. Carnahan JC. Low Dose Naltrexone (LDN): the Treatment you've never heard of. Int J Complement Alt Med 2016;4:3.
73. Madisch A, Vinson BR, Abdel-Aziz H, et al. Modulation of gastrointestinal motility beyond metoclopramide and domperidone. Wien Med Wochenschr 2017; 167(7–8):160–8.
74. Lazzini S, Polinelli W, Riva A, et al. The effect of ginger (Zingiber officinalis) and artichoke (Cynara cardunculus) extract supplementation on gastric motility: a pi-lot randomized study in healthy volunteers. Eur Rev Med Pharmacol 2016;20(1): 146–9.

Dietary Approaches to Treating Multiple Sclerosis-Related Symptoms

Terry L. Wahls, MD, IFMCP[a,b,c],*

KEYWORDS

- Multiple sclerosis • Low-saturated-fat diet • Paleolithic diet • Mediterranean diet
- Fasting • Swank diet • Wahls diet • Calorie restriction

KEY POINTS

- Refer patients to a registered dietitian or other nutrition professional to develop a mutually agreed-upon plan for improving diet quality.
- Offer dietary patterns that have preliminary data documenting efficacy in reducing MS-related symptoms (low-fat, modified Paleolithic, low-fat vegan, gluten-free, Mediterranean, intermittent fasting, ketogenic, intermittent calorie restriction) or have documented effectiveness to prevent or treat insulin resistance, obesity, diabetes, and other significant comorbidities (Mediterranean).
- Consider a trial of gluten-free/casein-free diet or food sensitivity testing to identify patients with unrecognized abnormal immune response to specific foods, which may be contributing to MS-related symptoms.
- Refer patient to registered dietitians, health psychologists, and/or health coaches with expertise in motivational interviewing and helping patients address the key facilitators and barriers to successfully adopting and then sustaining a new dietary plan.

INTRODUCTION

Approximately 2.5 million people have multiple sclerosis (MS) worldwide. Disease-modifying drug treatment is the standard of care to reduce the number of relapses and the number of enhancing lesions on MRI. Although the precise cause of MS remains elusive, it is being increasingly recognized that environmental factors, including lifestyle factors such as smoking, exercise level, and dietary patterns impact the risk of

[a] Department of Internal Medicine, University of Iowa, Carver College of Medicine, 200 Hawkins Drive, Iowa City, IA 52245, USA; [b] Department of Neurology, University of Iowa, Carver College of Medicine, 200 Hawkins Drive, Iowa City, IA 52245, USA; [c] Department of Epidemiology, University of Iowa, Carver College of Medicine, 200 Hawkins Drive, Iowa City, IA 52245, USA
* Department of Internal Medicine, University of Iowa, Carver College of Medicine, 200 Hawkins Drive, Iowa City, IA 52245.
E-mail address: terry-wahls@uiowa.edu

Phys Med Rehabil Clin N Am 33 (2022) 605–620
https://doi.org/10.1016/j.pmr.2022.04.004
1047-9651/22/© 2022 Elsevier Inc. All rights reserved.
pmr.theclinics.com

developing MS and affect the disease course, including the development of enhancing lesions and brain volume loss.[1] Patients with MS are increasingly using complementary and alternative medicine treatments, including diet, nutraceuticals, and exercise[2–4] with more than 40% reporting that they are using a specific dietary pattern as part of their disease management strategy.[4] Patients with MS often seek dietary guidance,[5,6] but neurologists rarely feel adequately trained to provide such guidance.[7] This article reviews the mechanisms by which diet may impact disease course, the status of the research, and dietary strategies with pilot data documenting efficacy for reducing MS-related symptoms or effectiveness for preventing or treating important comorbidities.

MECHANISMS OF DIET

Diet may influence the risk of developing MS and affect the disease course in several ways.[8] Diet will impact the risk of developing comorbid diagnoses that accelerate the development of disability. Diet also has a strong relationship with the risk of developing excessive body weight and the development of high blood pressure, obesity, diabetes, and heart disease. Maintaining a healthy body weight is associated with a lower risk of important comorbidities, MS disease activity, and development of disability.[9–11] Furthermore, the presence of morbid obesity, high blood pressure, diabetes, and/or heart disease is associated with more aggressive disease course and worse disability.[12–14] Diets that have been investigated specifically in the setting of MS to reduce MS-related symptoms, improve quality of life, and address important comorbidities are highlighted in **Table 1**.

The American Heart Association and the American Diabetes Association recommend restricting added sugar, cholesterol, total fat, and saturated fat.[15,16] Meta-analyses of Mediterranean[17–19] and Paleolithic[20–22] eating patterns are associated with favorable improvements in insulin sensitivity, glycemic control, and cardiovascular risk factors, which are important comorbid diagnoses in the MS population. Persons with MS report consuming diets of low quality with insufficient intake of fruits and vegetables, consistent with the average American diet, and significantly below US Departments of Health and Human Services and Agriculture guidelines.[2] However, the Dietary Guidelines for Americans[23] are developed for healthy Americans and may not address the nutritional needs for patients with complex, chronic diseases such as MS.

The role of gut microbiome in immune and brain health is increasingly recognized as an important factor in MS disease processes.[24–27] Both the composition of diet early in life and long-term and recent dietary patterns are major determinants in the patient's current microbiome composition.[28] Furthermore, microbial metabolites of the dietary components influence microbial activity in experimental autoimmune encephalitis (EAE), the animal model of MS.[29] Thus, a patient's previous and current dietary patterns are likely important factors in determining the risk for developing a health-promoting or inflammation-promoting microbiome, which may contribute to developing overly reactive microglia, leading to optic neuritis, clinically isolated syndrome, MS, and continued disease activity.

PRECLINICAL AND OBSERVATIONAL STUDIES

Animal model studies have investigated several nutritional interventions in the setting of EAE and the cuprizone model of demyelination. In an EAE model, diets with increased dietary fiber delayed onset and severity of symptoms.[30] Butyrate, a by-product of bacterial fermentation of soluble fiber, is associated with reduced

Table 1		
Multiple sclerosis-specific diets, benefits, and quality of evidence		
Diet	**Main Features**	**Benefit and Quality of Evidence**
Swank	• Low saturated fat (<15 g) • 4 servings of grain of which 50% is whole grain • 4 servings of vegetables • Red meat excluded the first year • White poultry meat, white fish	• Fatigue reduction, improved quality of life (B1) • Survival (C2)
McDougall	• Low fat vegan, stresses starchy plant foods • 10% of calories from fat • 14% of calories from protein • 76% of calories from carbohydrates • Meat, eggs, and dairy excluded	Improved body mass index, fatigue reduction (B1)
Wahls modified Paleolithic	• Moderate amount of meat (6–12 oz) • 9 daily servings of vegetables and berries • Gluten-containing grain, dairy, and eggs excluded • Starchy foods limited to 2 servings per week • Fermented foods, seaweed, algae and nutritional yeast, and omega-3 oils encouraged	• Fatigue reduction, improved quality of life (B1) • Improved cognition, mood, motor function (C2)
Wahls elimination	• In addition to Wahls guidelines, nightshades, all grain, and legumes excluded • After 3-month exclusion, patients may reintroduce nightshades, legumes, and nongluten grains, one food ingredient at a time each week to assess for worsening of symptoms	Fatigue reduction, improved quality of life, longer walking distance (B1)
Gluten-free, casein-free, elimination[a]	Careful exclusion of gluten- and casein-containing foodstuffs	• Fatigue reduction, improved quality of life (B2) • Reduced disease activity (C2)
Calorie restriction	• Reduction of daily calorie intake to 20%–30% below the basal metabolic rate daily, or periodic greater caloric restriction (60%–100%) followed by days of 0% calorie restriction • Example: 5 d of 0% calorie restriction without increasing calories consumed above basal metabolic rate and 2 d of 75% calorie restriction	Fatigue reduction, improved quality of life (B1)

(continued on next page)

Table 1 (continued)		
Diet	**Main Features**	**Benefit and Quality of Evidence**
Mediterranean	• Increased consumption of vegetables, legumes, whole grains, nuts, fish, olive oil • Reduced consumption of red meat	• Incident risk reduction (C1) • Fatigue reduction, improved function (B1) • Improved survival and reduced morbidity unrelated to MS (A1)
Ketogenic	• Dairy based • 90% fat with 25 g of carbohydrate diet • Medium-chain triglyceride ketogenic diet is 60%–70% fat and allows 50 g of daily carbohydrates	Fatigue reduction, reduced depression, improved body mass index (B1)
Fasting mimicking diet	• Periodic calorie restriction for 7 d with 300–800 calories provided by additional omega-3 fatty acids and a multivitamin • Followed by a Mediterranean diet	Improved quality of life (B1)

All studies are preliminary due to relatively small sample size and/or short duration. All diets listed eliminate or restrict added sugar, processed foods, and hydrogenated fats. Many also maximize nonstarchy vegetable and fiber intake.

^a No studies of a diet guided by food sensitivity testing have been reported in the setting of MS.

demyelination and improved remyelination. Several studies have found reduced butyrate and other short chain fatty acids coupled with altered immune function are present in patients with relapsing-remitting MS (RRMS) and secondary progressive MS (SPMS).[31,32] Increasing dietary fiber to increase production of short-chain fatty acids by gut bacteria has been proposed as a strategy to alter gut microbiota and favorably impact MS disease course.[33] Using a cuprizone mouse model of demyelination, a salmon-based diet was superior to either cod liver oil- or soybean oil-supplemented mouse chow groups in terms of cognitive performance,[33,34] and had less demyelination and brain volume loss as measured by both MRI and anatomic pathology.[34,35] Studies of calorie restriction and intermittent fasting in EAE animal models have demonstrated reduced disease severity; favorable changes in IL-10, tumor necrosis factor-alpha,[36] and T-regulatory cells; and favorable shifts in the microbiome.[37] Studies of the fasting mimicking diet in EAE have reported clinical regression of disease activity, induction of oligodendrocyte precursor cells, increased T-regulatory cells, and reduced numbers of TH1 and TH17 cells.[38] High salt intake was associated with activation of TH17 and TH1, worsening of EAE,[39] and worsening of MS in an observational study.[40] However, a 5-year study that followed urinary sodium, a reliable method of assessing sodium intake, found no relationship between sodium intake and risk of relapse or disease activity as measured by MRI.[41]

Observational studies using cross-sectional surveys of patients with MS have linked higher diet quality scores with better mood and quality of life[42–44] as well as less disability burden and slower rates of disease progression.[43,45–47] A pilot cross-sectional study that examined the dietary intake of 20 adults with mild-to-moderate MS found a significant correlation between improved ambulation, daily function, and quality of life with increased fat intake, increased saturated fat intake, decreased carbohydrate intake, and increased intake of the micronutrients cholesterol, folate, iron, and magnesium.[48] Patients with MS have consistently failed to meet the recommended daily intake of fruits and vegetables.[2] In a large longitudinal survey of lifestyle factors and function, more than 80% of respondents reported inadequate intake of fruits and vegetables.[45]

Casein and gluten have been investigated for their roles in MS. Dairy intake of these proteins has been associated with higher rates of MS and more severe symptoms.[43,49,50] Individuals who have an abnormal immune response to casein may also have an abnormal response to gluten.[51,52] Celiac disease is an autoimmune disease causing villous atrophy of the small bowel mucosa and malabsorption of fat, minerals, and other nutrients, and is often associated with more neuropsychiatric symptoms and enhancing central nervous system lesions than age-matched healthy controls.[53] Furthermore, abnormal immune response to gluten may also be associated with similar neuropsychiatric symptoms and enhancing lesions, which have been shown to resolve with meticulous exclusion of dietary gluten in the absence of any gut-related symptoms or pathology.[54] The precise role of gluten and the frequency of celiac disease and gluten sensitivity in the patient with MS is not completely understood. Two reviews of the role of gluten exclusion to treat MS symptoms found many case reports and case series documenting clinical improvement after excluding gluten from the diet.[55,56] However, the rates of celiac disease in patients with MS, and studies of the rates of elevated abnormal transglutaminase and antigliadin antibodies in patients with MS relative to controls, were mixed with both increased rates of gluten sensitivity and rates that are equivalent to the general population.[49] An observational study found consuming whole grains protective,[2] but several small prospective studies that excluded gluten were associated with reduced MS-related symptoms.[36,37,57] Although gluten and/or casein sensitivity may contribute to the development of neurologic symptoms and enhancing lesions in some patients with MS, the frequency with which this occurs is not known.

CHALLENGES OF DIETARY INTERVENTION STUDIES

Prospective dietary intervention trials to assess the impact of specific dietary patterns to favorably impact disease course, relapse rate, and brain structure and improve quality of life are needed to assess effectiveness. However, rigorous dietary intervention studies are challenging. Patients must begin a new dietary pattern that often requires them to discontinue familiar, enjoyable foods, including foods that have been part of a family or cultural tradition, and consume new, unfamiliar foods. In addition, the new eating pattern must be sustained over sufficient time so that changes in symptoms, relapse rate, and brain imaging can be observed.

Participants may require more teaching to grow internal motivation to do the work required with adopting the dietary intervention. Patients may need to learn menu planning, shopping, recipes, and cooking strategies to successfully adopt and sustain the new dietary pattern. Patients may experience cravings and withdrawal symptoms from reducing added sugars and processed foods.[38,58] New recommended foodstuffs may be more expensive than packaged foods containing processed corn, wheat, and soybeans, all of which receive governmental subsidies to lower the cost of production. Vegetables, which are not subsidized, are more expensive than grain- and soybean-based products. If vitamin and/or nutraceutical supplements are included in a dietary intervention, further additional costs are incurred. Participants in dietary intervention trials (and in clinical practice) often need substantially more support than participants in other types of clinical trials to successfully adopt and then sustain the assigned dietary pattern, leading to increased personnel costs to conduct the study.

STRENGTHS AND LIMITATIONS OF DIETARY INTERVENTION CLINICAL TRIALS

Dietary intervention studies to date have been small in size. Clinical research may be either observational or clinical trial; clinical trials are stronger evidence of the effectiveness of the intervention. Observational study may find associations but cannot determine causation. When evaluating the strength of a particular study it is important to consider the size of the study, duration, presence of a control group, use of blinding, randomization, and levels of adherence to the intervention. Higher sample size increases confidence in the findings. A longer duration increases confidence that the intervention can be sustained. A control group provides a comparison group. Use of randomization and blinding reduce the risk of bias. Measurement of adherence to the dietary intervention assesses the degree to which participants followed the assigned study diet. All reported studies to date are considered preliminary because they were observational, single arm, of brief duration, or had a relatively small sample size. The strength and quality of the research supporting each dietary plan reviewed here is summarized at the end of this article.

At present, no prospective clinical trials have documented the effectiveness of a specific dietary pattern to reduce the relapse rate or the number of enhancing lesions documented on brain imaging studies in patients with MS. Several small pilot dietary studies have been reported, demonstrating reduction in fatigue, improvement in quality of life, or improvement in biomarkers of important comorbid diseases.

LOW SATURATED FAT (SWANK DIET)

Based on epidemiologic evidence that regions with higher saturated fat intake had higher incidence of MS,[59] Dr Roy Swank began recommending his patients consume a diet low in saturated fat, and followed them for up to 50 years.[60–67] His cohort of patients was originally 264, and 120 were lost to follow-up. Swank compared those who consumed less than 15 g of saturated fat per day with those who consumed greater than 15 g. He observed that those who consumed less saturated fat experienced fewer relapses, were more likely to continue working and ambulate with or without unilateral/bilateral support, and had less risk of mortality. Diet instruction was provided via registered dietitian, and dietary adherence was assessed by registered dietitian interview at 12-month follow-up. Assessments were not blinded, but were completed by clinical staff and review of the medical records. The weakness of the study is the absence of a control arm, lack of blinded assessors, lack of randomization, and high attrition rate. The strength of the study is the 50-year duration and relatively large cohort size.

A recent prospective, randomized, parallel group study compared the Swank diet with a low lectin modified Paleolithic elimination diet (Wahls elimination) in patients with relapsing-remitting MS with moderate fatigue (87 were randomized with 72 completing all study visits).[68,69] After a 12-week observation period while consuming the usual diet, patients were randomized and trained on the assigned study diet and supported from the study dietitian for a portion of the study. Both the Swank and Wahls elimination diets were associated with clinically and statistically significantly reduced fatigue severity, and improved quality of life, and statistically improved walking distance and cognitive processing speed compared with baseline visits, with the Wahls elimination group having clinically and statistically significantly greater improvements in some measures (MS Quality of Life physical health and mental health subscales).

LOW FAT VEGAN (McDougall)

The McDougall diet supports a low-fat vegan diet to treat complex chronic disease states, including MS. One prospective, randomized, blinded clinical trial of 61 patients with relapsing-remitting MS has been reported.[70] Patients were randomized to receive training in the diet via a 10-day residential training program. Ten percent of calories were derived from fat, 15% from protein, and 75% from carbohydrates. Meat, fish, eggs, dairy, and vegetable oils (such as corn and olive oil) were prohibited. The control arm was a wait list control, with participants continuing their usual diet. Diet adherence was measured using monthly food frequency questionnaires. If patient consumed less than 20% fat in 10 or more months, they were considered adherent to the study diet. There was no difference in relapse rate, number of enhancing brain lesions, or brain volume loss between the 2 groups. There was a clinically and statistically significant reduction in fatigue severity as measured by Modified Fatigue Impact Scale scores in the intervention group when compared with the control group. There was also clinically and statistically significant reduction in body mass index, total cholesterol, and low-density lipoprotein (LDL) cholesterol in the intervention arm when compared with the control arm. The strength of the study is the randomization, blinded assessors, and measures of dietary adherence. The limitation is the small sample size and 1-year duration.

MODIFIED PALEOLITHIC (WAHLS) AND LOW LECTIN MODIFIED PALEOLITHIC (WAHLS ELIMINATION)

The Wahls diet is a modified Paleolithic diet that advocates for a moderate amount of meat, encourages 9 servings of vegetables and berries, and excludes gluten, casein, and eggs. The Wahls elimination diet adds exclusion of nightshade vegetables (peppers, tomatoes, eggplant, and potatoes), legumes, and grains for 3 months, with a gradual reintroduction of the nightshades, legumes, and gluten-free gains, 1 ingredient at a time, to assess tolerance to the reintroduced proteins. See the Swank diet section for a discussion on the recent study (n = 72 who completed 24 weeks of dietary intervention) examining the effects of both the Swank and Wahls elimination diets. The Wahls elimination diet intervention arm had clinically and statistically significant reduction in fatigue and improvement in MS Quality of Life score.[71,72]

Two small single-arm studies[36,37,71] and 2 small randomized studies[72,73] of the modified Paleolithic diet have been reported. The single-arm blinded studies (n = 10, n = 20, n = 20) used stress reduction, exercise, electrical stimulation of muscles, targeted supplements, and a modified Paleolithic diet in the setting of progressive MS. The diet eliminated gluten-containing grains, dairy (ghee was permitted), and eggs and limited meat to 6 to 12 oz/d. Nine or more daily servings of leafy green vegetables, sulfur-rich vegetables, and deeply colored vegetables and berries was encouraged. Patients were also encouraged to consume fermented foods, organ meats, algae, and seaweed. Nutraceuticals including vitamin D, fish oil, and B vitamins were also provided. Over 12 months, average adherence to the study diet exceeded 90%. Clinically and statistically significant reductions in fatigue severity and improvement in the quality of life were observed. Reductions in anxiety and depression and improvement in verbal and nonverbal reasoning were also observed.[74] Improvement in walking function was observed in half of the participants in the progressive population where a 10% to 20% annual decline in function would be anticipated in patients with progressive MS.[75] Reduction in level of total cholesterol and elevation of level of high-density cholesterol was reported.[76] The limitations of both of these studies is the lack of a control group and small sample size.

A small, 12-week, randomized, blinded, wait list control study (n = 34) of a modified Paleolithic diet in patients with relapsing-remitting MS was reported.[72] Clinically and statistically significant reduction in fatigue severity and improvement in quality of life were observed in the control arm compared with the wait list controls. In a similar study comparing the modified Paleolithic diet and the medium-chain triglyceride keto-genic diet the modified Paleolithic diet group had greater reduction in fatigue severity and improvement in quality of life than the wait list control or the medium-chain triglyc-eride ketogenic diet.[73]

GLUTEN-FREE DIET

A gluten-free diet eliminates gluten-containing grains (eg, wheat, rye, barley, and other grains containing gluten). Other foodstuffs are not restricted. Patients are taught to read labels to avoid accidental gluten exposure in the diet. A recent systematic review of studies investigating the role of gluten in MS found 3 prospective studies demon-strating benefits of a gluten-free diet; 17 studies demonstrating the incidence of gluten sensitivity biomarkers in the setting of MS, with inconsistent results; and 4 studies that did not find a higher rate of celiac disease in patients with MS when compared with the general population.[56] A total of 105 consecutive patients with relapsing-remitting MS were evaluated for potential gluten sensitivity with anti-tissue transglutaminase, ge-netic markers for DQ2 and DQ8, and duodenal biopsy [57]; 72 continued in the study and were followed for a mean of 4.5 years. All were trained in a gluten-free diet, of which 36 adhered closely and 36 did not. Participants were interviewed for the pres-ence of other autoimmune conditions, interval relapses since prior visit, number of enhancing lesions on MRI, and Expanded Disability Status Scale score. The frequency of DQ2, DQ8, anti-tissue transglutaminase, and anti-gliadin antibody; the number of autoimmune conditions; and annual relapse rate were the same for both groups. How-ever, the number of enhancing lesions on MRI and the Expanded Disability Status score was less for those who adhered to the gluten-free diet than those who did not, that is, regular diet group. The strength of the study is the 4.5-year duration, whereas the limitations are lack of randomization and absence of blinded assessors.

CALORIE RESTRICTION AND INTERMITTENT CALORIE RESTRICTION

Calorie-restricted and intermittent calorie-restricted diets reduce the calorie intake below the daily caloric requirement as specified by the person's basal metabolic rate. The restriction may be the same each day with a 20% to 30% daily reduction or a more severe reduction (60%–100%) for a specified number of days each week followed by a day of consuming the daily caloric requirement without increase. No food groups are eliminated. A small (n = 36) 8-week randomized, assessor-blinded trial compared daily calorie restriction, intermittent calorie restriction, and zero calorie restriction in patients with relapsing-remitting MS.[77] Patients were randomized to 1 of 3 diets: (1) a 22% calorie restriction every day, (2) 25% of calorie needs for 2 consec-utive days followed by 100% of calorie needs for 5 days in repeating cycles each week, or (3) 100% of calorie needs every day. Primary outcome was safety, and sec-ondary measures included fasting lipids, body weight, and mood. No serious adverse events were reported; however, hunger was frequently reported in both calorie-restricted groups. Weight loss, reduction in body fat, and reduction in total cholesterol were observed in both the calorie restriction and intermittent calorie restriction groups compared with controls, but were not different between groups. Emotional well-being as measured by the Functional Assessment in Multiple Sclerosis scale improved in both calorie-restricted groups when compared with the control group.[77]

Another small (n = 15), randomized study of 15 days tested the safety, feasibility, and immunomodulatory effects in relapsing-remitting MS.[37] Patients were assigned to usual diet (control) or less than 500 calories every other day to assess impact on adipokines and the microbiome. No serious adverse events were reported. Significant weight loss occurred in the intermittent fasting group compared with the control group, but no significant differences in microbiome or blood adipokine levels between groups were reported. Although these studies were randomized and assessor blinded, they were small and very brief.

MODIFIED MEDITERRANEAN DIET

The Mediterranean diet is based on dietary patterns in the Mediterranean region. Although there are several variations, the common themes for the Mediterranean diet stress vegetables, legumes, whole grains, fish, nuts, and olive oil and reduce red meat intake. A case-control study examined the association between dietary components and risk of MS in patients with MS versus matched controls.[78] Patients and controls were interviewed by dietitians using a food frequency questionnaire to identify dietary patterns in the previous year. Adherence to a Mediterranean diet was assessed using a standardized Mediterranean dietary score.[79] Univariate and multivariate analyses were conducted to calculate odds ratios between the components of the Mediterranean diet pattern and risk of MS and found that a higher intake of fruits and vegetables was significantly associated with a lower MS risk.

A small (n = 36) randomized 6-month study of patients with relapsing-remitting MS consuming a modified Mediterranean diet reported reduced fatigue, improved quality of life, and decreased Expanded Disability Status scale scores compared with controls on regular diet.[80] The modified Mediterranean diet stressed vegetables, legumes, nuts, fish, olive oil, and avocados and the avoidance of added sugar, meats (including red meat and poultry), dairy, white grains, and processed foods. Patients in the intervention arm participated in monthly support calls designed to keep patients engaged and adherent to the study diet. The usual diet arm received monthly seminars about MS that were not diet focused. The Mediterranean arm experienced reduced fatigue, improved quality of life, and decreased Disability Status score when compared with the control arm. The strengths of the study are the 90% adherence rate, randomization, and blinded assessors, although the study population was small.

KETOGENIC DIET

A small (n = 20) single-arm study of a modified Atkins ketogenic diet was conducted in patients with relapsing-remitting MS.[81] Patients were trained on the modified Atkins diet by a registered dietitian with expertise in ketogenic diets. The carbohydrate intake was restricted to less than 20 g. The dietitian met with participants at months 1, 3, and 6. One-third reported no side effects. The side effects reported included constipation, menstrual irregularities, and diarrhea. Significant weight loss and reduced abdominal circumference was reported, but no patients became underweight. Clinically and statistically significant reduction in fatigue, depression, and anxiety were reported. Clinically and statistically significant reduction in hemoglobinA_{1c} and insulin were observed. Total cholesterol and LDL cholesterol levels significantly increased at 3 months, but declined at 6 months and were not statistically different from baseline values. Expanded disability scores were reduced at 6 months due the favorable changes in bowel and bladder function.[81]

A small (n = 27) quasiexperimental (nonrandomized) trial was conducted, duration 4 months, using a modified ketogenic Mediterranean diet. The aim of the study was to determine changes in body composition and satiety markers. The macronutrient composition was 20% protein, 40% carbohydrates, and 40% fat. To facilitate ketone generation, patients were also given 30 mL coconut oil twice daily, a rich source of medium-chain triglycerides, which produce more ketones per gram than other fat sources. Nutritional ketosis was achieved. In addition, patients experienced decreased hunger and increased satiety. Patients experienced a significant increase in lean body mass and decrease in fat mass.[82] No MS-specific measures were obtained. Weakness in these studies is the lack of randomization.

FASTING MIMICKING AND OTHER FASTING DIETS

Periodic fasting (water only), intermittent calorie restriction, time-restricted feeding, and the fasting mimicking diet all use a period of reduced caloric intake and have been associated with favorable changes inflammatory markers, insulin sensitivity, blood lipid levels, blood pressure, and body weight in animal and human studies of aging and age-related degenerative diseases.[83,84] The fasting mimicking diet has been investigated in the setting of MS and is a periodic, 5- to 7-day restriction of calories, followed by a less restrictive diet. The frequency of the periodic calorie restriction varies. The fasting mimicking diet in animal models of autoimmunity is associated with improved T regulatory cells, cytokine profiles, and increased circulating stem cells, leading to reduced autoimmune disease activity, improved function, and increased remyelination.[85] In both EAE and cuprizone models, the fasting mimicking diet was associated with improved cytokine profiles, increased T regulatory cells, increased oligodendrocyte precursor activity, reduced demyelination, and improved remyelination.[38] A small (n = 60), 6-month, blinded and randomized study demonstrated clinically and statistically higher physical and mental health quality of life scores in groups on ketogenic or intermittent fasting mimicking diets when compared with controls.[38] The fasting mimicking diet restricted calories for 7 days followed by a Mediterranean diet that stressed vegetables, fish, legumes, nuts, and olive oil. The ketogenic diet provided greater than 160 g fat, less than 50 g carbohydrates, and less than 100 g protein.

Several dietary patterns have prospectively demonstrated reduced perceived fatigue severity and improvements in quality of life or biomarkers of disease activity in common comorbid diagnoses. Common themes across many of the dietary patterns reported to date include reduction or elimination of added sugars, processed foods, high-glycemic-index foods and trans fats. Most of these diets also stress nonstarchy vegetables. The amount and types of fat vary, but all reduce trans fats and many reduce high-glycemic-index carbohydrates.

KEY RECOMMENDATIONS

Although there is no single dietary pattern than has been proven effective for reducing number of relapses or enhancing lesions in patients with MS, several pilot studies have demonstrated efficacy of diet to reduce MS-related symptoms. Before any dietary changes are instituted, patients should be evaluated for comorbid diagnoses including obesity, high blood pressure, insulin resistance, diabetes, dyslipidemia, and other comorbidities. Recommendations in instituting a new dietary pattern with preliminary data demonstrating efficacy include:

- Reduction of added sugar, processed foods, and trans fats
- Removal of restricted or eliminated foods from the eating environment

- Trial of a gluten-free/casein-free diet or food sensitivity testing to identify patients with abnormal immune response to specific food proteins
- Referral to a registered dietitian or other qualified nutrition professional for nutrition education and support for improving diet quality
- Patient preferences and motivations for successfully adopting a specialized therapeutic dietary pattern
- Adoption of the new eating pattern by the patient's family with mutually agreed-upon goals
- Motivational interviewing and ongoing support through the use of cooking classes, support groups, and peer mentors

GENERAL RECOMMENDATIONS FOR PATIENTS

- Read food labels
- Increase consumption of nonstarchy vegetables (5+ servings daily) and non-starchy fruit (1–2 servings daily) if not following a ketogenic dietary pattern
- Eliminate or reduce high-glycemic-index foods
- If consuming grains, select whole grains
- Eliminate or reduce added sugars and sweetened beverages
- Eliminate or reduce processed meats
- Consider a diet relatively high in omega-3, polyunsaturated fatty acids such as cold-water fish, grass-fed or grass-finished meats, walnuts, and flax, chia, and hemp seeds
- Consume daily recommendation of 25 g or more of fiber, sufficient for 1 to 3 soft, easily passed daily bowel movements

RATING OF THE EVIDENCE

Evidence for the various diet plan studies described here has been rated using the following framework:

1. Randomized controlled trial (RCT)
2. Quasi-experimental, systemic review of a combination of RCTs or quasi-experimental only
3. Nonexperimental studies, qualitative study, or systematic review
   A. Consistent, generalizable results; consistent recommendations based on comprehensive literature review that includes thorough reference to scientific evidence
   B. Reasonably consistent results, sufficient sample size for the results, some control, reasonably consistent recommendations based on literature review
   C. Little evidence with inconsistent results, insufficient sample size for the study design, conclusions cannot be drawn

DISCLOSURE

Dr. Terry Wahls has completed grant funding from the National Multiple Sclerosis Society RG-1506-04312, private charity funding from Direct Multiple Sclerosis Charity, the Dillon Foundation and in kind funding from DJO Inc. and TZ Press. She has current funding from the Carter Chaman Shreve Family Foundation and in kind funding from Keto-Mojo Inc. and Dr. Terry Wahls LLC. Dr. Terry Wahls has equity interest in the following companies: Dr. Terry Wahls LLC; TZ Press LLC; The Wahls Institute, PLC; FBB Biomed Inc., and the website http://www.terrywahls.com. She also owns the copyright to the books Minding My Mitochondria (2nd Edition) and The Wahls

Protocol, The Wahls Protocol Cooking for Life, and the trademarks The Wahls Protocol® and Wahls™ diet, Wahls Paleo™ diet, and Wahls Paleo Plus™ diets. She has financial relationships with BioCeuticals, MCG Health LLC, Genova Diagnostics, Vibrant America LLC, and the Institute for Functional Medicine. She receives royalty payments from Penguin Random House. Dr. Wahls has conflict of interest management plans in place with the University of Iowa and the Iowa City Veteran's Affairs Medical Center.

REFERENCES

1. Jakimovski D, Weinstock-Guttman B, Gandhi S, et al. Dietary and lifestyle factors in multiple sclerosis progression: results from a 5-year longitudinal MRI study. J Neurol 2019;266(4):866–75.
2. Fitzgerald KC, Tyry T, Salter A, et al. A survey of dietary characteristics in a large population of people with multiple sclerosis. Mult Scler Relat Disord 2018; 22:12–8.
3. Schwarz S, Knorr C, Geiger H, et al. Complementary and alternative medicine for multiple sclerosis. Mult Scler 2008;14(8):1113–9.
4. Silbermann E, Senders A, Wooliscroft L, et al. Cross-sectional survey of complementary and alternative medicine used in Oregon and Southwest Washington to treat multiple sclerosis: A 17-Year update. Mult Scler Relat Disord 2020;41: 102041.
5. Apel A, Greim B, Konig N, et al. Frequency of current utilisation of complementary and alternative medicine by patients with multiple sclerosis. J Neurol 2006; 253(10):1331–6.
6. Kochs L, Wegener S, Suhnel A, et al. The use of complementary and alternative medicine in patients with multiple sclerosis: A longitudinal study. Complement Therapies Med 2014;22(1):166–72.
7. Russell RD, Black LJ, Begley A. The unresolved role of the neurologist in providing dietary advice to people with multiple sclerosis. Mult Scler Relat Disord 2020;44:102304.
8. Katz Sand I. The role of diet in multiple sclerosis: mechanistic connections and current evidence. Curr Nutr Rep 2018;7(3):150–60.
9. Stampanoni Bassi M, Iezzi E, Buttari F, et al. Obesity worsens central inflammation and disability in multiple sclerosis. Mult Scler 2019;Sep;26:1237–46. https://doi.org/10.1177/1352458519853473.
10. Pilutti LA, Motl RW. Body composition and disability in people with multiple sclerosis: A dual-energy x-ray absorptiometry study. Mult Scler Relat Disord 2019; 29:41–7.
11. Briggs FBS, Thompson NR, Conway DS. Prognostic factors of disability in relapsing remitting multiple sclerosis. Mult Scler Relat Disord 2019;30:9–16.
12. Marck CH, Neate SL, Taylor KL, et al. Prevalence of comorbidities, overweight and obesity in an international sample of people with multiple sclerosis and associations with modifiable lifestyle factors. PLoS One 2016;11(2):e0148573.
13. Jakimovski D, Gandhi S, Paunkoski I, et al. Hypertension and heart disease are associated with development of brain atrophy in multiple sclerosis: a 5-year longitudinal study. Eur J Neurol 2019;26(1):87–e88.
14. Zhang T, Tremlett H, Zhu F, et al. Effects of physical comorbidities on disability progression in multiple sclerosis. Neurology 2018;90(5):e419–27.
15. Arnett DK, Blumenthal RS, Albert MA, et al. 2019 ACC/AHA guideline on the primary prevention of cardiovascular disease: a report of the american college of

cardiology/american heart association task force on clinical practice guidelines. Circulation 2019;140(11):e596–646.

16. Garvey WT, Mechanick JI, Brett EM, et al. American association of clinical endo-crinologists and american college of endocrinology comprehensive clinical prac-tice guidelines for medical care of patients with obesity. Endocr Pract 2016; 22(Suppl 3):1–203.

17. Becerra-Tomas N, Blanco Mejia S, Viguiliouk E, et al. Mediterranean diet, cardio-vascular disease and mortality in diabetes: a systematic review and meta-analysis of prospective cohort studies and randomized clinical trials. Crit Rev Food Sci Nutr 2020;60(7):1207–27.

18. Chareonrungrueangchai K, Wongkawinwoot K, Anothaisintawee T, et al. Dietary factors and risks of cardiovascular diseases: an umbrella review. Nutrients 2020;12(4):1088.

19. Kahleova H, Salas-Salvado J, Rahelic D, et al. Dietary patterns and cardiometa-bolic outcomes in diabetes: a summary of systematic reviews and meta-ana-lyses. Nutrients 2019;11(9):2209.

20. de Menezes EVA, Sampaio HAC, Carioca AAF, et al. Influence of Paleolithic diet on anthropometric markers in chronic diseases: systematic review and meta-analysis. Nutr J 2019;18(1):41.

21. Dinu M, Pagliai G, Angelino D, et al. Effects of popular diets on anthropometric and cardiometabolic parameters: an umbrella review of meta-analyses of ran-domized controlled trials. Adv Nutr 2020;11(4):815–33.

22. Jamka M, Kulczynski B, Juruc A, et al. The effect of the paleolithic diet vs. healthy diets on glucose and insulin homeostasis: a systematic review and meta-analysis of randomized controlled trials. J Clin Med 2020;9(2):296.

23. U.S. Department of Health and Human Services and U.S. Department of Agri-culture. 2015 – 2020 Dietary Guidelines for Americans. 8th Edition. December 2015. Available at https://health.gov/our-work/food-nutrition/previous-dietary-guidelines/2015.

24. Moles L, Otaegui D. The impact of diet on microbiota evolution and human health. is diet an adequate tool for microbiota modulation? Nutrients 2020;12(6):1654.

25. Kumar M, Singh P, Murugesan S, et al. Microbiome as an Immunological Modifier. Methods Mol Biol 2020;2055:595–638.

26. Cryan JF, O'Riordan KJ, Sandhu K, et al. The gut microbiome in neurological dis-orders. Lancet Neurol 2020;19(2):179–94.

27. Tremlett H, Bauer KC, Appel-Cresswell S, et al. The gut microbiome in human neurological disease: a review. Ann Neurol 2017;81(3):369–82.

28. Hills RD Jr, Pontefract BA, Mishcon HR, et al. Gut microbiome: profound implica-tions for diet and disease. Nutrients 2019;11(7):1613.

29. Rothhammer V, Borucki DM, Tjon EC, et al. Microglial control of astrocytes in response to microbial metabolites. Nature 2018;557(7707):724–8.

30. Berer K, Martinez I, Walker A, et al. Dietary non-fermentable fiber prevents auto-immune neurological disease by changing gut metabolic and immune status. Sci Rep 2018;8(1):10431.

31. Takewaki D, Suda W, Sato W, et al. Alterations of the gut ecological and functional microenvironment in different stages of multiple sclerosis. Proc Natl Acad Sci U S A 2020;117(36):22402–12.

32. Zeng Q, Junli G, Liu X, et al. Gut dysbiosis and lack of short chain fatty acids in a Chinese cohort of patients with multiple sclerosis. Neurochem Int 2019;129: 104468.

33. Fan Y, Zhang J. Dietary modulation of intestinal microbiota: future opportunities in experimental autoimmune encephalomyelitis and multiple Sclerosis. Front Microbiol 2019;10:740.

34. Torkildsen O, Brunborg LA, Milde AM, et al. A salmon based diet protects mice from behavioural changes in the cuprizone model for demyelination. Clin Nutr 2009;28(1):83–7.

35. Torkildsen O, Brunborg LA, Thorsen F, et al. Effects of dietary intervention on MRI activity, de- and remyelination in the cuprizone model for demyelination. Exp Neurol 2009;215(1):160–6.

36. Razeghi Jahromi S, Ghaemi A, Alizadeh A, et al. Effects of intermittent fasting on experimental autoimmune encephalomyelitis in C57BL/6 mice. Iran J Allergy Asthma Immunol 2016;15(3):212–9.

37. Cignarella F, Cantoni C, Ghezzi L, et al. Intermittent fasting confers protection in CNS autoimmunity by altering the gut microbiota. Cell Metab 2018;27(6): 1222–1235 e1226.

38. Choi IY, Piccio L, Childress P, et al. A diet mimicking fasting promotes regeneration and reduces autoimmunity and multiple sclerosis symptoms. Cell Rep 2016; 15(10):2136–46.

39. Kleinewietfeld M, Manzel A, Titze J, et al. Sodium chloride drives autoimmune disease by the induction of pathogenic TH17 cells. Nature 2013;496(7446):518–22.

40. Farez MF, Fiol MP, Gaitan MI, et al. Sodium intake is associated with increased disease activity in multiple sclerosis. J Neurol Neurosurg Psychiatry 2015;86(1): 26–31.

41. Fitzgerald KC, Munger KL, Hartung HP, et al. Sodium intake and multiple sclerosis activity and progression in BENEFIT. Ann Neurol 2017;82(1):20–9.

42. Taylor KL, Simpson S Jr, Jelinek GA, et al. Longitudinal associations of modifiable lifestyle factors with positive depression-screen over 2.5-years in an international cohort of people living with multiple sclerosis. Front Psychiatry 2018;9:526.

43. Hadgkiss EJ, Jelinek GA, Weiland TJ, et al. The association of diet with quality of life, disability, and relapse rate in an international sample of people with multiple sclerosis. Nutr Neurosci 2015;18(3):125–36.

44. Taylor KL, Hadgkiss EJ, Jelinek GA, et al. Lifestyle factors, demographics and medications associated with depression risk in an international sample of people with multiple sclerosis. BMC Psychiatry 2014;14:327.

45. Marck CH, Aitken Z, Simpson S, et al. Does a modifiable risk factor score predict disability worsening in people with multiple sclerosis? Mult Scler J Exp Transl Clin 2019;5(4). 2055217319881769.

46. Jelinek GA, De Livera AM, Marck CH, et al. Associations of lifestyle, medication, and socio-demographic factors with disability in people with multiple sclerosis: an international cross-sectional study. PLoS One 2016;11(8):e0161701.

47. Fitzgerald KC, Tyry T, Salter A, et al. Diet quality is associated with disability and symptom severity in multiple sclerosis. Neurology 2018;90(1):e1–11.

48. Bromley L, Horvath PJ, Bennett SE, et al. Impact of nutritional intake on function in people with mild-to-moderate multiple sclerosis. Int J MS Care 2019;21(1):1–9.

49. Malosse D, Perron H, Sasco A, et al. Correlation between milk and dairy product consumption and multiple sclerosis prevalence: a worldwide study. Neuroepidemiology 1992;11(4–6):304–12.

50. Munger KL, Chitnis T, Frazier AL, et al. Dietary intake of vitamin D during adolescence and risk of multiple sclerosis. J Neurol 2011;258(3):479–85.

51. Garcia-Peris M, Donat Aliaga E, Roca Llorens M, et al. [Anti-tissue transglutaminase antibodies not related to gluten intake]. An Pediatr (Engl Ed) 2018;89(5): 279–85.

52. Suomalainen H, Isolauri E, Kaila M, et al. Cow's milk provocation induces an immune response to unrelated dietary antigens. Gut 1992;33(9):1179–83.

53. Croall ID, Sanders DS, Hadjivassiliou M, et al. Cognitive deficit and white matter changes in persons with celiac disease: a population-based study. Gastroenterology 2020;158(8):2112–22.

54. Hadjivassiliou M, Sanders DS, Grunewald RA, et al. Gluten sensitivity: from gut to brain. Lancet Neurol 2010;9(3):318–30.

55. Passali M, Josefsen K, Frederiksen JL, et al. Current Evidence on the Efficacy of Gluten-Free Diets in Multiple Sclerosis, Psoriasis, Type 1 Diabetes and Autoimmune Thyroid Diseases. Nutrients 2020;12(8):2316.

56. Thomsen HL, Jessen EB, Passali M, et al. The role of gluten in multiple sclerosis: a systematic review. Mult Scler Relat Disord 2019;27:156–63.

57. Rorigo LH-LC, Fuentes D, Mauri G, et al. Randomized clinical trial comparing the efficacy of a gluten free diet to a regular diet in a series of relapsing-remitting multiple sclerosis patients. Int J Neurol Neurotherapy 2014;1(1):6.

58. Carlier N, Marshe VS, Cmorejova J, et al. Genetic similarities between compulsive overeating and addiction phenotypes: a case for "food addiction. Curr Psychiatry Rep 2015;17(12):96.

59. Swank RL, Lerstad O, Strom A, et al. Multiple sclerosis in rural Norway its geographic and occupational incidence in relation to nutrition. N Engl J Med 1952;246(19):722–8.

60. Swank RL, Grimsgaard A. Multiple sclerosis: the lipid relationship. Am J Clin Nutr 1988;48(6):1387–93.

61. Swank RL, Goodwin J. Review of MS patient survival on a Swank low saturated fat diet. Nutrition 2003;19(2):161–2.

62. Swank RL, Dugan BB. Effect of low saturated fat diet in early and late cases of multiple sclerosis. Lancet 1990;336(8706):37–9.

63. Swank RL. Multiple sclerosis: fat-oil relationship. Nutrition 1991;7(5):368–76.

64. Swank RL. Multiple sclerosis: twenty years on low fat diet. Arch Neurol 1970; 23(5):460–74.

65. Swank RL. Treatment of multiple sclerosis with low-fat diet: result of seven years' experience. Ann Intern Med 1956;45(5):812–24.

66. Swank RL. Treatment of multiple sclerosis with low-fat diet; results of five and one-half years' experience. AMA Arch Neurol Psychiatry 1955;73(6):631–44.

67. Swank RL. Treatment of multiple sclerosis with low-fat diet. AMA Arch Neurol Psychiatry 1953;69(1):91–103.

68. Wahls T, Hoth K, Kamholz J, Rubenstein L, Ten Eyck P, Bisht B, Titcomb T, Snetselaar L Effects of wahls elimination and swank dietary patterns on multiple sclerosis related fatigue, quality of life, processing speed and walking distance. . Poster presentation presented at 8th Joint Americas Committee on Treatment and Research in Multiple Sclerosis - European Committee on Treatment and Research in Multiple Sclerosis September 11, 2020 2020 MS Virtual 2020.

69. Wahls TL, Titcomb TJ, Bisht B, et al. Impact of the Swank and Wahls elimination dietary interventions on fatigue and quality of life in relapsing-remitting multiple sclerosis: The WAVES randomized parallel-arm clinical trial. Mult Scler J Exp Transl Clin 2021;7(3). 20552173211035399.

70. Yadav V, Marracci G, Kim E, et al. Low-fat, plant-based diet in multiple sclerosis: A randomized controlled trial. Mult Scler Relat Disord 2016;9:80–90.

71. Lee JE, Bisht B, Hall MJ, et al. A multimodal, nonpharmacologic intervention improves mood and cognitive function in people with multiple sclerosis. J Am Coll Nutr 2017;36(3):150–68.

72. Irish AKEC, Wahls TL, Stenselaar LG, et al. Randomized control trial evaluation of a modified Paleolithic dietary intervention in the treatment of relapsing-remitting multiple sclerosis: a pilot study. Degenerative Neurol Neuromuscul Dis 2017; 2017:18.

73. Lee JE, Titcomb TJ, Bisht B, et al. A modified MCT-based ketogenic diet increases plasma beta-hydroxybutyrate but has less effect on fatigue and quality of life in people with multiple sclerosis compared to a modified paleolithic diet: a waitlist-controlled, randomized pilot study. J Am Coll Nutr 2020;1–13.

74. Lee JEBB, Hall MJ, Rubenstein LM, et al. A multimodal, nonpharamacologic intervention improves mood and cognition function in people with multiple sclerosis-Mar-Apr. American College of Nutrition; 2017. p. 150–68.

75. Bisht B, Darling WG, White EC, et al. Effects of a multimodal intervention on gait and balance of subjects with progressive multiple sclerosis: a prospective longitudinal pilot study. Degener Neurol Neuromuscul Dis 2017;7:79–93.

76. Fellows Maxwell K, Wahls T, Browne RW, et al. Lipid profile is associated with decreased fatigue in individuals with progressive multiple sclerosis following a diet-based intervention: Results from a pilot study. PLoS One 2019;14(6): e0218075.

77. Fitzgerald KC, Vizthum D, Henry-Barron B, et al. Effect of intermittent vs. daily calorie restriction on changes in weight and patient-reported outcomes in people with multiple sclerosis. Mult Scler Relat Disord 2018;23:33–9.

78. Sedaghat F, Jessri M, Behrooz M, et al. Mediterranean diet adherence and risk of multiple sclerosis: a case-control study. Asia Pac J Clin Nutr 2016;25(2):377–84.

79. Trichopoulou A, Costacou T, Bamia C, et al. Adherence to a Mediterranean diet and survival in a Greek population. N Engl J Med 2003;348(26):2599–608.

80. Katz Sand I, Benn EKT, Fabian M, et al. Randomized-controlled trial of a modified Mediterranean dietary program for multiple sclerosis: A pilot study. Mult Scler Relat Disord 2019;36:101403.

81. Brenton JN, Banwell B, Bergqvist AGC, et al. Pilot study of a ketogenic diet in relapsing-remitting MS. Neurol Neuroimmunol Neuroinflamm 2019;6(4):e565.

82. Benlloch M, Lopez-Rodriguez MM, Cuerda-Ballester M, et al. Satiating effect of a ketogenic diet and its impact on muscle improvement and oxidation state in multiple sclerosis patients. Nutrients 2019;11(5):1156.

83. Longo VD, Panda S. Fasting, circadian rhythms, and time-restricted feeding in healthy lifespan. Cell Metab 2016;23(6):1048–59.

84. Mattson MP, Longo VD, Harvie M. Impact of intermittent fasting on health and disease processes. Ageing Res Rev 2017;39:46–58.

85. Choi IY, Lee C, Longo VD. Nutrition and fasting mimicking diets in the prevention and treatment of autoimmune diseases and immunosenescence. Mol Cell Endocrinol 2017;455:4–12.

Women: Diet, Cardiometabolic Health, and Functional Medicine

Sara Gottfried, MD[a,b]

KEYWORDS

- Women • Women's health • Perimenopause • Menopause • Hormone therapy
- Nutrition • Metabolism • Metabolic health

KEY POINTS

- Our aim is to help clinicians to recognize the value added by a functional medicine approach in the assessment of women in physical medicine and rehabilitation care, vis-à-vis relevant cardiometabolic pathways, phenotypes, and differences in risk compared with men.
- We will cover the chronic conditions for which a systems biology approach is particularly effective, such as polycystic ovary syndrome, autoimmune disease, perimenopause, and menopause, and other nontraditional risk factors for cardiometabolic dysfunction.
- We will cover several of the tools that we use in a functional medicine evaluation of a woman, including the timeline and matrix, as well as customized protocols that may reduce the burden of cardiometabolic disease and indications for physical medicine and rehabilitation, or may hasten recovery once a patient has established care.
- We will review novel biomarkers used in the functional medicine assessment of women, with emphasis on changes in hormonal signaling that involve production, transportation, sensitivity, and detoxification, particularly of the traditional and novel estrogen receptors. Emerging biomarkers, ranging from genomics to lipoprotein fractionation and beyond, may provide a more effective strategy to risk stratify women into those who most benefit from menopausal hormone therapy versus those who may be at the greatest risk.
- We will summarize the latest evidence of the effect of menopausal hormone therapy on cardiometabolic disease, including our aggregate understanding of the critical window hypothesis, for primary and secondary prevention of coronary heart disease, stroke, venous thromboembolism (VTE), and dementia.

[a] Marcus Institute of Integrative Health, 789 E Lancaster Avenue, Suite 110, Villanova, PA 19085, USA; [b] Department of Integrative Medicine and Nutritional Sciences, Sidney Kimmel Medical College, Thomas Jefferson University, Philadelphia, PA, USA
E-mail address: Sara.Gottfried@Jefferson.edu
Twitter: @DrGottfried (S.G.)

Phys Med Rehabil Clin N Am 33 (2022) 621–645
https://doi.org/10.1016/j.pmr.2022.04.005
1047-9651/22/© 2022 Elsevier Inc. All rights reserved.

INTRODUCTION

Functional medicine provides a unique model of care to promote health, reverse disease, and optimize function.[1–3] In the functional medicine evaluation of women, we address many disease states that are commonly encountered in physical medicine and rehabilitation, such as the greater prevalence in women of autoimmune disease and chronic pain across the lifespan, as well as the role of female aging on cardiometabolic disease, the leading killer of women, which broadly encompasses the risk of coronary heart disease, heart failure, diabetes, and even breast cancer and Alzheimer's disease.

Sex and gender differences underlie most of the gaps we see in women who present for physical medicine and rehabilitation, including the following.

- Women have smaller coronary arteries than men. Women show lower prevalence of anatomically obstructive coronary artery disease but higher rates of myocardial ischemia and mortality compared with men.[4–7] Overall, women have a similar or slightly higher prevalence of angina than men.[8]
- Sex-based comparisons demonstrate that women have more microvascular dysfunction,[9] abnormal coronary reactivity,[10] and plaque erosion/distal microembolization[11–13] as the root cause of female-specific loss of function.
- As a result, women experience more subtle and nonspecific symptoms of coronary heart disease,[14–17] and standard diagnostic algorithms may be less accurate for women.[18] Bias toward angiographically defined obstructive coronary artery disease still exists, leading to underdiagnosis of the unique aspects of female pathophysiology, and thereby less aggressive recommendation of lifestyle-based solutions. The net effect is suboptimal treatment of women, poorer outcomes compared with men, and a sex-based mortality gap.[19–22]

Other sex differences related to cardiometabolic function include the following.

- While response to medical treatment may differ in women, they are less represented in clinical trials[23–27]
- Women have greater risk of diastolic dysfunction[28–31] and risk is compounded in certain autoimmune diseases.[32]
- Women experience higher cardiovascular mortality compared with men despite assumptions to the contrary.[15]
- Complications, for example, cardiogenic shock and reinfarction, are more frequent in women than in men. Older women with acute coronary syndromes demonstrate increased frailty and readmissions than men.[33]
- Females demonstrate greater stress responsivity,[34] and increased prevalence of mood disorders and posttraumatic stress disorder.[35]
- Perhaps related to cardiometabolic health, as well as other potential root causes, women account for two-thirds of cases of Alzheimer's disease.[36,37]
- Women have a higher prevalence of autoimmune disease, which may relate to sex differences in gut, immune, and hormone function.
- Women across the lifespan show increased rates of orthorexia[38] and other disordered eating patterns,[39] including at midlife.[40]
- The female athletic triad, associated with energy deficiency (with or without disordered eating), menstrual disturbance (often, amenorrhea), with increased risk of bone loss and osteoporosis.[41,42]
- Women tend to underutilize rehabilitation services,[43] and greater women-focused rehabilitative care may be one solution.[44]

On the other hand, women experience certain advantages over their male counterparts. Women have greater genetic stability, longer telomeres, and increased life expectancy at birth of 80.2 years in women versus 74.5 years in men based on the data from 2020.[45] Women and men age differently, though the exact mechanisms are still under investigation. Some of the factors may be behavioral, such as a woman being more likely to seek health care when sick and tend to put effort into healthy habits. Other differences seem to be genomic and biological. Overall, women have lower rates of cancer. The female proteome is more stable—when the blood is examined of women aged 65 to 95, women's protein levels experience 277 significant changes, compared with 600 significant changes for men.[46] Women have a significant dynamic range with cardiac output, with increases of up to 20% throughout the menstrual cycle and in pregnancy, leading to the protection of the "jogging" female heart and greater organ reserves to accommodate pregnancy and lactation.[47] Women demonstrate differences in the microbiome, leading the term "microgenderome" to describe the greater microbial diversity and to account for sex differences in autoimmunity.[48] Women have more favorable fat distribution until perimenopause when more visceral fat accumulates and total body fat increases, associated with a decline in estradiol and increased follicle-stimulating hormone.[49–51]

In this article, we will describe how functional medicine provides an understanding of these gaps from a systems biology framework, which can serve as a broader foundation for adding value with targeted treatments that address the root cause of dysfunction rather than symptom management.[52] Systems biology is a method of analysis and modeling of complex biological systems and serves as the basis for a functional medicine evaluation of an individual patient, as well as clusters of similar chronic conditions and syndromes. According to the definition by the National Institutes of Health, it is a "biology-based interdisciplinary field of study that focuses on complex interactions within biological systems, using a holistic approach to biological research."[53] We will challenge the flawed assumptions that women do not experience cardiometabolic disease until they are past menopause nor that they experience as serious sequelae as men. We will highlight new evidence that is appropriate for clinical application as well as the key knowledge gaps that limit optimal cardiometabolic care for women.

We will focus on the role of functional medicine in the changing cardiometabolic landscape as a woman ages, including issues for which a systems biology approach is particularly effective, such as polycystic ovary syndrome, autoimmune disease, perimenopause, and menopause, and other nontraditional risk factors for cardiometabolic dysfunction. We will include novel biomarkers that we use in the functional medicine assessment of women, with emphasis on changes in hormonal signaling that involve production, transportation, sensitivity, and detoxification, particularly of the traditional and novel estrogen receptors. Emerging biomarkers, ranging from genomics to lipoprotein fractionation and beyond, may provide a more effective strategy to risk stratify women into those who most benefit from menopausal hormone therapy versus those who may be at the greatest risk.

The purpose of this article is to help clinicians, whether you practice functional medicine or not, to recognize the benefit of a systems biology approach to health and disease vis-à-vis relevant cardiometabolic pathways, phenotypes, and risk profiling in women compared with men. We will apply several of the tools that we use in a functional medicine evaluation of a woman, including the matrix, as well as the type of assessment and analysis that can be used to create customized protocols designed to reduce the burden of cardiometabolic disease and relevant indications for physical medicine and rehabilitation, or may hasten recovery once a patient has established care.

Background

In functional medicine, we seek the root cause of the symptoms that a patient is facing. Throughout a woman's lifecycle, cardiometabolic dysfunction is a primary driver of chronic disease, morbidity, and mortality, though women experience a significant uptick in pregnancy, perimenopause, and menopause.

Regarding cardiometabolic conditions, both predisease and disease are underrecognized and underdiagnosed in women. Half of the women in developed countries will die of mostly preventable heart disease or stroke. While it was previously believed that men and women share the same cardiovascular risk factors, we now know that there are dozens of factors that affect women exclusively and that some traditional risk factors are more deleterious in women, which we will review in a functional medicine framework.

Moreover, awareness among women is declining. Recent evidence highlights that women are less aware of their risk of cardiovascular disease than they were 1 decade ago, despite public service campaigns such as "Go Red for Women."[54] Overall, less than half of women identify cardiovascular disease as the leading cause of death. They are not alone: only half of primary care physicians identify cardiovascular disease as a top concern after breast health and weight.

Regarding cardiovascular disease in women, one woman dies of cardiovascular disease every 80 seconds in the United States, a tragedy driven primarily by coronary heart disease and stroke.[55] For most of the past century, cardiovascular disease was considered primarily a problem for men, despite more women than men dying from a cardiovascular cause year after year. Mortality from coronary heart disease is higher in women than men, even though the prevalence is higher in men for all age groups except 20 to 39. Women experience delays in receiving care,[56–59] poorer outcomes when treated by male physicians,[60] and lower rates of guideline-based medical therapy than men.[61] These data confirm a sex and gender gap in the cardiovascular care of women.

There are cardiometabolic risk factors that occur in both men and women, such as smoking, hypertension, hyperlipidemia, and certain psychosocial factors, but pose a unique or differential risk to women. Traditional risk factors, such as insulin resistance, hypertension, and tobacco use, are more deleterious in women—and at equal age, women have more cardiovascular risk factors than men. When considered along with sex differences in the manifestations and clinical presentation of cardiometabolic disease, a discrepancy emerges that is not sufficiently captured in recent guidelines such that the risk of women remains underestimated. Other unique and nontraditional factors that affect women but not men include polycystic ovary syndrome for which the excess testosterone is most predictive of future cardiometabolic dysfunction.[62]

Mapping the Matrix of Cardiometabolic Disease in Women

The timeline and matrix are tools that help us organize and assess the patient's story. One example is the "Cardiometabolic Matrix" as published by the Institute of Functional Medicine (**Fig. 1**). Note that the Institute for Functional Medicine provides continuing medical education on how to organize the patient's narrative into the matrix. In this article, we will review how our understanding of the matrix in cardiometabolic disease can be adapted for women's unique experiences.

Antecedents, Triggers, and Mediators

In mapping the matrix, we begin with the identification of core factors involved in the patient's experience of health and disease, including antecedents, triggers, and mediators (ATMs).[63,64]

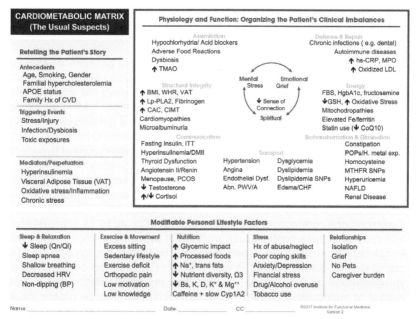

Fig. 1. Cardiometabolic Matrix from the Institute for Functional Medicine. (*Used with permission from* The Institute for Functional Medicine (IFM), the global leader in Functional Medicine and a collaborator in the transformation of healthcare.)

Antecedents are genes and the factors controlling their expression that may predispose them to health or illness. Regarding cardiometabolic disease in women, there are clear sex differences in the genetic predisposition of coronary heart disease, with genetic risk scores conferring greater risk in men.[65] Age affects the risk of cardiometabolic disease differently in women versus men, as we will discuss. Current evidence suggests that genetic risk scores should not be assumed to apply equally to men and women. Further, the Y chromosome seems to play an important role in the heritability of coronary heart disease risk and atherosclerosis.[66] Women receive some age-related protection from the interaction of sex chromosomes with sex hormones,[67] but that markedly decreases when endogenous estradiol levels fall—however, the effect may be mitigated with early hormone therapy within 6 to 10 years of menopause.[68,69] Other factors to consider in cardiometabolic disease are intrauterine stressors and transgenerational epigenetic influence. One example of intrauterine stress affecting an offspring's future metabolic health is "Project Ice Storm," the research performed on women who were pregnant during the Canadian ice storm of 1998 that affected residents from Ontario to Nova Scotia. The vicious storm with severe subzero weather was associated with power outages and extreme cold exposure in people's homes for weeks. Researchers tracked pregnant women and their children 18 years later to see what type of genetic tags they had placed by the toxic stressor. They found that maternal hardship predicted the degree of methylation of DNA in the T cells of offspring in genes involved in metabolism, obesity, and insulin signaling, as well as adolescent BMI and central adiposity.[70–76]

Triggers are discrete events or factors that initiate the symptoms and signs of illness. Host factors combine with the trigger to create disease. Common triggers in women for cardiometabolic dysfunction include trauma, microbes, use of oral contraceptives, disordered eating, nutrition, environmental toxin exposure, pregnancy, perimenopause, and menopause. Examples relevant to physical medicine and rehabilitation include the following.

- Mercury has numerous effects on the body and may be more deleterious to women at lower doses of exposure. Mercury induces mitochondrial dysfunction, depletes glutathione, raises oxidative stress, and lowers the effectiveness of metalloenzymes, with a net result of vascular damage.[77] Mercury exposure may be associated in a nonlinear dose-response with a greater risk of hypertension though data are limited and mixed.[77-79] Women seem to be more vulnerable to the effects of mercury exposure to men and show higher odds of hypertension compared with men when estimates are reported separately.[80-82]
- Pregnancy is a risk factor for spontaneous coronary artery dissection,[83,84] an uncommon cause of myocardial infarction in younger women. (Pregnancy-related complications are described more fully in the next section.)
- Combined oral contraceptives increase the risk of acute MI by approximately 5-fold in an older case-control study, primarily in women with known cardiovascular risk factors, such as age, hypertension, or smoking.[85] Though data are limited, combined oral contraceptives as well as another contraceptives, depot medroxyprogesterone acetate, lower brachial flow-mediated dilation, an important marker of endothelial function.[86] Another mechanism may be greater oxidized low-density lipoprotein in women on combined oral contraceptives.[87]
- Women are more likely to experience trauma, such as adverse childhood experiences (ACEs), which are associated with later risk of cardiometabolic disease.[88-90] One's sensitivity to triggers can vary even among women with similar conditions, such as among women with autoimmune disease.

Mediators are factors that produce damage to the body, symptoms, or behaviors associated with illness. They are biochemical or psychosocial factors that contribute to responses, and there are multiple interacting mediators involved in disease. Examples of biochemical mediators include endogenous and exogenous hormones, neurotransmitters, peptides, cytokines, free radicals, and transcription factors. Other mediators include electromagnetic fields, fear, beliefs, habits such as cigarette smoking, social determinants of health, and other forms of toxic stress.

Certain mediators have differential effects on women versus men. For example, smoking confers a 25% greater risk of coronary heart disease in women versus men,[91] which can be compounded by combined oral contraceptives as mentioned previously.

To summarize, women experience unique or more prevalent ATMs that predispose them to cardiometabolic health or disease, including polycystic ovary syndrome (PCOS), pregnancy-related complications and weight gain, perimenopause and menopause, autoimmune disease, breast cancer treatment, trauma, depression, and insomnia.

Changes in homeostasis underlie the transition from health to predisease to disease. ATMs form a network that can alter homeostasis, thereby predisposing to illness, initiating or provoking dysfunction, and/or modulating the role of mediators through complex mechanisms.[64]

Pregnancy as a Stress Test

In addition to the traditional risk factors for coronary heart disease, women with complications associated with pregnancy—such as chronic hypertension, preeclampsia, gestational diabetes, prematurity, abruption, preterm delivery, and low birth weight for gestational age—are at greater risk of future development of cardiometabolic disease. Pregnancy provides a critical window for many women regarding future endothelial and vascular function and chronic cardiometabolic disease, pregnancy can be viewed as an underutilized opportunity for early intervention. Highlights include the following.

- Hypertensive disorders of pregnancy (HDPs) have been increasing in prevalence, from 8 to 11% of pregnancies from 2004 to 2014 based on more than 44 million hospitalizations. This group includes chronic hypertension, preeclampsia, eclampsia, superimposed preeclampsia on chronic hypertension, and gestational hypertension.[92]
- Chronic hypertension with superimposed preeclampsia is associated with the greatest future risk, including a 7.8-fold increased risk of stroke 7.8-, 5.2-fold risk of MI, and 4.4-fold risk of peripartum cardiomyopathy 4.4-, 4.6-fold preterm birth, and 2.2-fold risk of abruption compared with women without HDP.
- Gestational diabetes increases the risk of the future diagnosis of type 2 diabetes by 4-fold.[93]
- Left ventricular diastolic dysfunction is higher in women with multiparity (3 or more pregnancies) compared with women with lower parity.[94] Multiparity is associated with a greater risk of future diastolic dysfunction, whereby the myocardium doesn't fully relax. The cardinal sign of diastolic dysfunction is shortness of breath.
- Women with signs and symptoms of ischemia without obstructive coronary artery disease are more likely to have a history of adverse pregnancy outcomes. Additionally, these women demonstrate reduced coronary flow reserve, indicative of coronary microvascular dysfunction.[95]

Modifiable personalized lifestyle factors

In functional medicine, we complete a timeline and matrix for each patient. When considering the matrix, the modifiable personal lifestyle factors along the bottom row show sex and gender differences as indicated later in discussion.

- *Insomnia* is 50% more likely to occur in women compared with men. Current evidence links insomnia to an increased risk of incident hypertension, coronary heart disease, recurrent acute coronary syndrome, and heart failure.[96] Potential mechanisms include the dysregulation of the hypothalamic–pituitary axis, hyperarousal from heightened sympathetic nervous system activity, and higher levels of inflammation. Short sleep is one of the triggers of immunometabolic dysfunction that can lead to cardiometabolic disease and cancer.[97]
- *Heart rate variability*, a measure of cardiac autonomic activity, is overall reduced in women with spectral density showing less total power, and with lower mean RR interval and standard deviation of RR intervals.[98] Women have greater high frequency and less low-frequency power, and thereby a lower LF/HF ratio). Women show higher mean heart rate but greater vagal activity. In women who are status post myocardial infarction, all measures of HRV are lower than in men.[99]
- *Nondipping hypertension* increases 16-fold in postmenopausal women compared with premenopausal women.[100]
- *Sedentary lifestyle* affects women more than men, according to the World Health Organization.[101] Both sedentary time and long bouts of sedentary activity are associated in a dose–response manner with greater cardiometabolic risk, including impaired glucose control and coronary heart disease events.[102–104]
- *Low knowledge* is an additional factor as mentioned in the Background.
- *Trauma* is more prevalent in women compared with men as described earlier.
- *Stress.* Women have more white-coat hypertension,[105] and demonstrate more microvascular dysfunction after stress. Women show higher rates of mental

stress-induced-myocardial ischemia (MSIMI), and the sex difference is not explained by psychosocial or clinical risk factors.[106,107]

- *Anxiety and Depression.* Women experience higher lifetime risk of anxiety and depression compared with men.[108,109] In the NHANES I study, women with depression have a greater relative risk of coronary heart disease incidence compared with nondepressed women.[110] In some women, chest pain, shortness of breath, and tachycardia can be presenting symptoms of anxiety and depression as well as coronary heart disease or diastolic dysfunction, so a thorough and clinically appropriate cardiac evaluation is indicated.[111] The effect of anxiety and mood disorders may be bidirectional: complications after acute myocardial infarction are higher in depressed women compared with nondepressed women and are higher than in depressed men.[112] Once again, functional medicine is uniquely suited to address comorbid conditions such as depression in the setting of cardiometabolic disease.
- *Feminine personality traits and roles* may be linked to increased rates of recurrent acute coronary syndrome (ACS) and major adverse cardiac events (MACE) compared with traditional masculine characteristics.[113]
- *Caregiver burden.* One of the major gender differences is that women experience greater stress associated with social roles, particularly as primary caregivers. In the Study of Women's Health Across the Nation, a stressful social role at age 47 to 52 is linked to higher atherosclerotic burden later in life, as measured by carotid intima-media thickness.[114]

Clinical Imbalances

When mapping the matrix of cardiometabolic disease in women in functional medicine, we can consider 7 core areas: Assimilation, Defense and Repair, Energy, Biotransformation and Elimination, Transport, Communication, and Structural Integrity. Mental, emotional, and spiritual influences are important too and aspects have been addressed previously in this article. Key points regarding sex differences in cardiometabolic physiology and function are described later in discussion. Some areas, such as the dramatic hormonal changes that occur in the Communications node, have greater influence than others.

- *Assimilation.* Regarding digestion, absorption, and microbiota, women show greater microbial diversity compared with men but also more antibiotic resistance genes,[115] perhaps because women receive more antibiotic prescriptions.[116] In one study of primary care prescribing habits in England, among 4.57 million antibiotic prescriptions, female patients received 67% more prescriptions than men, and 43% more when excluding treatment of urinary tract infections. Gut microbiota are a novel modulator of cardiometabolic function and disease,[117,118] and antibiotic use is a common root cause of dysbiosis and immune dysregulation that can impact cardiometabolic risk—for example, azithromycin has been associated with a modest increase in cardiovascular death, noncardiovascular death, and all-cause mortality.[119,120] In another study of sex differences in the microbiome, composition is different overall, including a lower abundance of Bacteroidetes.[121] Body mass index is also associated with microbiome composition, and the relationship is stronger in women but not in men.
- *Defense and Repair.* Women experience a greater immune response compared with men.[122] For example, females respond more strongly to vaccines and have a lower risk of cancer, but the flip side is that women have a higher incidence of autoimmune disease.[123] Specifically, women show higher antibody responses

and have more adverse events following vaccination.[124] Similarly, women have lower COVID-19 mortality, likely related to sexual dimorphism in angiotensin-converting enzyme 2 (ACE2) expression, the main receptor used by SARS-CoV-2 to enter cells.[125–127]

- *Energy.* Women show adverse effects of elevated fasting glucose at lower thresholds than men.[128] Coronary heart disease risk increases substantially in women with fasting glucose greater than or equal to 110 mg/dL—and this lower cutoff should be considered carefully in female patients. It is well known that statin use can affect COQ10 levels, many more women compared with men develop side effects on statins, including weakness and myalgias.[129] In addition, the calcification of the coronaries[130] and diabetes,[131–133] may be problematic for women on long-term statin therapy. The risk of prediabetes and diabetes with statin therapy varies depending on baseline glucose and insulin pathways, dose, and statin potency, though many of the studies on statin use do not report sex-specific results.[133–135] One meta-analysis found that statin therapy increased coronary heart disease risk in women.[136] Efficacy of statin use in women versus men continues to be debated.

- *Biotransformation and Elimination.* Regarding toxicity and detoxification, constipation can affect homeostasis and is more common in women.[137] The root cause is multifactorial: women tend to have a longer colon,[138,139] are more likely to have a longer transit time, and are more likely to experience thyroid dysfunction which can slow transit time further.[140] Women seem to be particularly vulnerable to endocrine-disrupting chemicals (EDCs): over 15 EDCs have been associated with earlier menopause by 2 to 4 years,[141] and earlier menopause is linked to greater cardiometabolic risk. We have previously mentioned the increased vulnerability that women experience when exposed to mercury, particularly with regard to the downstream risk of hypertension.

- *Transport.* Sex differences exist in many of the clinical imbalances that affect transport, including endothelial dysfunction, hypertension, dyslipidemia, and dysglycemia. Regarding hypertension, men and women are sometimes treated similarly, but there are sex differences that need to be considered.[142] After smoking cessation, management of hypertension is the most important intervention to reduce the risk of future cardiovascular events in women. Life expectancy is nearly 5 years less for women 50 and older with hypertension compared with normotensive controls. In the elderly, high blood pressure affects more women than men and in general is under-diagnosed and under-treated. The risk of high systolic blood pressure (SBP) confers a greater risk in women compared with men: a 15-point rise in SBP is associated with a 56% increase in cardiovascular risk compared with 32% in men.[142] The SPRINT trial showed that aggressive treatment with target blood pressures less than 120 mm/Hg not only reduce cardiovascular events but the risk of death as well, though the data were significant when men and women were grouped together, and when men were considered separately, but was not significant in women.[143]

- *Communication.* The primary factor that differentiates men from women in terms of communication and signaling is the abrupt change in estrogen production and sensitivity that occurs in perimenopause and menopause. Endogenous estradiol acts in picomolar concentrations but dramatically protects women from cardiometabolic disease. Women lag 8 to 10 years behind men in terms of cardiometabolic disease, but gap closes by age 55 to 60 after menopause,[144–146] or in women with premature ovarian insufficiency, early menopause, or surgical menopause.[147,148] Specifically, menopause before age 40 is associated with a

55% greater risk of cardiovascular disease.[149] Estrogen is a primary regulator of the female body, and estradiol withdrawal is associated with loss of the benefits listed later in discussion. In premenopausal hypothalamic hypoestrogenemia, there is a 7-fold risk of coronary heart disease.[150] Further, women are exposed to other hormonal transitions that men do not experiences, such as pregnancy and the marked hormonal changes of perimenopause and menopause. Additionally, hormonal shifts mays modulate not just cardiometabolic health but also the risk of other chronic diseases, including Alzheimer's disease (AD). Researchers at Cornell have found from multimodal brain imaging that sex differences exist in the development of AD.[151] The preclinical phase of AD coincides with the endocrinological shift of perimenopause and seems to affect most of women after age 40. Specifically, they have found in the early AD-phenotype of women aged 40 to 60, decreased metabolic activity and increased brain amyloid-beta deposition compared with premenopausal women.[152] Once again, estrogen seems to be a primary driver of the decrement in glucose utilization in the female brain after age 40. Research suggests that the optimal window for intervention is early in the endocrinological shift of perimenopause.

Estradiol as Primary Regulator of Cardiometabolic Function

For cardiometabolic health, estradiol—the main and most potent form of estrogen—is a primary regulator. Endogenous estradiol plays a central role in cardiometabolic protection through the following mechanisms.
- Increases nitric oxide bioavailability[153]
- Improves plasma lipids[154,155]
- Antiinflammatory[156,157]
- Antiplatelet[158]
- Antioxidant[159]
- Antiapoptotic[159]
- Prevents arterial stiffening[160]
- Antiatherogenic: Inhibits monocyte adhesion to vascular endothelium via neural cell adhesion molecules[161]
- Regulates micro-RNA[159]
- Increases angiotensinogen levels and decreases renin levels, angiotensin-converting enzyme (ACE), angiotensin-1 receptor density, and aldosterone production[162]

- *Structural Integrity.* Many aspects of structure are different in women versus men, ranging from the length of telomeres and diastolic dysfunction to carotid intima medial thickness and fat distribution. Generally, telomeres are longer in women though the difference becomes significant only after age 50.[163] Diastolic dysfunction (DD) is a poorly understood pathologic condition affecting both men and women, and a key predisposing factor leading to systolic and eventually global left ventricular dysfunction. Diminished compliance leads to stiffening of the heart muscle. Most patients, women more than men, with DD have normal or near-normal left ventricular ejection fractions.[164,165] Many patients with DD experience the same signs and symptoms as patients with heart failure and reduced ejection fraction, leading to poor quality of life.[166,167] Overall, the prevalence of DD is increasing,[168] and associated with 3.5-fold increased risk of cardiovascular events or mortality.[169] Starting in puberty and occurring more significantly in perimenopause, women may notice changes in how and whereby body fat is stored,[170] as described in a previous section. Men have 50% more lean body mass and 13% lower fat mass than premenopausal women. Weight tends to climb for women as they age past the premenopausal years, including more central fat deposition.[171]

DISCUSSION

Functional medicine offers a systems biology approach that can close the sex and gender gaps underlying women's risk of cardiometabolic disease. As a result of the sex and gender differences in cardiometabolic health, women often experience more nonspecific symptoms of coronary heart disease, so we must maintain a high index of suspicion in women and consider more comprehensive functional testing (**Box 1**).

Functional Testing

Given that at equal age, women have more cardiovascular risk factors than men, we need to consider sex and gender differences when assessing and stratifying women by risk. In a review of risk scoring and tracking system for global cardiovascular risk calculation, we found the most highly validated for women is the Consortium for Southeast Healthcare Quality (COSEHC).[174–177]

Novel and more accurate evaluations of cardiometabolic subphenotypes in women are now available, including 24-h ambulatory blood pressure (ABM) results, advanced lipid profiles, advanced inflammatory markers (myeloperoxidase, Lp-PLA2, F_2-IsoPs, oxLDL, ADMA/SMDA, microalbumin, hsCRP, fibrinogen), redefined fasting and 2-h dysglycemia parameters (including defining glycotype on continuous glucose monitoring),[178] HDL function, retinal vascular imaging, a focus on visceral obesity and body composition, measurement of CIMT, and coronary artery calcium scoring. These are in addition to the more common functional tests that we perform in functional medicine, such as nutritional and micronutrient testing, heavy metal body burden, and genomics.

Women show increased rates of small intramyocardial vessel disease, which requires a different approach for imaging, particularly stress perfusion cardiac magnetic

---

Box 1
Symptoms of acute coronary syndrome in women

Women are more likely to experience atypical symptoms compared with men; therefore, provides must have a higher index of suspicion when atypical symptoms are encountered in women. Common symptoms include the following.[172,173]

- Nausea
- Dyspnea
- Fatigue
- Unexplained weakness
- Generally "unwell"
- Pain in upper back + neck
- Sense of foreboding
- Syncope

resonance imaging (CMRI).[179–181] CMRI may be especially helpful in women with signs and symptoms of angina but no obstructive coronary artery disease as it can reflect microvascular angina and reference values have been published for women.[182–184]

TREATMENT

Given the cardiometabolic changes that occur for women in premenopause and the endocrinological transition to menopause, a multimodal approach aimed at improving function is warranted. In functional medicine, once we organize the patient's story, assess modifiable personal lifestyle factors, and organize the core clinical imbalances, we then create a customized protocol that aligns with the matrix for each patient.

Beginning first with lifestyle modifications, we work with the patient to optimize sleep and relaxation, exercise and movement, toxic stress, relationships, and nutrition. Regarding nutrition, the most proven dietary approach is the Mediterranean diet, which we adapt to the individual. Specifically, we use the IFM Cardiometabolic Food Plan with our patients to improve cardiometabolic health, and anecdotally, we routinely find that it improves inflammatory, lipid, and metabolic profile.

Nutritional and Other Lifestyle Factors

- *Mediterranean diet (MedDiet).* When followed for 12 weeks, men experience more beneficial changes on the MedDiet than women, especially in metabolic profile.[185] Still, evidence suggests that the MedDiet may reduce vasomotor symptoms, high blood pressure, dysglycemia, mood disorders, depression, loss of bone density, and loss of cognitive function, though not all of these outcomes are supported by well-designed randomized trials that enrolled sufficient women.[186] While sex-based studies and/or reporting of the Mediterranean diet are limited, one small study showed that women on MedDiet decrease medium LDL but not small, dense LDL, which is the opposite trend observed in men.[187] Another small study suggests that MedDiet improves insulin homeostasis in men but not women.[188] Sexual dimorphism may depend on menopausal status.[189] In the PREDIMED trial, MedDIet supplemented with extra-virgin olive oil is associated with a lower risk of incident breast cancer compared with a low-fat diet.[190] From a functional medicine perspective, breast cancer and cardiometabolic disease share clinical imbalances. Further, women tend to be more compliant with the MedDiet compared with men and high compliance is associated with a lower risk of incident atrial fibrillation.[191] In aggregate, both men and women benefit from MedDiet, though men seem to benefit more and the existing data basis is not reliably separated by sex.
- *Microbiota manipulation.* Regarding the sex differences in microbiota, we need to consider the role that sex plays in response to treatments used commonly in functional medicine to modulate the gastrointestinal microbiota, including prebiotics, live biotherapeutics, and potentially even fecal transplant.[115] One example to track is the potential use of Akkermansia for blood sugar modulation.[192,193] Further sex-based study is needed.

Additional factors to consider include the role of pregnancy and postpartum period as an opportunity for risk stratification, as well as perimenopausal and menopausal hormone therapy.

- *Pregnancy.* We must identify women at risk earlier—pregnancy and postpartum are critical opportunity for more thorough functional assessment, referral, and follow-up. Ideally, women would be evaluated by a multidisciplinary team that can carry out the more advanced testing described previously. Additionally, there is the opportunity for counseling regarding future pregnancies and the key role of personalized nutritional counseling, sleep, stress management, physical activity, weight loss between pregnancies, and even the initiation of low-dose aspirin for women at risk for future preeclampsia and fetal growth restriction,[194] or possibly the use of progesterone for women at risk for preterm labor,[195,196] though data are mixed.[197,198] The link between pregnancy complications and future cardio-metabolic risk provides us with an important early opportunity for risk stratification and reduction.[199]

- *Bioidentical hormone therapy.* The consensus after the Women's Health Initiative (WHI) is that healthy women under the age of 60 or within 10 years of menopause may benefit from menopausal hormone therapy when risk versus benefit is considered.[200] The decision process requires careful phenotyping to identify the candidates most likely to benefit. However, the WHI, the largest randomized trial to date of conventional hormone therapy for the primary prevention of cardiovascular disease, and the Heart and Estrogen/progestin Replacement Study (HERS) which assess conventional hormone therapy for the secondary prevention of cardiovascular disease, have left us with the legacy that conjugated equine estrogen and medroxyprogesterone acetate does not have a role for primary or secondary cardiovascular prevention in women more than 60, though conventional treatment does reduce the risk of type 2 diabetes in healthy postmenopausal women.[201–204] While both WHI and HERS failed to demonstrate benefit, leading functional-medicine clinicians and similarly minded clinicians consider the timing hypothesis and the use of bioidentical hormones that are structurally the same as endogenous estradiol and progesterone to the treatment of common perimenopausal and menopausal symptoms. Women closer to menopausal onset on hormone therapy have a reduced risk of developing subclinical atherosclerosis and cardiovascular disease.[205,206] The ELITE trial suggests estradiol may be preferred for reducing CIMT though it did not demonstrate benefit on coronary artery calcium as measured by computed tomography.[207] In the right candidate, bioidentical hormone therapy can be safe and effective to treat perimenopausal and menopausal symptoms in younger women less than 10 years from menopause, though larger randomized trials are limited.

SUMMARY

We need to challenge the dogma that women are at lesser risk of cardiometabolic disease than men, or that their risk does not begin until they are 10 years or longer from menopause. We need to understand sex-based differences in chronic disease and in medical research, and translate our understanding of these differences into clinical practice. Functional medicine provides a framework from which to understand sex-based differences, particularly with cardiometabolic health, and to apply them in a systems biology approach that can address root cause and potentially mitigate adverse events that affect women seen in physical medicine and rehabilitation. Further, functional medicine allows for the organization of the complex clinical imbalances that alter homeostasis and affect cardiometabolic risk, thereby providing a framework for customized and precision protocols to reduce adverse outcomes. Ultimately, we need a collaborative approach that transcends silos of care to reconceptualize how we can identify the women at greatest risk from cardiometabolic disease starting at a younger age, and work together more collaboratively to close the gender gap.

CLINICS CARE POINTS

- Throughout a woman's lifecycle, cardiometabolic dysfunction is a primary driver of chronic disease, morbidity, and mortality, though women experience a significant uptick in pregnancy, perimenopause, and menopause.

- Women have smaller coronary arteries than men and lower prevalence of anatomically obstructive coronary artery disease but higher rates of myocardial ischemia and mortality compared with men. Sex-based comparisons demonstrate that women have more microvascular dysfunction, abnormal coronary reactivity, and plaque erosion/distal microembolization as the root cause of female-specific loss of function.

- Women experience more subtle and nonspecific symptoms of coronary heart disease, and standard diagnostic algorithms may be less accurate for women. Bias toward angiographically defined obstructive coronary artery disease still exists, leading to underdiagnosis of the unique aspects of female pathophysiology, and thereby less aggressive recommendation of lifestyle-based solutions. The net effect is suboptimal treatment of women, poorer outcomes compared with men, and a sex-based mortality gap.

- Triggers that may serve as nontraditional cardiometabolic risk factors in women include mercury exposure, pregnancy as a stress test, exposure to oral contraceptives, and trauma, such as adverse childhood experiences.

- In functional medicine, consider and address modifiable lifestyle factors as well as upstream clinical imbalances that may contribute to cardiometabolic disease.

DISCLOSURE

The author has nothing to disclose related to the article.

REFERENCES

1. Beidelschies M, Alejandro-Rodriguez M, Ji X, et al. Association of the functional medicine model of care with patient-reported health-related quality-of-life outcomes. JAMA Netw Open 2019;2(10):e1914017.
2. Beidelschies M, Alejandro-Rodriguez M, Guo N, et al. Patient outcomes and costs associated with functional medicine-based care in a shared versus individual setting for patients with chronic conditions: a retrospective cohort study. BMJ Open 2021;11(4):e048294.
3. Bland JS. Treatment adherence, compliance, and the success of integrative functional medicine. Integr Med (Encinitas) 2021;20(3):66–7.
4. Shaw LJ, Bairey Merz CN, Pepine C, et al. Insights from the NHLBI-Sponsored Women's Ischemia Syndrome Evaluation (WISE) Study: Part I: Gender differences in traditional and novel risk factors, symptom evaluation, and gender-optimized diagnostic strategies. J Am Coll Cardiol 2006;47(3 Suppl):S4–20.
5. Shaw LJ, Shaw RE, Merz CN, et al. Impact of ethnicity and gender differences on angiographic coronary artery disease prevalence and in-hospital mortality in the American College of Cardiology-National Cardiovascular Data Registry. Circulation 2008;117(14):1787–801.
6. Smilowitz NR, Sampson BA, Abrecht CR, et al. Women have less severe and extensive coronary atherosclerosis in fatal cases of ischemic heart disease: an autopsy study. Am Heart J 2011;161(4):681–8.
7. Bairey Merz CN, Shaw LJ, Reis SE, et al. Insights from the NHLBI-Sponsored Women's Ischemia Syndrome Evaluation (WISE) Study: Part II: gender differences in presentation, diagnosis, and outcome with regard to gender-based

pathophysiology of atherosclerosis and macrovascular and microvascular coronary disease. J Am Coll Cardiol 2006;47(3 Suppl):S21–9.

8. Hemingway H, Langenberg C, Damant J, et al. Prevalence of angina in women versus men: a systematic review and meta-analysis of international variations across 31 countries. Circulation 2008;117(12):1526–36.

9. Wong TY, Klein R, Sharrett AR, et al. Retinal arteriolar narrowing and risk of coronary heart disease in men and women. The Atherosclerosis Risk in Communities Study. JAMA 2002;287(9):1153–9.

10. von Mering GO, Arant CB, Wessel TR, et al. Abnormal coronary vasomotion as a prognostic indicator of cardiovascular events in women: Results from the National Heart, Lung, and Blood Institute-Sponsored Women's Ischemia Syndrome Evaluation (WISE). Circulation 2004;109(6):722–5.

11. Burke AP, Farb A, Malcom GT, et al. Effect of risk factors on the mechanism of acute thrombosis and sudden coronary death in women. Circulation 1998;97(21):2110–6.

12. Reynolds HR, Srichai MB, Iqbal SN, et al. Mechanisms of myocardial infarction in women without angiographically obstructive coronary artery disease. Circulation 2011;124(13):1414–25.

13. Libby P. Mechanisms of acute coronary syndromes and their implications for therapy. N Engl J Med 2013;368(21):2004–13.

14. Wenger NK, Speroff L, Packard B. Cardiovascular health and disease in women. N Engl J Med 1993;329(4):247–56.

15. Khamis RY, Ammari T, Mikhail GW. Gender differences in coronary heart disease. Heart 2016;102(14):1142–9.

16. Peña JM, Min JK. Coronary artery disease: Sex-related differences in CAD and plaque characteristics. Nat Rev Cardiol 2016;13(6):318–9.

17. Martínez-Sellés H, Martínez-Sellés D, Martínez-Sellés M. Sex, lies, and coronary artery disease. J Clin Med 2021;10(14):3114.

18. Zuchi C, Tritto I, Ambrosio G. Angina pectoris in women: focus on microvascular disease. Int J Cardiol 2013;163(2):132–40.

19. Daly C, Clemens F, Lopez Sendon JL, et al. Gender differences in the management and clinical outcome of stable angina. Circulation 2006;113(4):490–8.

20. Vaccarino V, Parsons L, Peterson ED, et al. Sex differences in mortality after acute myocardial infarction: changes from 1994 to 2006. Arch Intern Med 2009;169(19):1767–74.

21. Jneid H, Fonarow GC, Cannon CP, et al. Sex differences in medical care and early death after acute myocardial infarction. Circulation 2008;118(25):2803–10.

22. Blomkalns AL, Chen AY, Hochman JS, et al. Gender disparities in the diagnosis and treatment of non-ST-segment elevation acute coronary syndromes: large-scale observations from the CRUSADE (Can Rapid Risk Stratification of Unstable Angina Patients Suppress Adverse Outcomes With Early Implementation of the American College of Cardiology/American Heart Association Guidelines) National Quality Improvement Initiative. J Am Coll Cardiol 2005;45(6):832–7.

23. Heiat A, Gross CP, Krumholz HM. Representation of the elderly, women, and minorities in heart failure clinical trials. Arch Intern Med 2002;162(15):1682–8.

24. Farahani P. Sex/gender disparities in randomized controlled trials of statins: the impact of awareness efforts. Clin Invest Med 2014;37(3):E163.

25. Vitale C, Fini M, Spoletini I, et al. Under-representation of elderly and women in clinical trials. Int J Cardiol 2017;232:216–21.

26. Khan SU, Khan MZ, Raghu Subramanian C, et al. Participation of women and older participants in randomized clinical trials of lipid-lowering therapies: a systematic review. JAMA Netw Open 2020;3(5):e205202.

27. Gaudino M, Di Mauro M, Fremes SE, et al. Representation of women in randomized trials in cardiac surgery: a meta-analysis. J Am Heart Assoc 2021;10(16): e020513.

28. Scantlebury DC, Borlaug BA. Why are women more likely than men to develop heart failure with preserved ejection fraction? Curr Opin Cardiol 2011;26(6): 562–8.

29. Savarese G, D'Amario D. Sex differences in heart failure. Adv Exp Med Biol 2018;1065:529–44.

30. Bender SB. Linking coronary microvascular and cardiac diastolic dysfunction in diabetes: are women more vulnerable? Diabetes 2019;68(3):474–5.

31. Oneglia A, Nelson MD, Merz CNB. Sex differences in cardiovascular aging and heart failure. Curr Heart Fail Rep 2020;17(6):409–23.

32. Kim GH, Park YJ. Accelerated diastolic dysfunction in premenopausal women with rheumatoid arthritis. Arthritis Res Ther 2021;23(1):247.

33. Vicent L, Ariza-Solé A, Alegre O, et al. Octogenarian women with acute coronary syndrome present frailty and readmissions more frequently than men. Eur Heart J Acute Cardiovasc Care 2019;8(3):252–63.

34. Oyola MG, Handa RJ. Hypothalamic-pituitary-adrenal and hypothalamic-pituitary-gonadal axes: sex differences in regulation of stress responsivity. Stress 2017;20(5):476–94.

35. Swaab DF, Bao AM. Sex differences in stress-related disorders: major depressive disorder, bipolar disorder, and posttraumatic stress disorder. Handb Clin Neurol 2020;175:335–58.

36. Committee on family caregiving for older adults. In: Schulz R, Eden J, editors. Families caring for an aging America. . Washington, DC: National Academies Press (US); 2016.

37. Volgman AS, Bairey Merz CN, Aggarwal NT, et al. Sex differences in cardiovascular disease and cognitive impairment: another health disparity for women? J Am Heart Assoc 2019;8(19):e013154.

38. Strahler J. Sex differences in orthorexic eating behaviors: a systematic review and meta-analytical integration. Nutrition 2019;67-68:110534.

39. Culbert KM, Sisk CL, Klump KL. A narrative review of sex differences in eating disorders: is there a biological basis? Clin Ther 2021;43(1):95–111.

40. Mangweth-Matzek B, Hoek HW. Epidemiology and treatment of eating disorders in men and women of middle and older age. Curr Opin Psychiatry 2017;30(6): 446–51.

41. Sanborn CF, Jankowski CM. Physiologic considerations for women in sport. Clin Sports Med 1994;13(2):315–27.

42. Daily JP, Stumbo JR. Female athlete triad. Prim Care 2018;45(4):615–24.

43. Bittner V. Cardiac rehabilitation for women. Adv Exp Med Biol 2018;1065: 565–77.

44. Mamataz T, Ghisi GLM, Pakosh M, et al. Nature, availability, and utilization of women-focused cardiac rehabilitation: a systematic review. BMC Cardiovasc Disord 2021;21(1):459.

45. Arias VE, Tejada-Vera B, Ahmad F, et al. Provisional life expectancy estimates for 2020. 2021. Available at: https://www.cdc.gov/nchs/data/vsrr/vsrr015-508.pdf. Accessed November 16, 2021.

46. Lehallier B, Gate D, Schaum N, et al. Undulating changes in human plasma proteome profiles across the lifespan. Nat Med 2019;25(12):1843–50.
47. Eskes T, Haanen C. Why do women live longer than men? Eur J Obstet Gynecol Reprod Biol 2007;133(2):126–33.
48. Flak MB, Neves JF, Blumberg RS. Immunology. Welcome to the microgenderome. Science 2013;339(6123):1044–5.
49. Svendsen OL, Hassager C, Christiansen C. Age- and menopause-associated variations in body composition and fat distribution in healthy women as measured by dual-energy X-ray absorptiometry. Metabolism 1995;44(3): 369–73.
50. Lovejoy JC, Champagne CM, de Jonge L, et al. Increased visceral fat and decreased energy expenditure during the menopausal transition. Int J Obes (Lond) 2008;32(6):949–58.
51. Zaidi M, Lizneva D, Kim SM, et al. FSH, bone mass, body fat, and biological aging. Endocrinology 2018;159(10):3503–14.
52. Trachana K, Bargaje R, Glusman G, et al. Taking systems medicine to heart. Circ Res 2018;122(9):1276–89.
53. Wanjek C. Systems biology as defined by NIH: an intellectual resource for integrative biology. Available at: https://irp.nih.gov/catalyst/v19i6/systems-biology-as-defined-by-nih. Accessed November 16, 2021.
54. Cushman M, Shay CM, Howard VJ, et al. Ten-year differences in women's awareness related to coronary heart disease: results of the 2019 American Heart Association national survey: a special report from the American Heart Association. Circulation 2020;143(7):e239–e48.
55. Virani SS, Alonso A, Aparicio HJ, et al. American Heart Association Council on Epidemiology and Prevention Statistics Committee and Stroke Statistics Subcommittee. Heart disease and stroke statistics-2021 update: a report from the American Heart Association. Circulation 2021;143(8):e254–743.
56. Dreyer RP, Beltrame JF, Tavella R, et al. Evaluation of gender differences in door-to-balloon time in ST-elevation myocardial infarction. Heart Lung Circ 2013; 22(10):861–9.
57. Bugiardini R, Ricci B, Cenko E, et al. Delayed care and mortality among women and men with myocardial infarction. J Am Heart Assoc 2017;6(8):e005968.
58. Huded CP, Johnson M, Kravitz K, et al. 4-Step protocol for disparities in STEMI care and outcomes in women. J Am Coll Cardiol 2018;71:2122–32.
59. Hertler C, Seiler A, Gramatzki D, et al. Sex-specific and gender-specific aspects in patient-reported outcomes. Eur Soc Med Oncol Open 2020;5(Suppl 4): e000837.
60. Greenwood BN, Carnahan S, Huang L. Patient-physician gender concordance and increased mortality among female heart attack patients. Proc Natl Acad Sci United States America 2018;115(34):8569–74.
61. Liakos M, Parikh PB. Gender disparities in presentation, management, and outcomes of acute myocardial infarction. Curr Cardiol Rep 2018;20(8):64–73.
62. McCartney CR, Marshall JC. Clinical practice. Polycystic ovary syndrome. N Engl J Med 2016;375(1):54–64.
63. Galland L. Patient-centered care: antecedents, triggers, and mediators. Altern Ther Health Med 2006;12(4):62–70.
64. Jones DS. Textbook of functional medicine. Gig Harbor, Institute for Functional Medicine; 2010, pages 80-91.
65. Huang Y, Hui Q, Gwinn M, et al. Sexual differences in genetic predisposition of coronary artery disease. Circ Genom Precis Med 2021;14(1):e003147.

66. Den Ruijter H. Sex and gender matters to the heart. Front Cardiovasc Med 2020; 7:587888.
67. Arnold AP, Cassis LA, Eghbali M, et al. Sex hormones and sex chromosomes cause sex differences in the development of cardiovascular diseases. Arterioscler Thromb Vasc Biol 2017;37(5):746–56.
68. Hodis HN, Mack WJ, Henderson VW, et al. Vascular effects of early versus late postmenopausal treatment with estradiol. N Engl J Med 2016;374(13):1221–31.
69. Naftolin F, Friedenthal J, Nachtigall R, et al. Cardiovascular health and the menopausal woman: the role of estrogen and when to begin and end hormone treatment. F1000Res. 2019;8:F1000 Faculty Rev-1576.
70. Cao-Lei L, Massart R, Suderman MJ, et al. DNA methylation signatures triggered by prenatal maternal stress exposure to a natural disaster: Project Ice Storm. PLoS One 2014;9(9):e107653.
71. Cao-Lei L, Dancause KN, Elgbeili G, et al. Pregnant women's cognitive appraisal of a natural disaster affects their children's BMI and central adiposity via DNA methylation: Project Ice Storm. Early Hum Dev 2016;103:189–92.
72. Cao-Lei L, Veru F, Elgbeili G, et al. DNA methylation mediates the effect of exposure to prenatal maternal stress on cytokine production in children at age 13½ years: Project Ice Storm. Clin Epigenetics 2016;8:54.
73. Cao-Lei L, Dancause KN, Elgbeili G, et al. DNA methylation mediates the effect of maternal cognitive appraisal of a disaster in pregnancy on the child's C-peptide secretion in adolescence: Project Ice Storm. PLoS One 2018;13(2): e0192199.
74. Szyf M. The epigenetics of perinatal stress. Dialogues Clin Neurosci 2019;21(4): 369–78.
75. Cao-Lei L, Elgbeili G, Szyf M, et al. Differential genome-wide DNA methylation patterns in childhood obesity. BMC Res Notes 2019;12(1):174.
76. Cao-Lei L, de Rooij SR, King S, et al. Prenatal stress and epigenetics. Neurosci Biobehav Rev 2020;117:198–210.
77. Houston MC. Role of mercury toxicity in hypertension, cardiovascular disease, and stroke. J Clin Hypertens (Greenwich) 2011;13(8):621–7.
78. Mozaffarian D, Shi P, Morris JS, et al. Mercury exposure and risk of hypertension in US men and women in 2 prospective cohorts. Hypertension 2012;60(3): 645–52.
79. Hu XF, Singh K, Chan HM. Mercury exposure, blood pressure, and hypertension: A systematic review and dose-response meta-analysis. Environ Health Perspect 2018;126(7):076002.
80. Yorifuji T, Tsuda T, Kashima S, et al. Long-term exposure to methylmercury and its effects on hypertension in Minamata. Environ Res 2010;110(1):40–6.
81. Nielsen AB, Davidsen M, Bjerregaard P. The association between blood pressure and whole blood methylmercury in a cross-sectional study among Inuit in Greenland. Environ Health 2012;11:44.
82. Choi B, Yeum KJ, Park SJ, et al. Elevated serum ferritin and mercury concentrations are associated with hypertension; analysis of the fourth and fifth Korea national health and nutrition examination survey (KNHANES IV-2, 3, 2008-2009 and V-1, 2010). Environ Toxicol 2015;30(1):101–8.
83. Tweet MS, Hayes SN, Codsi E, et al. Spontaneous coronary artery dissection associated with pregnancy. J Am Coll Cardiol 2017;70(4):426–35.
84. Hayes SN, Tweet MS, Adlam D, et al. Spontaneous coronary artery dissection: JACC State-of-the-Art Review. J Am Coll Cardiol 2020;76(8):961–84.

85. Acute myocardial infarction and combined oral contraceptives: results of an international multicentre case-control study. WHO Collaborative Study of Cardiovascular Disease and Steroid Hormone Contraception. Lancet 1997;349(9060): 1202–9.

86. Lizarelli PM, Martins WP, Vieira CS, et al. Both a combined oral contraceptive and depot medroxyprogesterone acetate impair endothelial function in young women. Contraception 2009;79(1):35–40.

87. Santos ACND, Petto J, Diogo DP, et al. Elevation of oxidized lipoprotein of low density in users of combined oral contraceptives. Arq Bras Cardiol 2018; 111(6):764–70.

88. Felitti VJ, Anda RF, Nordenberg D, et al. Relationship of childhood abuse and household dysfunction to many of the leading causes of death in adults. The Adverse Childhood Experiences (ACE) Study. Am J Prev Med 1998;14(4): 245–58.

89. Felitti VJ, Anda RF. The relationship of adverse childhood experiences to adult medical disease, psychiatric disorders, and sexual behavior: implications for healthcare. In: Lanius RA, Vermetten E, Pain C, editors. The impact of early life trauma on health and disease. The hidden epidemic. Cambridge, UK: Cambridge University Press; 2010. p. 77–87.

90. Stork BR, Akselberg NJ, Qin Y, et al. Adverse childhood experiences (ACEs) and community physicians: What we've learned. Perm J 2020;24:19–099.

91. Huxley RR, Woodward M. Cigarette smoking as a risk factor for coronary heart disease in women compared with men: a systematic review and meta-analysis of prospective cohort studies. Lancet 2011;378(9799):1297–305.

92. Wu P, Chew-Graham CA, Maas AH, et al. Temporal changes in hypertensive disorders of pregnancy and impact on cardiovascular and obstetric outcomes. Am J Cardiol 2020;125(10):1508–16.

93. Tobias DK, Stuart JJ, Li S, et al. Association of history of gestational diabetes with long-term cardiovascular disease risk in a large prospective cohort of US women. JAMA Intern Med 2017;177(12):1735–42.

94. Kim HJ, Kim MA, Kim HL, et al. Effects of multiparity on left ventricular diastolic dysfunction in women: cross-sectional study of the Korean Women's chest pain registry (KoROSE). BMJ Open 2018;8(12):e026968.

95. Park K, Quesada O, Cook-Wiens G, et al. Adverse pregnancy outcomes are associated with reduced coronary flow reserve in women with signs and symptoms of ischemia without obstructive coronary artery disease: a report from the Women's Ischemia Syndrome Evaluation-Coronary Vascular Dysfunction Study. J Womens Health 2020;29(4):487–92.

96. Javaheri S, Redline S. Insomnia and risk of cardiovascular disease. Chest 2017; 152(2):435–44.

97. Kravitz HM, Kazlauskaite R, Joffe H. Sleep, health, and metabolism in midlife women and menopause: Food for thought. Obstet Gynecol Clin North Am 2018;45(4):679–94.

98. Koenig J, Thayer JF. Sex differences in healthy human heart rate variability: a meta-analysis. Neurosci Biobehav Rev 2016;64:288–310.

99. Pinheiro Ade O, Pereira VL Jr, Baltatu OC, et al. Cardiac autonomic dysfunction in elderly women with myocardial infarction. Curr Med Res Opin 2015;31(10): 1849–54.

100. Routledge FS, McFetridge-Durdle JA, Dean CR. Stress, menopausal status and nocturnal blood pressure dipping patterns among hypertensive women. Can J Cardiol 2009;25(6):e157–63.

101. Physical Activity and Women In: Global Strategy on Diet, Physical Activity and Health. Available at: https://www.who.int/dietphysicalactivity/factsheet_women/en/#:~:text=Despite%20this%2C%20physical%20inactivity%20is,women%20than%20their%20male%20counterparts. Accessed December 3, 2021.

102. Chastin SF, Egerton T, Leask C, et al. Meta-analysis of the relationship between breaks in sedentary behavior and cardiometabolic health. Obesity 2015;23(9):1800–10.

103. Brocklebank LA, Falconer CL, Page AS, et al. Accelerometer-measured sedentary time and cardiometabolic biomarkers: A systematic review. Prev Med 2015;76:92–102.

104. Bellettiere J, LaMonte MJ, Evenson KR, et al. Sedentary behavior and cardiovascular disease in older women: The Objective Physical Activity and Cardiovascular Health (OPACH) Study. Circulation 2019;139(8):1036–46.

105. Song JJ, Ma Z, Wang J, et al. Gender differences in hypertension. J Cardiovasc Translational Res 2019;3(1):47–54.

106. Vaccarino V, Sullivan S, Hammadah M, et al. Mental stress-induced-myocardial ischemia in young patients with recent myocardial infarction: Sex differences and mechanisms. Circulation 2018;137(8):794–805.

107. Pimple P, Hammadah M, Wilmot K, et al. Chest pain and Mental Stress-Induced Myocardial Ischemia: Sex differences. Am J Med 2018;131(5):540–7.e1.

108. Faravelli C, Alessandra Scarpato M, Castellini G, et al. Gender differences in depression and anxiety: the role of age. Psychiatry Res 2013;210(3):1301–3.

109. Albert PR. Why is depression more prevalent in women? J Psychiatry Neurosci 2015;40(4):219–21.

110. Ferketich AK, Schwartzbaum JA, Frid DJ, et al. Depression as an antecedent to heart disease among women and men in the NHANES I study. National Health and Nutrition Examination Survey. Arch Intern Med 2000;160(9):1261–8.

111. Saeed A, Kampangkaew J, Nambi V. Prevention of cardiovascular disease in women. Methodist Debakey Cardiovasc J 2017;13(4):185–92.

112. AbuRuz ME, Al-Dweik G. Depressive symptoms and complications early after acute myocardial infarction: Gender differences. Open Nurs J 2018;12:205–14.

113. Pelletier R, Khan NA, Cox J, et al. Sex versus gender-related characteristics: which predicts outcome after acute coronary syndrome in the young? J Am Coll Cardiol 2016;67(2):127–35.

114. Stewart AL, Barinas-Mitchell E, Matthews KA, et al. Social role-related stress and social role-related reward as related to subsequent subclinical cardiovascular disease in a longitudinal study of midlife women: The Study of Women's Health Across the Nation. Psychosom Med 2019;81(9):821–32.

115. Vemuri R, Sylvia KE, Klein SL, et al. The microgenderome revealed: sex differences in bidirectional interactions between the microbiota, hormones, immunity and disease susceptibility. Semin Immunopathol 2019;41(2):265–75.

116. Smith DRM, Dolk FCK, Smieszek T, et al. Understanding the gender gap in antibiotic prescribing: a cross-sectional analysis of English primary care. BMJ Open 2018;8(2):e020203.

117. Battson ML, Lee DM, Weir TL, et al. The gut microbiota as a novel regulator of cardiovascular function and disease. J Nutr Biochem 2018;56:1–15.

118. Witkowski M, Weeks TL, Hazen SL. Gut microbiota and cardiovascular disease. Circ Res 2020;127(4):553–70.

119. Ray WA, Murray KT, Hall K, et al. Azithromycin and the risk of cardiovascular death. N Engl J Med 2012;366(20):1881–90.

120. Zaroff JG, Cheetham TC, Palmetto N, et al. Association of azithromycin use with cardiovascular mortality. JAMA Netw Open 2020;3(6):e208199.
121. Dominianni C, Sinha R, Goedert JJ, et al. Sex, body mass index, and dietary fiber intake influence the human gut microbiome. PLoS One 2015;10(4): e0124599.
122. Klein SL, Flanagan KL. Sex differences in immune responses. Nat Rev Immunol 2016;16(10):626–38.
123. Ortona E, Pierdominici M, Maselli A, et al. Sex-based differences in autoimmune diseases. Ann Ist Super Sanita 2016;52(2):205–12.
124. Fischinger S, Boudreau CM, Butler AL, et al. Sex differences in vaccine-induced humoral immunity. Semin Immunopathol 2019;41(2):239–49.
125. Bienvenu LA, Noonan J, Wang X, et al. Higher mortality of COVID-19 in males: sex differences in immune response and cardiovascular comorbidities. Cardiovasc Res 2020;116(14):2197–206.
126. Arulkumaran N, Snow TAC, Kulkarni A, et al. Sex differences in immunological responses to COVID-19: a cross-sectional analysis of a single-centre cohort. Br J Anaesth 2021;127(2):e75–8.
127. Viveiros A, Rasmuson J, Vu J, et al. Sex differences in COVID-19: candidate pathways, genetics of ACE2, and sex hormones. Am J Physiol Heart Circ Physiol 2021;320(1):H296–304.
128. Ahn SV, Kim HC, Nam CM, et al. Sex difference in the effect of the fasting serum glucose level on the risk of coronary heart disease. J Cardiol 2018;71(2):149–54.
129. Golomb BA, Evans MA. Statin adverse effects: a review of the literature and evidence for a mitochondrial mechanism. Am J Cardiovasc Drugs 2008;8: 373–418.
130. Hecht HS, Harman SM. Relation of aggressiveness of lipid-lowering treatment to changes in calcified plaque burden by electron beam tomography. J Am Coll Cardiol 2003;92(3):334–6.
131. de Lorgeril M, Salen P, Abramson J, et al. Cholesterol lowering, cardiovascular diseases, and the rosuvastatin-JUPITER controversy: A critical reappraisal. Arch Intern Med 2010;170(12):1032–6.
132. Jones M, Tett S, Geeske M, et al. New-onset diabetes after statin exposure in elderly women: the Australian longitudinal study on women's health. Drugs & Aging 2017;34(3):203.
133. Ma Y, Culver A, Rossouw J, et al. Statin therapy and the risk for diabetes among adult women: do the benefits outweigh the risk? Ther Adv Cardiovasc Dis 2013; 7(1):41–4.
134. Jones M, Tett S, Peeters GM, et al. New-onset diabetes after statin exposure in elderly women: The Australian Longitudinal Study on Women's Health. Drugs & Aging 2017;34(3):203–9.
135. Faubion SS, Kapoor E, Moyer AM, et al. Statin therapy: does sex matter? Menopause 2019 2021;26(12):1425–35. Erratum in: Menopause 28(2):228.
136. Sattar N, Preiss D, Murray HM, et al. Statins and risk of incident diabetes: A collaborative meta-analysis of randomized statin trials. Lancet 2010;375: 735–42.
137. Black CJ, Ford AC. Chronic idiopathic constipation in adults: epidemiology, pathophysiology, diagnosis and clinical management. Med J Aust 2018; 209(2):86–91.
138. Khashab MA, Pickhardt PJ, Kim DH, et al. Colorectal anatomy in adults at computed tomography colonography: normal distribution and the effect of age, sex, and body mass index. Endoscopy 2009;41:674–8.

139. Saunders BP, Fukumoto M, Halligan S, et al. Why is colonoscopy more difficult in women? Gastrointest Endosc 1996;43:124–6.
140. Wilson SA, Stem LA, Bruehlman RD. Hypothyroidism: diagnosis and treatment. Am Fam Physician 2021;103(10):605–13.
141. Grindler NM, Allsworth JE, Macones GA, et al. Persistent organic pollutants and early menopause in U.S. women. PLoS One 2015;10(1):e0116057.
142. Engberding N, Wenger NK. Management of hypertension in women. Hypertens Res 2012;35:251–60.
143. SPRINT Research Group, Wright JT Jr, Williamson JD, et al. A randomized trial of intensive versus standard blood-pressure control. N Engl J Med 2015; 373(22):2103–16.
144. Kannel WB, Hjortland MC, McNamara PM, et al. Menopause and risk of cardiovascular disease: the Framingham study. Ann Intern Med 1976;85(4):447–52.
145. Ford ES, Ajani UA, Croft JB, et al. Explaining the decrease in U.S. deaths from coronary disease, 1980-2000. N Engl J Med 2007;356(23):2388–98.
146. El Khoudary SR, Aggarwal B, Beckie TM, et al. Menopause transition and cardiovascular disease risk: implications for timing of early prevention: a scientific statement from the American Heart Association. Circulation 2020;142(25): e506–32.
147. Tsiligiannis S, Panay N, Stevenson JC. Premature ovarian insufficiency and long-term health consequences. Curr Vasc Pharmacol 2019;17(6):604–9.
148. Young L, Cho L. Unique cardiovascular risk factors in women. Heart 2019; 105(21):1656–60.
149. Zhu D, Chung HF, Dobson AJ, et al. Age at natural menopause and risk of incident cardiovascular disease: a pooled analysis of individual patient data. Lancet Public Health 2019;4(11):e553–64.
150. Bairey Merz CN, Johnson BD, Sharaf BL, et al. Hypoestrogenemia of hypothalamic origin and coronary artery disease in premenopausal women: a report from the NHLBI-sponsored WISE study. J Am Coll Cardiol 2003;41(3):413–9.
151. Mosconi L, Berti V, Quinn C, et al. Sex differences in Alzheimer risk: Brain imaging of endocrine vs chronologic aging. Neurology 2017;89(13):1382–90.
152. Scheyer O, Rahman A, Hristov H, et al. Female sex and Alzheimer's risk: The menopause connection. J Prev Alzheimers Dis 2018;5(4):225–30.
153. Somani YB, Pawelczyk JA, De Souza MJ, et al. Aging women and their endothelium: probing the relative role of estrogen on vasodilator function. Am J Physiol Heart Circ Physiol 2019;317(2):H395–404.
154. Guetta V, Cannon RO III. Cardiovascular effects of estrogen and lipid-lowering therapies in postmenopausal women. Circulation 1996;93(10):1928–37.
155. Fåhraeus L. The effects of estradiol on blood lipids and lipoproteins in postmenopausal women. Obstet Gynecol 1988;72(5 Suppl):18S–22S.
156. Kovats S. Estrogen receptors regulate innate immune cells and signaling pathways. Cell Immunol 2015;294(2):63–9.
157. Song CH, Kim N, Sohn SH, et al. Effects of 17β-estradiol on colonic permeability and inflammation in an azoxymethane/dextran sulfate sodium-induced colitis mouse model. Gut and Liver 2018;12(6):682.
158. Miller VM, Lahr BD, Bailey KR, et al. Longitudinal effects of menopausal hormone treatments on platelet characteristics and cell-derived microvesicles. Platelets 2016;27(1):32–42.
159. Ramesh SS, Christopher R, Indira Devi B, et al. The vascular protective role of oestradiol: a focus on postmenopausal oestradiol deficiency and aneurysmal subarachnoid haemorrhage. Biol Rev 2019;94(6):1897–917.

160. Westendorp IC, Bots ML, Grobbee DE, et al. Menopausal status and distensibility of the common carotid artery. Arterioscler Thromb Vasc Biol 1999;19(3): 713–7.
161. Lephart ED, Naftolin F, Friedenthal J, et al. Cardiovascular health and the menopausal woman: the role of estrogen and when to begin and end hormone treatment. F1000Research 2019;8.
162. O'Donnell E, Floras JS, Harvey PJ. Estrogen status and the renin angiotensin aldosterone system. Am J Physiol Regul Integr Comp Physiol 2014;307(5): R498–500.
163. Lapham K, Kvale MN, Lin J, et al. Automated assay of telomere length measurement and informatics for 100,000 subjects in the Genetic Epidemiology Research on Adult Health and Aging (GERA) Cohort. Genetics 2015;200(4): 1061–72.
164. Owan TE, Hodge DO, Herges RM, et al. Trends in prevalence and outcome of heart failure with preserved ejection fraction. New Engl J Med 2006;355:251–9.
165. Bhatia RS, Tu JV, Lee DS, et al. Outcome of heart failure with preserved ejection fraction in a population-based study. New Engl J Med 2006;355:260–9.
166. Redfield MM, Jacobsen SJ, Burnett JC, et al. Burden of systolic and diastolic ventricular dysfunction in the community: appreciating the scope of the heart failure epidemic. J Am Med Assoc 2003;289:194–202.
167. Hoekstra T, Lesman-Leegte I, van Veldhuisen DJ, et al. Quality of life is impaired similarly in heart failure patients with preserved and reduced ejection fraction. Eur J Heart Fail 2011;13:1013–8.
168. Upadhya B, Kitzman DW. Heart failure with preserved ejection fraction: new approaches to diagnosis and management. Clin Cardiol 2019;43(2):145–55.
169. Ladeiras-Lopes R, Araújo M, Sampaio F, et al. The impact of diastolic dysfunction as a predictor of cardiovascular events: A systematic review and meta-analysis. Revista Portuguesa de Cardiologis 2019;38(11):789–804.
170. Pulit SL, Karaderi T, Lindgren CM. Sexual dimorphisms in genetic loci linked to body fat distribution. Biosci Rep 2017;37(1):BSR20160184.
171. Karvonen-Gutierrez C, Kim C. Association of mid-life changes in body size, body composition and obesity status with the menopausal transition. Healthcare (Basel) 2016;4(3):42.
172. Chamsi-Pasha MA, Kurrelmeyer KM. Noninvasive evaluation of symptomatic women with suspected coronary artery disease. Methodist Debakey Cardiovasc J 2017;13(4):193–200.
173. Shufelt CL, Pacheco C, Tweet MS, et al. Sex-specific physiology and cardiovascular disease. Adv Exp Med Biol 2018;1065:433–54.
174. Ferrario CM, Moore MA, Bestermann W Jr, et al. COSEHC global vascular risk management quality improvement program: rationale and design. Vasc Health Risk Manag 2010;6:1135–45.
175. Ferrario CM, Joyner J, Colby C, et al. The COSEHC™ Global Vascular Risk Management quality improvement program: first follow-up report. Vasc Health Risk Manag 2013;9:391–400.
176. Joyner J, Moore MA, Simmons DR, et al. Impact of performance improvement continuing medical education on cardiometabolic risk factor control: the COSEHC initiative. J Contin Educ Health Prof 2014;34(1):25–36.
177. Gottfried SE, Houston MC. Women and heart disease: best practices in screening and diagnosis, poster American Medical Women's Association. In: 106th annual Meeting, March 25 – 28. 2021. Available at: https://vimeo.com/ 521231326. Accessed December 5, 2021.

178. Hall H, Perelman D, Breschi A, et al. Glucotypes reveal new patterns of glucose dysregulation. Plos Biol 2018;16(7):e2005143.
179. Cardona A, Zareba KM, Raman SV. The role of stress cardiac magnetic resonance in women. J Nucl Cardiol 2016;23(5):1036–40.
180. Kwong RY, Ge Y, Steel K, et al. Cardiac magnetic resonance stress perfusion imaging for evaluation of patients with chest pain. J Am Coll Cardiol 2019; 74(14):1741–55.
181. Antiochos P, Ge Y, Steel K, et al. Evaluation of stress cardiac magnetic resonance imaging in risk reclassification of patients with suspected coronary artery disease. JAMA Cardiol 2020;5(12):1401–9.
182. Bakir M, Wei J, Nelson MD, et al. Cardiac magnetic resonance imaging for myocardial perfusion and diastolic function-reference control values for women. Cardiovasc Diagn Ther 2016;6(1):78–86.
183. Jalnapurkar S, Zarrini P, Mehta PK, et al. Role of stress cardiac magnetic resonance imaging in women with suspected ischemia but no obstructive coronary artery disease. J Radiol Nurs 2017;36(3):180–3.
184. Honigberg MC, Pirruccello JP, Aragam K, et al. Menopausal age and left ventricular remodeling by cardiac magnetic resonance imaging among 14,550 women. Am Heart J 2020;229:138–43.
185. Leblanc V, Bégin C, Hudon AM, et al. Gender differences in the long-term effects of a nutritional intervention program promoting the Mediterranean diet: changes in dietary intakes, eating behaviors, anthropometric and metabolic variables. Nutr J 2014;13:107.
186. Cano A, Marshall S, Zolfaroli I, et al. The Mediterranean diet and menopausal health: an EMAS position statement. Maturitas 2020;139:90–7.
187. Bédard A, Corneau L, Lamarche B, et al. Sex differences in the impact of the Mediterranean diet on LDL particle size distribution and oxidation. Nutrients 2015;7(5):3705–23.
188. Bédard A, Riverin M, Dodin S, et al. Sex differences in the impact of the Mediterranean diet on cardiovascular risk profile. Br J Nutr 2012;108(8):1428–34.
189. Goossens GH, Jocken JWE, Blaak EE. Sexual dimorphism in cardiometabolic health: the role of adipose tissue, muscle and liver. Nat Rev Endocrinol 2021; 17(1):47–66.
190. Toledo E, Salas-Salvadó J, Donat-Vargas C, et al. Mediterranean diet and invasive breast cancer risk among women at high cardiovascular risk in the PRE-DIMED Trial: a randomized clinical trial. JAMA Intern Med 2015;175(11): 1752–60.
191. Mattioli AV, Pennella S, Pedrazzi P, et al. Gender differences in adherence to Mediterranean diet and risk of atrial fibrillation. J Hypertens Cardiol 2015; 1(4):4–13.
192. Dao MC, Everard A, Aron-Wisnewsky J, et al. Akkermansia muciniphila and improved metabolic health during a dietary intervention in obesity: relationship with gut microbiome richness and ecology. Gut 2016;65(3):426–36.
193. Depommier C, Everard A, Druart C, et al. Supplementation with Akkermansia muciniphila in overweight and obese human volunteers: a proof-of-concept exploratory study. Nat Med 2019;25(7):1096–103.
194. Rolnik DL, Wright D, Poon LC, et al. Aspirin versus placebo in pregnancies at high risk for preterm preeclampsia. N Engl J Med 2017;377(7):613–22.
195. Norman JE. Progesterone and preterm birth. Int J Gynaecol Obstet 2020;150(1): 24–30.

196. Romero R, Conde-Agudelo A, Da Fonseca E, et al. Vaginal progesterone for preventing preterm birth and adverse perinatal outcomes in singleton gestations with a short cervix: a meta-analysis of individual patient data. Am J Obstet Gynecol 2018;218(2):161–80.

197. Blackwell SC, Gyamfi-Bannerman C, Biggio JR Jr, et al. 17-OHPC to prevent recurrent preterm birth in singleton gestations (PROLONG Study): a multicenter, international, randomized double-blind trial. Am J Perinatol 2020;37(2):127–36.

198. Norman JE, Marlow N, Messow CM, et al. Vaginal progesterone prophylaxis for preterm birth (the OPPTIMUM study): a multicentre, randomised, double-blind trial. Lancet 2016;387(10033):2106–16.

199. Smith GN, Louis JM, Saade GR. Pregnancy and the postpartum period as an opportunity for cardiovascular risk identification and management. Obstet Gynecol 2019;134(4):851–62.

200. Zaw JJ, Howe PR, Wong RH. Postmenopausal health interventions: time to move on from the Women's Health Initiative? Ageing Res Rev 2018;48:79–86.

201. Rossouw JE, Anderson GL, Prentice RL, et al. for the Writing Group for the Women's Health Initiative Investigators. Risks and benefits of estrogen plus progestin in healthy postmenopausal women: principal results from the Women's Health Initiative randomized controlled trial. JAMA 2002;288:321–33.

202. Hulley S, Grady D, Bush T, et al. for the Heart and Estrogen/progestin Replacement Study (HERS) Research Group. Trial of estrogen plus progestin for secondary prevention of coronary heart disease in postmenopausal women. JAMA 1998;280:605–13.

203. Committee on Gynecologic Practice. ACOG Committee Opinion No. 565: hormone therapy and heart disease. Obstet Gynecol 2013;121:1407–10.

204. Cho L, Davis M, Elgendy I, et al. Summary of updated recommendations for primary prevention of cardiovascular disease in women: JACC state-of-the-art review. J Am Coll Cardiol 2020;75(20):2602–18.

205. Rossouw JE, Prentice RL, Manson JE, et al. Postmenopausal hormone therapy and risk of cardiovascular disease by age and years since menopause. JAMA 2007;297:1465–77.

206. Manson JE, Allison MA, Rossouw JE, et al. for the WHI and WHI-CACS Investigators. Estrogen therapy and coronary-artery calcification. N Engl J Med 2007;356:2591–602.

207. Hodis HN, Mack WJ, Henderson VW, et al. for the ELITE Research Group. Vascular effects of early versus late postmenopausal treatment with estradiol. N Engl J Med 2016;374:1221–31.

Mycotoxin Illness: Recognition and Management from Functional Medicine Perspective

Alice Prescott Sullivan, DO

KEYWORDS

- Environmental toxins • Mold • Mycotoxins • mold illness • ochratoxin • aflatoxin
- detoxification

KEY POINTS

- Mold toxins are in our everyday environment and are relevant to our health.
- Mold toxins may contribute and/or exacerbate many common progressive conditions affecting health such as asthma, digestive disorders, and systemic inflammation.
- Recognition of symptoms of mold toxins is important in order for testing to be ordered and confirmed.
- Treatment is straightforward from a functional medicine perspective: recognition and remediation or avoidance of environmental exposures, along with quality nutritional and detoxification strategies.;

INTRODUCTION

Mold toxin exposure by inhalation and ingestion has significant health consequences for humans. In this article, we discuss the sources of these everyday toxins and their relevance to patient health. The effects of mycotoxins can present across all body systems, and the resulting symptoms can be acute, cumulative, and chronic. These effects can occur discretely, but they can also present alongside other clinical entities. It is important for the clinician to recognize the phenomenon of mycotoxin illness because, as a primary cause, it does not resolve with current standards of care for conditions secondary to it.

The aims of this article are to aid the clinician in the recognition of symptoms that may be due to mycotoxin exposure, suggest an established convenient method of testing for mycotoxins, and propose a reliable treatment approach using functional medicine principles.

Collectively, mold toxins can be pantecedents to illness as well as triggers and mediators per the functional medicine paradigm, and affect all aspects of the functional medicine matrix.

Center for Functional Medicine, Cleveland Clinic, 9500 Carnegie Avenue, Q2-1 Glickman Tower, Cleveland, OH 44195, USA
E-mail address: prescottsullivan@protonmail.com

Phys Med Rehabil Clin N Am 33 (2022) 647–663
https://doi.org/10.1016/j.pmr.2022.04.006
1047-9651/22/© 2022 Elsevier Inc. All rights reserved.

BACKGROUND

Mold toxicity is defined as exposure to mycotoxins or "natural products produced by fungi that evoke a toxic response when introduced in low concentration to higher vertebrates and other animals by a natural route."[1] The deleterious health effects of mold and mold toxins (aka mycotoxins) in the home were recognized in biblical times.[2] In the Middle Ages, the consumption of grains, flour, or bread contaminated by ergot alkaloids caused the condition known as St Anthony's fire or "ergotism."[3] Since then, the primary intervention has been to reduce and prevent mycotoxin contamination by optimizing handling and storage of grains. Modern research into mycotoxins began in earnest with the discovery of aflatoxins, following the deaths of 100,000 young turkeys in the UK in 1960. Mold and their mycotoxins are ubiquitous in our environment,[4] evident and tested in our food supply,[5–7] housing, and workplaces.[8,9] Exposure routes for humans include ingestion, inhalation, and/or absorption by dermal contact.[10] From anthe agricultural perspective, mycotoxins permeate the food supply at the crop stage, whether freshly harvested or postprocessed, or stored or exposed to the elements for any length of time. With the changing environmental landscape due to global warming, the ability to mitigate mold and the resulting mycotoxin burden in the food supply is becoming increasingly challenging.[11,12] Heat and humidity[13] as well as rain late in the harvesting season[14] can potentiate mold growth on crops. Contaminated crops may then be fed to livestock or used as part of their housing, exposing both livestock them as well as consumers.[15] When contaminated crops make it to the consumer, *mold toxins persist even when their parent spores are destroyed with cooking.* Because of the known deleterious effects of mycotoxins, several of these are regulated by the food industry. These regulated mycotoxins include, but are not limited to aflatoxins, fumonisins, trichothecenes, ochratoxin, and zearalenone.[16] Despite this surveillance, there is evidence that there is a regular occurrence of elevated mycotoxins in the diets of people living in developed countries.[17,18]

From the perspective of buildings and indoor air, it is estimated that 20% to 40% of all dwellings and workplaces have significant mold populations.[9] Major mycotoxin producing genera in indoor environments include Aspergillus, Penicillium, Stachybotrys, and Chaetomium.[19] Dampness is often the rate-limiting factor for mold growth, and different species favor different ranges of temperature and humidity. Indoor toxigenic molds favor higher humidity levels.[20–22] Water damage by leaks or flooding are often the catalyst for the exponential growth of indoor molds, whether visible to casual inspection or hidden beneath appliances, in air ducts or behind walls. Multiple studies have measured significant mold counts within air handling and AC units, revealing the persisting necessity for better engineering of our air optimization strategy.[23,24] Residents and workers inside water-damaged buildings may inhale mold spores as well as airborne mycotoxins.[25] In recent years, there has been increasing interest in the health impact of inhaled mycotoxins in water-damage buildings caused by stronger and more frequent storms that result in flooding.[26–28] Residential dampness and mold are associated with substantial and statistically significant increases in allergic rhinitis, upper respiratory infections, asthma, and bronchitis.[29] A recent systematic review linked water-damaged buildings to the deleterious health of inhabitants or workers; the studies reviewed reported respiratory, neurologic, immunologic (allergic and non-IgE mediated), cognitive, ophthalmologic, and dermatologic effects.[30] The issue of water damage disproportionately impacts underserved populations who may not have adequate resources to repair their homes to prevent water intrusion, or to remediate their water-damaged homes once colonized with mold. Despite the available evidence, some believe the associations of indoor mold and human disease to be unsupported; however, evidence is mounting in the unbiased reviews by government agencies and educational institutions of indoor air quality and the impact of various indoor air pollutants including mold on human health.[9,26,31]

Fungal colonization of the upper respiratory tract has been established[32,33] in both controls and patients with allergic rhinitis. It is widely accepted among ENT and pulmonology specialists that steroids and other immune suppressants may encourage aggressive habits of some fungal organisms and that a patient may be colonized in an immune-competent state but later, through the use of steroids or other immune suppressants, become immune-compromised leading to an invasive fungal infection by the formerly latent colonization. Overgrowth of Candida and Alternaria have even been noted in several immune-competent individuals using steroid nasal sprays.[34,35]

Mold toxins had not been thought to be secreted significantly by colonized fungal organisms; Brewer[1] contended that because Aspergillus and other molds release toxins maximally at 20 to 30°C (aflatoxin production is optimal at 25–33°C), their secretion would, therefore, not be relevant to human physiology at 37°C. This assertion has failed to hold. The temperature of the nasal mucosa during the respiratory cycle has been measured between 28 and 34°C.[36] Furthermore, cell cultures of aspergillus fumigatus have shown significant gliotoxin secretion at 37°C with attendant effects on PMNs and monocytes.[37] Ochratoxins have been measured also in the nares of patients with chronic rhinosinusitis.[38] Fusarium and Aspergillus are known for expressing mycotoxins and can secrete them at the temperature of the nasal mucosa. These genera are frequent causes of common allergic fungal rhinosinusitis.[39] A small study of patients with candida vaginitis showed that gliotoxin was present in the vagina along with candida, but not present in patients without vaginal yeast.[40]

Significantly, the pathologic effects of molds and their toxins are not yet covered in US medical school curricula. According to Pitt,[41] "acute toxicity is rare: toxicity due to mycotoxins is almost always insidious, without any overt indication of effects on health in the short term. For this reason, the health effects of mycotoxins are among the most neglected areas of medical science."

Impact of Mycotoxins on Health

Mold and their mycotoxins are known causes of human illness by a variety of biological mechanisms which can be classified into 4 groups: (1) allergic or hypersensitivity reactions, (2) irritant reactions, (3) toxic reactions, and (4) infections.[31] The research cataloging effects of mycotoxins show a widely varied impact on the organism, the cell, and on intracellular and mitochondrial chemistry. Mold toxins are now known to affect multiple systems in the body, ranging from the obvious, such as respiratory and gastrointestinal, to deeper systems causing immune, nerve, and endocrine disruptions.[42,43] Additionally, the health effects of mycotoxins are potentiated in contexts of multiple mycotoxin exposures.[44–46]

Patient's Timeline

When exposed to mold toxins, patients may present with single or multiple symptoms due to various system insults. Symptoms may accumulate in sequence or present spontaneously together.[47] When taking a patient history, a timeline is useful for noting the start of symptoms relative to water damage, a move, or a change of workplace. It is important to note that a lag may follow the initial exposure to develop symptoms or that an unknown leak may occur years after a move, confounding the interviewer and patient to correlate symptom onset with the source of mycotoxins. Patients may be unaware of their exposure as toxic mold colonies can be out of sight in air ducts, in the dry wall behind walls, under appliances, in carpeting, or under mattresses.

Presentation: Symptoms and Conditions

Respiratory effects

Sinus irritation from mold spores and mycotoxins is common. While the topical use of nasal steroids may suppress a local immune response to molds, it is not a successful approach to removing mycotoxins, which can be absorbed through the respiratory mucosa. One research group found that concurrent use of methylprednisolone in the context of gliotoxin exposure actually *increased* reactive oxygen species in granulocytes.[48]

Exposure to mycotoxin or other dampness-related agents augments the risk for the development of asthma symptoms among those with rhinosinusitis symptoms.[49] Approximately 4.6 million cases of asthma in America in 1 year were due to mold exposure in the home.[50] While patients with preexisting asthma can be triggered by mycotoxin exposure, just the exposure itself can be a singular cause of the initiation and persistence of asthma.[51]

Respiratory effects beyond sinusitis and asthma can be quite varied and profound. Vocal cord dysfunction was found in 2 office workers who were working in a water-damaged building; they also had concurrent cough, wheeze, hoarseness, and dyspnea.[52] One investigation identified a high prevalence of new-onset sarcoidosis, as well as asthma, among workers of a water-damaged building with a history of indoor environmental quality complaints.[53] Mycotoxins including patulin and citrinin cause oxidative stress and glutathione depletion effects in respiratory tissues.[54,55]

Pneumonitis and pulmonary hemorrhage in infants have been caused by exposure to stachybotrys and other fungi.[56,57] Pulmonary infection by inhaled mold spores is known to occur with certain mold species, including but not limited to the genera Mucor, Histoplasma, Blastomyces, Aspergillus, and Fusarium.[58,59]

Digestive disturbances

Mold toxins can compromise several key functions of the gastrointestinal tract including nutrient absorption, modulation of nutrient transporters, barrier integrity, and microbiome stability.[60–62] Destruction of enterocytes can limit nutrient absorption in the intestine and result in malnutrition.[42] Some mycotoxins facilitate the persistence of intestinal pathogens and potentiate intestinal inflammation.[15] Effects between mycotoxins and intestinal flora are bidirectional, as mycotoxins disrupt the intestinal microbiome, and normal intestinal flora detoxify and absorb mycotoxins.[63,64]

Fatigue

Fatigue is a recognized secondary effect of mycotoxin exposure.[65,66] Wang and colleagues[67] made an interesting connection between mold exposure, secondary snoring, and daytime sleepiness. This would suggest that mold, by way of triggering inflammation in the upper airway, may cause sleep apnea or hypopnea. But fatigue could also be a result of mast cell activation, ,as discussed under "immune effects" below, or a result of mitochondrial dysfunction, as several mycotoxins are directly toxic to mitochondria.[68,69]

Immune effects

Allergic symptoms in skin, eyes, and upper/lower respiratory tissues are common effects of molds in general and may wax and wane with exposure. Minimally, mycotoxins as allergens can cause itching,[70] inflame nasal epithelial cells,[71] and irritate corneal cells.[72] However, mast cell activation in mold-exposed individuals can lead to hypersensitivity conditions that present as chronic irritation of not only the eyes and respiratory tract, that is, recurrent sinusitis, bronchitis, and cough, but also with neurologic manifestations, such as fatigue, nausea, headaches, and brain fog.[73] Many mycotoxins are inflammatory as well as immunosuppressive.[74] One such example is mycophenolic acid, under the brand name CellCept, which has been purified to prevent organ rejection in transplant recipients. Immunosuppression has been demonstrated in studies of other mycotoxins as well, including ochratoxin, trichothecenes, zearalenone, and gliotoxin.[37,75–78]

Hepatotoxicity

Aflatoxins are well-known for their toxic effects on the liver. Phase I detoxification of aflatoxin B1 results in an epoxide that creates DNA adducts. Due to the oxidative stress of this epoxide and other metabolites, there are many other cellular effects including the degranulation of endoplasmic reticulum, increased hepatic lipid peroxides, glutathione depletion, mitochondrial dysfunction, and reduction of enzymatic and nonenzymatic antioxidants.[68,79] Clinically, aflatoxins may cause nausea, abdominal pain, jaundice, ascites, and produce testable elevation of liver enzymes.[80] However, their effects can be insidious, without signs or symptoms. The classic result of cumulative aflatoxicosis is liver carcinoma, cited and studied extensively in humans and animals.[81–83]

Renal toxicity

Ochratoxins from penicillium and aspergillus species have been studied extensively for their effects on the kidney, including tubular adenomas, necrosis, and renal cell carcinoma. Balkan endemic nephropathy has been shown to arise from excessive exposure to ochratoxin from aspergillus and penicillium species.[84,85]

Neurologic effects

Neurologic symptoms of mycotoxins include brain fog, inability to focus/concentrate, poor short-term memory, and poor comprehension.[86,87] IQ scores of children growing up in moldy environments show the effect on cognitive function and learning capacity.[88] Mold exposure with traumatic brain injury contributes to cognitive symptoms, imperiling patients further than with TBI alone.[89] Tremors and seizures are possible presentations described in human case reports.[90,91] Stachybotrys spores have been shown to adversely affect behavior and memory in mice.[92] Ochratoxin, which is a product of certain Aspergillus and Penicillium species, has been shown to affect hippocampus neuroprogenitor cells of mouse brain.[93,94]

Additional late effects

In addition to aflatoxins and ochratoxin, multiple other mycotoxins are known to cause cancer, including trichothecenes, zearalenone, ochratoxin, fumonisin, and deoxynivalenol.[81–83,95] Zearalenone has estrogen receptor affinity, causing multiple downstream effects such as infertility,[96,97] as well as enhancement of breast tumor cell proliferation.[98]

Diagnostic Strategy

Patient assessment

Testing the symptomatic patient is helpful to make the diagnosis of mycotoxin illness. At the time of this writing, there is no universal standard for ascribing a patient's presentation to a level of mold toxin in blood or urine. There are urine tests available commercially, using either mass spectrometry (Great Plains Laboratory: GPL) or ELISA (Real-time Laboratory), to assess levels of urinary concentration of specific mycotoxins. The ELISA test by Real-Time Laboratories has met standards for CLIA certification.

It is recommended once patients are diagnosed with a positive urine test that they investigate potential current sources in their living and/or working spaces. Relief of symptoms by leaving or remediating affected premises may be sufficient for a diagnosis in retrospect. Elevated risk of mold presence is seen in areas of high humidity, near water, or having central air intake from the basement for redistribution to the rest of the building. Social determinants such as poverty, living in the housing of poor construction, or delaying repair of or tolerating evident leaks, are also risk factors for mold exposure. These risks should be cues to the clinician that the patient is likely to have significant mold exposure.

The expression and penetrance of mycotoxin illness has a wide spectrum, and this presentation in any individual will depend on each exposed individual's detoxification genetics, nutritional status, gut microbiome, proximity to the mold overgrowth in living/working space, duration of exposure, and concurrent physiologic stressors.[1,47] In an environment where there are many individuals exposed but only one apparently affected, the affected individual is often singled out as inordinately sensitive in their family or work cohort. Since their symptoms may cause disruptions in family life or work productivity, their symptoms are generally unwelcome. However, as the effects of mold toxins are often insidious the symptoms of the sensitive person may be helpful to recognize an air quality issue in their environment. If toxic mold is found and , remediation is done promptly, others who are similarly exposed will be prevented from silently developing late effects such as infertility or cancer.

Detoxification, Biotransformation, and Elimination

The liver plays a critical role in detoxifying mycotoxins. There are two phases of detoxification. Phase I converts lipophilic toxins via oxidation, reduction, or hydroxylation in the cytochrome P450 system. The result of this conversion is a highly unstable molecule that then quickly undergoes Phase II detoxification, which is conjugation with small deactivating molecules, such as glucuronide, glutathione, sulfate, glycine, taurine, acetyl or methyl moieties [99]. If there is a temporal gap between phases I and II, the free radical products of phase I are likely to cause damage to surrounding tissue.

The following discussion reviews the major detoxification pathways for several prominent mycotoxins considered relevant to human health.

Detoxification of aflatoxins requires both phase I and phase II detoxification pathways. In phase I, aflatoxins are detoxified using the aldo-keto reductase pathway in the CYP 450 system. This creates an intermediate molecule that can cause DNA adducts known to cause hepatocellular cancer.[100,101] An increased risk for hepatocellular cancer results from the aflatoxin itself as well as the intermediary created in biotransformation. Glutathione conjugation is one of the phase II detoxication conjugates for aflatoxin, and oral glutathione can improve detoxification.[101]

Ochratoxin is detoxified by phase II, per the work of Muñoz and colleagues[102]; its conjugates have been directly measured in urine, as OTA bound to N-acetyl cysteine and to glutathione.[103] Conjugates have also been indirectly assessed in the urine by the addition of hydrolyzing agent,[104] or addition of beta-glucuronidase,[105] which have significantly enhanced urinary assessment of ochratoxin excretion. Ochratoxin has a very long half-life, about 35 days as studied in one fasting subject.[104] This is likely due to ochratoxin binding extensively to albumin[106] as only the free ochratoxin is available for detoxification, and primary detoxification pathways requiring phase II glucuronidation would be slowed during a fast. Follow-up studies with 8 individuals showed significantly different and fluctuating ochratoxin levels with the same exposure.[105]

Zearalenone, mycophenolate, and deoxynivalenol are primarily detoxified through the glucuronidation pathway.[107]

Citrinin is transformed to dihydrocitrinin as the primary detoxification pathway by hepatic transformation, then is filtered by kidneys or released through bile. Enterohepatic circulation is evident in the study of citrinin.[108]

Treatment Strategy

It is expected that symptomatic mycotoxin illness may require weeks or months of detoxification before resolution. Symptoms deriving from *toxicity* from molds may take much longer to clear than *allergic* symptoms. In the functional medicine paradigm, assisting the detoxification processes of the body to remove the root cause of the problem contributes significantly to the restoration of patients to their former level of health. The following strategy will assist the patient in the detoxification of mycotoxins. Clearance in cases of underlying colonization will likely require further treatment beyond detoxification.

1. Hydration. Adequate hydration is essential to detoxification. Water improves kidney clearance of water-soluble toxins and is protective of the kidneys.[109] Water dilutes toxins within the lymphatics and assists in flushing. Appropriate hydration supports bowel regularity which reduces transit time and therefore reduces mold toxin absorption and resorption. Current recommendations for daily water intake are 2.7 L per day for women and 3.7 L per day for men.[110]
2. Sauna. Sauna therapy supports the removal of toxins and provides symptomatic relief for the patient. There are no studies that have measured mold toxin release by sweating, but Rea has published studies showing success in detoxifying patients suffering from mycotoxin illness with sauna.[111] Rea's study may have illustrated that patients improve from excreting mycotoxins directly in their sweat, or that release of other toxins through sweat enables faster elimination of mycotoxins through other channels. There are other recent studies that have demonstrated significant parallel rates of secretion of heavy metals and organochlorinated pesticides in human sweat and urine.[112,113]
3. Antioxidants. Mycotoxins have been shown to cause oxidative stress. Effects of oxidative stress can be mitigated by the consumption of antioxidants. Glutathione, polyphenols, carotenoids, vitamin C, sulforaphane, ubiquinol, and other antioxidants can all help reduce the burden of oxidative stress.[114] Resveratrol has been shown to ameliorate the effects of ochratoxin in the kidney.[115]
4. Antiinflammatories. Antiinflammatories have been shown to be helpful in mitigating symptoms of mold exposure. Curcumin,[116] quercetin,[117] Omega-3 essential fatty acids,[118] and luteolin[119] can be helpful.[120]
5. Liver support. Phase II support can be enhanced with various foods and supplements. Sulforaphane from cruciferous veges are protective.[121] The presence of a functional glutathione S-transferase mu 1 (GSTM1) allele has been shown to provide protection again aflatoxin-B DNA damage in human liver.[69] This suggests that glutathione is helpful in the clearance of aflatoxins and their metabolites. Provision of supplemental NAC and glutathione can increase available phase II conjugates and thereby assist in phase II conjugation of mycotoxins.[103,122]
6. Optimizing bowel habits. As adsorption and resorption of mycotoxins through the GI tract is the major vehicle for mycotoxin penetrance, it is important to establish bowel regularity in affected patients. Constipation is to be avoided as increased transit time

causes increased absorption of newly ingested mycotoxins. Furthermore, prolonged intestinal transit time provides an opportunity for gut bacteria to deconjugate processed mycotoxins.[123] Magnesium glycinate is recommended to promote bowel motility gently, while also providing glycine for phase II conjugation and for glutathione production. Glucomannan may be helpful with constipation.[124,125]

7. The foundational step in mold detoxification is the use of various binding agents, taken orally. The mycotoxins adhere to these binders thereby preventing their resorption through the intestinal mucosa. The binders may prevent the absorption of recently ingested mycotoxins as well as the resorption of processed mycotoxins coming from the liver released through the bile.[126] As binders can cause constipation, maintaining bowel regularity is critical. Charcoal, clay, yeast cell walls, and lactobacilli have all been studied for their effectiveness to bind various mycotoxins.[127–134] Chlorophyll has also been shown to effectively reduce urinary aflatoxin gene adducts in a placebo-controlled study.[135] Nonorganic binders such as clay and charcoal are recommended to be taken 2 hours away from meals and medications because their binding qualities are global and nonspecific; the effectiveness of binders is enhanced by consuming them with fat.

8. Probiotics. Probiotics have been studied extensively with respect to their ability to absorb and inactivate mycotoxins. Lactobacilli, Bifidobacteria, and Saccharomyces have been used to moderate the effects of mold contamination of grain and studies show they help maintain the health of animals at risk for ingesting contaminated grain. These beneficial organisms can be taken liberally by patients to effectively metabolize and/or bind mycotoxins in the GI tract.[136–139]

9. Avoidance in diet. Patients are advised to take measures to reduce potential mold content in their diets, especially during treatment. Common foods such as cereals and dairy products are especially prone to molding, due to processing and removal of protective natural antifungal properties.

10. Nasal rinses. Nasal colonization by mold species is nearly universal. Fungal species have been cultured in 100%, 97%, and 93% of nares of control patients tested in 3 separate studies, respectively.[32,140,141] Daily nasal irrigation is safe and helpful for rhinitis symptoms.[142] Nasal irrigation assists in reducing the effects of current exposures, as well as discouraging further colonization by potentially aggressive spores.[143]

11. Remediation. It is recommended to patients that they determine potential current sources of mold toxins through food and/or environment and remediate as necessary.[144] Home testing can be conducted with commercially available air sampling, mold plates, and/or environmental relative mold index (ERMI) testing. It is recommended to work with a mold-certified inspector with knowledge of environmental health to remediate the home safely and efficiently. As stated previously, cereal grains and dairy products are common sources of mold in food and so it is encouraged to reduce or eliminate these, as well as freezing leftovers rather than refrigerating them.

12. Treatment of Colonization. As fungal species are present in the nares and occasionally the sinuses, it is often helpful to treat this potential source of mold toxins with intranasal antifungal therapy. Treatment of enteric yeast overgrowth, as a source of gliotoxin, is also recommended.

SUMMARY

As mold and their mycotoxins are present in our food and environment, it is prudent to consider their high potential for adverse effects on our patients. A good history and review of symptoms will help lead the clinician to consider the possibility of exposure, order available testing, and establish the relevance of mold toxin exposure in the perspective of the patient's case. The symptoms resulting from mold exposure may present on a spectrum from mundane allergy to profound fatigue and cognitive effects. Missing thecause for these symptoms will prolong the suffering of the patient. Furthermore, myriad secondary conditions such as rhinitis, diarrhea, asthma, and mast cell activation, to give a few examples, may be erroneously treated as primary phenomena withsuppressive medications such as steroids and antimotility agents which may worsen the true underlying problem if due to mold toxins. Neglecting the cause may result in a cognitive decline for some patients, and cancer in others. The exposed patient's detoxification genetics, nutritional status, gut microbiome, proximity to the mold overgrowth in the living/working space, duration of exposure, and concurrent physiologic stressors will all contribute to the severity of mycotoxin illness. The complexity of these interacting variables does explain how and why there can be a singular affected patient within an otherwise asymptomatic family or working cohort in the same environment. Confirming the patient's exposure by testing urine mycotoxins is therefore important to uncover this root cause of illness, both fot the individual and those who share their environment. Detoxification using a functional medicine approach can help restore function and improve symptom burden. Support of the various detoxification routes using binders and other available nutraceuticals is critical to helping patients recover from mycotoxin illness.

CLINICS CARE POINTS

- Consider mold toxicity in any patient's history when a move precipitated a new set of symptoms.
- Presentation of asthma is commonly caused by mold exposure. Asthmatics should avoid or remediate areas of known mold exposure.
- Consistent hydration, sauna, movement, and probiotics are good hygiene practice for anyone, and especially for someone with mold exposure, to assist with detoxification.
- Remediation and/or avoidance of exposure is recommended as a minimal step to prevent further progression of mycotoxin-induced illness, but by itself, remediation/avoidance will likely be insufficient as a single intervention to resolve long-term mycotoxin exposure.
- There are many governmental organizations with sound, practical advice for homeowners and renters, which can be invaluable resources to help the patient determine if their home or workplace is a source of mold exposure.

DISCLOSURE

The author has nothing to disclose.

REFERENCES

1. Bennett JW, Klich M. Mycotoxins, editor(s): Moselio Schaechter, . Encyclopedia of Microbiology. 3rd edition. Oxford: Academic Press; 2009. p. 559–65.
2. Leviticus 14; 33-47.
3. CR Armendáriz et al, 2014. Mycotoxins, encyclopedia of toxicology (3rd Edition). 424–7.
4. Marin S, Ramos AJ, Cano-Sancho G, et al. Mycotoxins: occurrence, toxicology, and exposure assessment. Food Chem Toxicol 2013;60:218–37.

5. EPA. "Mold Course, chapter 2". Available at: Epa.gov/mold/mold-course-chapter-2

6. WHO. Guidelines for indoor for indoor air quality: dampness and mould. Available at https://apps.who.int/iris/handle/10665/164348, 2009

7. Peraica M, Radić B, Lucić A, et al. Toxic effects of mycotoxins in humans. Bull World Health Organ 1999;77(9):754.

8. Miller JD. Mycotoxins in small grains and maize: old problems, new challenges. Food Addit Contam Part A Chem Anal Control Expo Risk Assess 2008;25(2):219–30.

9. EPA. "Mold Course, chapter 1". Available at Epa.gov/mold/mold-course-chapter-1

10. FDA. BAM Chapter 18: Yeasts, Molds and Mycotoxins. Available at: https://www.fda.gov/food/laboratory-methods-food/bam-chapter-18-yeasts-molds-and-mycotoxins, 2017

11. Schatzmayr G, Streit E. Global occurrence of mycotoxins in the food and feed chain: facts and figures. World Mycotoxin J 2013;6(3):213–22.

12. Perrone G, Ferrara M, Medina A, et al. Toxigenic fungi and mycotoxins in a climate change scenario: Ecology, genomics, distribution, prediction and prevention of the risk. Microorganisms 2020;8(10):1496.

13. Pitt JI, Miller JD. A concise history of mycotoxin research. J Agric Food Chem 2017;65(33):7021–33.

14. Gornall J, Betts R, Burke E, et al. Implications of climate change for agricultural productivity in the early twenty-first century. Philosophical Trans R Soc B Biol Sci 2010;365(1554):2973–89.

15. Grenier B, Applegate TJ. Modulation of intestinal functions following mycotoxin ingestion: Meta-analysis of published experiments in animals. Toxins 2013;5(2):396–430.

16. Logrieco AF, Miller JD, Eskola M, et al. The mycotox charter: increasing awareness of, and concerted action for, minimizing mycotoxin exposure worldwide. Toxins 2018;10(4):149.

17. Sundheim L, Brodal G, Hofgaard IS, et al. Temporal variation of mycotoxin producing fungi in Norwegian cereals. Microorganisms 2013;1(1):188–98.

18. BIOMIN Mycotoxin Survey in US and Canada: January 2021 Update. Available at: https://www.biomin.net/us/science-hub/biomin-mycotoxin-survey-in-us-and-canada-january-2021-update/. Accessed January 2, 2022.

19. Nielsen KF. Mycotoxin production by indoor molds. Fungal Genet Biol 2003;39(2):103–17.

20. EPA. "A Brief Guide to Mold, Moisture, and Your Home". Available at epa.gov/mold/brief-guide-mold-moisture-and-your-home, 2021

21. Norbäck D, Cai GH. Fungal DNA in hotel rooms in Europe and Asia—associations with latitude, precipitation, building data, room characteristics and hotel ranking. J Environ Monit 2011;13(10):2895–903.

22. Cai GH, Bröms K, Mälarstig B, et al. Quantitative PCR analysis of fungal DNA in Swedish day care centers and comparison with building characteristics and allergen levels. Indoor Air 2009;19(5):392–400.

23. Wilson SC, Palmatier RN, Andriychuk LA, et al. Mold contamination and air handling units. J Occup Environ Hyg 2007;4(7):483–91.

24. Bakker A, Siegel JA, Mendell MJ, et al. Bacterial and fungal ecology on air conditioning cooling coils is influenced by climate and building factors. Indoor Air 2020;30(2):326–34.

25. Clark N, Ammann HM, Brunekreef B, et al. Damp indoor spaces and health. Washington, DC: Institute of Medicine of the National Academies; 2004.

26. FEMA. "Mold & Mildew: Cleaning Up Your Flood-Damaged Home", FEMA B-606/July 2008. 2008. Available at: http://dnrc.mt.gov/divisions/water/operations/floodplain-management/disaster-and-recovery/MoldandMildrew.pdf. Accessed January 2, 2022.

27. CDC. "Mold After a Disaster". 2020. Available at: https://www.cdc.gov/disasters/mold/index.html. Accessed December 16, 2021.

28. Khan NN, Wilson BL. An environmental assessment of mold concentrations and potential mycotoxin exposures in the greater Southeast Texas area. J Environ Sci Health A 2003;38(12):2759–72.

29. Baxi SN, Portnoy JM, Larenas-Linnemann D, et al. Exposure and health effects of fungi on humans. J Allergy Clin Immunol Pract 2016;4(3):396–404.

30. Dooley M, McMahon S. A comprehensive review of mold research literature from 2011-2018. Int Med Rev 2020;6:1.

31. Storey E, Dangman KH, Schenck P, et al. Guidance for clinicians on the recognition and management of health effects related to mold exposure and moisture indoors. Farmington (CT): University of Connecticut Health Center; 2004. p. 1–206.

32. Ponikau JU, Sherris DA, Kern EB, et al. The diagnosis and incidence of allergic fungal sinusitis. In: Mayo clinic proceedings, vol. 74. Elsevier; 1999. p. 877–84. The American Rhinologic Society at the Combined Otolaryngology Spring Meetings, May 11, 1998.San Francisco (California).

33. Braun H, Buzina W, Freudenschuss K, et al. 'Eosinophilic fungal rhinosinusitis': a common disorder in Europe? Laryngoscope 2003;113(2):264–9.

34. Chang GH, Wang WH. Intranasal fungal (Alternaria) infection related to nasal steroid spray. Am J Otolaryngol 2013;34(6):743–5.

35. Wang T, Zhang L, Hu C, et al. Clinical features of chronic invasive fungal rhinosinusitis in 16 cases. Ear Nose Throat J 2020;99(3):167–72.

36. Bailey RS, Casey KP, Pawar SS, et al. Correlation of nasal mucosal temperature with subjective nasal patency in healthy individuals. JAMA Facial Plast Surg 2017;19(1):46–52.

37. Stanzani M, Orciuolo E, Lewis R, et al. Aspergillus fumigatus suppresses the human cellular immune response via gliotoxin-mediated apoptosis of monocytes. Blood 2005;105(6):2258–65.

38. Lieberman SM, Jacobs JB, Lebowitz RA, et al. Measurement of mycotoxins in patients with chronic rhinosinusitis. Otolaryngol Head Neck Surg 2011;145(2):327–9.

39. Montone KT, Livolsi VA, Feldman MD, et al. Fungal rhinosinusitis: a retrospective microbiologic and pathologic review of 400 patients at a single university medical center. Int J Otolaryngol 2012;2012:1–9. https://doi.org/10.1155/2012/684835.

40. Shah DT, Glover DD, Larsen B. In situ mycotoxin production by Candida albicans in women with vaginitis. Gynecol Obstet Invest 1995;39(1):67–9.

41. Pitt JI, Taniwaki MH, Cole MB. Mycotoxin production in major crops as influenced by growing, harvesting, storage and processing, with emphasis on the achievement of Food Safety Objectives. Food Control 2013;32(1):205–15.

42. Milićević DR, Škrinjar M, Baltić T. Real and perceived risks for mycotoxin contamination in foods and feeds: challenges for food safety control. Toxins 2010;2(4):572–92.

43. Liew WPP, Mohd-Redzwan S. Mycotoxin: its impact on gut health and microbiota. Front Cell Infect Microbiol 2018;8:60.

44. Gao YN, Wang JQ, Li SL, et al. Aflatoxin M1 cytotoxicity against human intestinal Caco-2 cells is enhanced in the presence of other mycotoxins. Food Chem Toxicol 2016;96:79–89.

45. Torres O, Matute J, Gelineau-van Waes J, et al. Human health implications from co-exposure to aflatoxins and fumonisins in maize-based foods in Latin America: Guatemala as a case study. World Mycotoxin J 2015;8(2):143–59.

46. Mueller A, Schlink U, Wichmann G, et al. Individual and combined effects of mycotoxins from typical indoor moulds. Toxicol Vitro 2013;27(6):1970–8.

47. Ráduly Z, Szabó L, Madar A, et al. Toxicological and medical aspects of Aspergillus-derived mycotoxins entering the feed and food chain. Front Microbiol 2020;10:2908.

48. Orciuolo E, Stanzani M, Canestraro M, et al. Effects of Aspergillus fumigatus gliotoxin and methylprednisolone on human neutrophils: implications for the pathogenesis of invasive aspergillosis. J Leukoc Biol 2007;82(4):839–48.

49. Park JH, Kreiss K, Cox-Ganser JM. Rhinosinusitis and mold as risk factors for asthma symptoms in occupants of a water-damaged building. Indoor Air 2012;22(5):396–404.

50. Mudarri D, Fisk WJ. Public health and economic impact of dampness and mold. Indoor Air 2007;17(3):226–35.

51. Zhang Z, Reponen T, Hershey GKK. Fungal exposure and asthma: IgE and non-IgE-mediated mechanisms. Curr Allergy Asthma Rep 2016;16(12):1–12.

52. Cummings KJ, Fink JN, Vasudev M, et al. Vocal cord dysfunction related to water-damaged buildings. J Allergy Clin Immunol Pract 2013;1(1):46–50.

53. Laney AS, Cragin LA, Blevins LZ, et al. Sarcoidosis, asthma, and asthma-like symptoms among occupants of a historically water-damaged office building. Indoor Air 2009;19(1):83.

54. Luft P, Oostingh GJ, Gruijthuijsen Y, et al. Patulin influences the expression of Th1/Th2 cytokines by activated peripheral blood mononuclear cells and T cells through depletion of intracellular glutathione. Environ Toxicol 2008;23(1):84–95.

55. Johannessen LN, Nilsen AM, Løvik M. Mycotoxin-induced depletion of intracellular glutathione and altered cytokine production in the human alveolar epithelial cell line A549. Toxicol Lett 2007;168(2):103–12.

56. Novotny WE, Dixit A. Pulmonary hemorrhage in an infant following 2 weeks of fungal exposure. Arch Pediatr Adolesc Med 2000;154(3):271–5.

57. Etzel RA, Montana E, Sorenson WG, et al. Acute pulmonary hemorrhage in infants associated with exposure to Stachybotrys atra and other fungi. Arch Pediatr Adolesc Med 1998;152(8):757–62.

58. Baumgardner DJ. Use of urine antigen testing for Blastomyces in an integrated health system. J Patient-Centered Res Rev 2018;5(2):176.

59. CDC. "Fungal diseases". Available at: CDC.gov/fungal/diseases/index.html, 2019

60. Gonkowski S, Gajęcka M, Makowska K. Mycotoxins and the enteric nervous system. Toxins 2020;12(7):461.

61. Robert H, Payros D, Pinton P, et al. Impact of mycotoxins on the intestine: are mucus and microbiota new targets? J Toxicol Environ Health B 2017;20(5):249–75.

62. Wang X, Yu H, Shan A, et al. Toxic effects of Zearalenone on intestinal microflora and intestinal mucosal immunity in mice. Food Agric Immunol 2018;29(1): 1002–11.

63. Jin J, Beekmann K, Ringø E, et al. Interaction between food-borne mycotoxins and gut microbiota: a review126. Food Control; 2021. p. 1–13, 107998.

64. Guerre P. Mycotoxin and gut microbiota interactions. Toxins 2020;12(12):769.

65. Chester AC, Levine PH. Concurrent sick building syndrome and chronic fatigue syndrome: Epidemic neuromyasthenia revisited. Clin Infect Dis 1994; 18(Supplement_1):S43–8.

66. Brewer JH, Thrasher JD, Straus DC, et al. Detection of mycotoxins in patients with chronic fatigue syndrome. Toxins 2013;5(4):605–17.

67. Wang J, Janson C, Lindberg E, et al. Dampness and mold at home and at work and onset of insomnia symptoms, snoring and excessive daytime sleepiness. Environ Int 2020;139:105691.

68. Doherty WP, Campbell TC. Aflatoxin inhibition of rat liver mitochondria. Chem Biol Interact 1973;7(2):63–77.

69. Ribeiro SM, Chagas GM, Campello AP, et al. Mechanism of citrinin-induced dysfunction of mitochondria. V. Effect on the homeostasis of the reactive oxygen species. Cell Biochem Funct 1997;15(3):203–9.

70. Aihara R, Ookawara T, Morimoto A, et al. Acute and subacute oral administration of mycotoxin deoxynivalenol exacerbates the pro-inflammatory and pro-pruritic responses in a mouse model of allergic dermatitis. Arch Toxicol 2020;94(12): 4197–207.

71. Cremer B, Soja A, Sauer JA, et al. Pro-inflammatory effects of ochratoxin A on nasal epithelial cells. Eur Arch Otorhinolaryngol 2012;269(4):1155–61.

72. Bossou YM, Serssar Y, Allou A, et al. Impact of mycotoxins secreted by Aspergillus molds on the inflammatory response of human corneal epithelial cells. Toxins 2017;9(7):197.

73. Lauritano D, Conti P. Impact of mold on mast cell-cytokine immune response. J Biol Regul Homeost Agents 2018;32(4):763–8.

74. Corrier DE. Mycotoxicosis: mechanisms of immunosuppression. Vet Immunol Immunopathol 1991;30(1):73–87.

75. Cooray R. Effects of some mycotoxins on mitogen-induced blastogenesis and SCE frequency in human lymphocytes. Food Chem Toxicol 1984;22(7):529–34.

76. Pahl HL, Krauss B, Schulze-Osthoff K, et al. The immunosuppressive fungal metabolite gliotoxin specifically inhibits transcription factor NF-kappaB. J Exp Med 1996;183(4):1829–40.

77. Yamada A, Kataoka T, Nagai K. The fungal metabolite gliotoxin: immunosuppressive activity on CTL-mediated cytotoxicity. Immunol Lett 2000;71(1):27–32.

78. Eichner RD, Al Salami M, Wood PR, et al. The effect of gliotoxin upon macrophage function. Int J Immunopharmacol 1986;8(7):789–97.

79. Mary VS, Theumer MG, Arias SL, et al. Reactive oxygen species sources and biomolecular oxidative damage induced by aflatoxin B1 and fumonisin B1 in rat spleen mononuclear cells. Toxicology 2012;302(2–3):299–307.

80. Kamala A, Shirima C, Jani B, et al, investigation team. Outbreak of an acute aflatoxicosis in Tanzania during 2016. World Mycotoxin J 2018;11(3):311–20.

81. Khan SA, Carmichael PL, Taylor-Robinson SD, et al. DNA adducts, detected by 32P postlabelling, in human cholangiocarcinoma. Gut 2003;52(4):586–91.

82. Kew MC. Aflatoxins as a cause of hepatocellular carcinoma. J Gastrointest Liver Dis 2013;22(3).

83. Wogan GN. Aflatoxins as risk factors for hepatocellular carcinoma in humans. Cancer Res 1992;52(7 Supplement):2114s–8s.
84. Malir F, Ostry V, Pfohl-Leszkowicz A, et al. Ochratoxin A: 50 years of research. Toxins 2016;8(7):191.
85. Castegnaro M, Canadas D, Vrabcheva T, et al. Balkan endemic nephropathy: role of ochratoxins A through biomarkers. Mol Nutr Food Res 2006;50(6): 519–29.
86. Baldo JV, Ahmad L, Ruff R. Neuropsychological performance of patients following mold exposure. Appl Neuropsychol 2002;9(4):193–202.
87. Empting LD. Neurologic and neuropsychiatric syndrome features of mold and mycotoxin exposure. Toxicol Ind Health 2009;25(9–10):577–81.
88. Jedrychowski W, Maugeri U, Perera F, et al. Cognitive function of 6-year old children exposed to mold-contaminated homes in early postnatal period. Prospective birth cohort study in Poland. Physiol Behav 2011;104(5):989–95.
89. Gordon WA, Cantor JB, Johanning E, et al. Cognitive impairment associated with toxigenic fungal exposure: a replication and extension of previous findings. Appl Neuropsychol 2004;11(2):65–74.
90. Lewis PR, Donoghue MB, Cook L, et al. Tremor syndrome associated with a fungal toxin: sequelae of food contamination. Med J Aust 2005;182(11):582–4.
91. Kushnir-Sukhov NM. A novel link between early life allergen exposure and neuroimmune development in children. J Clin Exp Immunol 2020;5(4):188.
92. Harding CF, Pytte CL, Page KG, et al. Mold inhalation causes innate immune activation, neural, cognitive and emotional dysfunction. Brain Behav Immun 2020;87:218–28.
93. Sava V, Reunova O, Velasquez A, et al. Acute neurotoxic effects of the fungal metabolite ochratoxin-A. Neurotoxicology 2006;27(1):82–92.
94. Sava V, Velasquez A, Song S, et al. Adult hippocampal neural stem/progenitor cells in vitro are vulnerable to the mycotoxin ochratoxin-A. Toxicol Sci 2007; 98(1):187–97.
95. Ahmed Adam MA, Tabana YM, Musa KB, et al. Effects of different mycotoxins on humans, cell genome and their involvement in cancer. Oncol Rep 2017;37(3): 1321–36.
96. Pang J, Cao QF, Sun ZY. Impact of zearalenone on male fertility: an update. Zhonghua Nan Ke Xue 2016;22(11):1034–7.
97. Minervini F, Dell'Aquila ME, Maritato F, et al. Toxic effects of the mycotoxin zearalenone and its derivatives on in vitro maturation of bovine oocytes and 17β-estradiol levels in mural granulosa cell cultures. Toxicol Vitro 2001; 15(4–5):489–95.
98. Martin PM, Horwitz KB, Ryan DS, et al. Phytoestrogen interaction with estrogen receptors in human breast cancer cells. Endocrinology 1978;103(5):1860–7.
99. Liska, D., Lyon, M., and Jones, D.S. 2005. Detoxification and Biotransformation Imbalances. Textbook of Functional Medicine, Chapter 22, pp 277-279.
100. Hamid AS, Tesfamariam IG, Zhang Y, et al. Aflatoxin B1-induced hepatocellular carcinoma in developing countries: Geographical distribution, mechanism of action and prevention. Oncol Lett 2013;5(4):1087–92.
101. Raney KD, Meyer DJ, Ketterer B, et al. Glutathione conjugation of aflatoxin B1 exo-and endo-epoxides by rat and human glutathione S-transferases. Chem Res Toxicol 1992;5(4):470–8.
102. Muñoz K, Cramer B, Dopstadt J, et al. Evidence of ochratoxin A conjugates in urine samples from infants and adults. Mycotoxin Res 2017;33(1):39–47.

103. Sueck F, Specht J, Cramer B, et al. Identification of ochratoxin-N-acetyl-L-cysteine as a new ochratoxin A metabolite and potential biomarker in human urine. Mycotoxin Res 2020;36(1):1–10.

104. Al Ayoubi M, Salman M, Gambacorta L, et al. Assessment of Dietary Exposure to Ochratoxin A in Lebanese Students and Its Urinary Biomarker Analysis. Toxins 2021;13(11):795.

105. Studer-Rohr I, Schlatter J, Dietrich DR. Kinetic parameters and intraindividual fluctuations of ochratoxin A plasma levels in humans. Arch Toxicol 2000;74(9):499–510.

106. Marquardt RR, Frohlich AA. A review of recent advances in understanding ochratoxicosis. J Anim Sci 1992;70(12):3968–88.

107. Warth B, Sulyok M, Berthiller F, et al. New insights into the human metabolism of the Fusarium mycotoxins deoxynivalenol and zearalenone. Toxicol Lett 2013;220(1):88–94.

108. Ali N, Blaszkewicz M, Degen GH. Occurrence of the mycotoxin citrinin and its metabolite dihydrocitrinone in urines of German adults. Arch Toxicol 2015;89(4):573–8.

109. Nakamura Y, Watanabe H, Tanaka A, et al. Effect of increased daily water intake and hydration on health in japanese adults. Nutrients 2020;12(4):1191.

110. Mayo Clinic Staff. Water: How much should you drink every day? Mayo Clinic website. 2021. Available at: https://www.mayoclinic.org/healthy-lifestyle/nutrition-and-healthy-eating/in-depth/water/art-20044256. Accessed December 16, 2021.

111. Rea WJ. A large case-series of successful treatment of patients exposed to mold and mycotoxin. Clin Ther 2018;40(6):889–93.

112. Genuis SJ, Birkholz D, Rodushkin I, et al. Blood, urine, and sweat (BUS) study: monitoring and elimination of bioaccumulated toxic elements. Arch Environ Contam Toxicol 2011;61(2):344–57.

113. Genuis SJ, Lane K, Birkholz D. Human elimination of organochlorine pesticides: blood, urine, and sweat study16. BioMed Research International; 2016. p. 1–10.

114. Tan BL, Norhaizan ME, Liew WPP, et al. Antioxidant and oxidative stress: a mutual interplay in age-related diseases. Front Pharmacol 2018;9:1162.

115. Raghubeer S, Nagiah S, Phulukdaree A, et al. The phytoalexin resveratrol ameliorates ochratoxin A toxicity in human embryonic kidney (HEK293) cells. J Cell Biochem 2015;116(12):2947–55.

116. Mohajeri M, Behnam B, Cicero AF, et al. Protective effects of curcumin against aflatoxicosis: A comprehensive review. J Cell Physiol 2018;233(4):3552–77.

117. Gugliandolo E, Peritore AF, D'Amico R, et al. Evaluation of neuroprotective effects of quercetin against aflatoxin B1-intoxicated mice. Animals 2020;10(5):898.

118. Hutchinson AN, Tingö L, Brummer RJ. The potential effects of probiotics and ω-3 fatty acids on chronic low-grade inflammation. Nutrients 2020;12(8):2402.

119. Liu M, Cheng C, Li X, et al. Luteolin alleviates ochratoxin A induced oxidative stress by regulating Nrf2 and HIF-1α pathways in NRK-52E rat kidney cells. Food Chem Toxicol 2020;141:111436.

120. Ghazi T, Arumugam T, Foolchand A, et al. The Impact of Natural Dietary Compounds and Food-Borne Mycotoxins on DNA Methylation and Cancer. Cells 2020;9(9):2004.

121. Gross-Steinmeyer K, Stapleton PL, Tracy JH, et al. Sulforaphane-and phenethyl isothiocyanate–induced inhibition of aflatoxin B1–mediated genotoxicity in

human hepatocytes: Role of GSTM1 genotype and CYP3A4 gene expression. Toxicol Sci 2010;116(2):422–32.

122. Fuchs R, Hult K. Ochratoxin A in blood and its pharmacokinetic properties. Food Chem Toxicol 1992;30(3):201–4.

123. Chen HL, Cheng HC, Wu WT, et al. Supplementation of konjac glucomannan into a low-fiber Chinese diet promoted bowel movement and improved colonic ecology in constipated adults: a placebo-controlled, diet-controlled trial. J Am Coll Nutr 2008;27(1):102–8.

124. Janani F, Changaee F. The effect of glucomannan on pregnancy constipation. J Fam Med Prim Care 2018;7(5):903.

125. Roberts MS, Magnusson BM, Burczynski FJ, et al. Enterohepatic circulation. Clin Pharmacokinet 2002;41(10):751–90.

126. Avantaggiato G, Havenaar R, Visconti A. Assessing the zearalenone-binding activity of adsorbent materials during passage through a dynamic in vitro gastrointestinal model. Food Chem Toxicol 2003;41(10):1283–90.

127. Plank G, Bauer J, Grünkemeier A, et al. The protective effect of adsorbents against ochratoxin A in swine. Tierarztl Prax 1990;18(5):483–9.

128. Abbès S, Salah-Abbès JB, Ouanes Z, et al. Preventive role of phyllosilicate clay on the immunological and biochemical toxicity of zearalenone in Balb/c mice. Int Immunopharmacol 2006;6(8):1251–8.

129. Phillips TD, Lemke SL, Grant PG. Characterization of clay-based enterosorbents for the prevention of aflatoxicosis. Mycotoxins Food Saf 2002;504:157–71.

130. Bordini JG, Borsato D, Oliveira AS, et al. In vitro zearalenone adsorption by a mixture of organic and inorganic adsorbents: Application of the Box Behnken approach. World Mycotoxin J 2015;8(3):291–9.

131. Haskard CA, El-Nezami HS, Kankaanpää PE, et al. Surface binding of aflatoxin B1 by lactic acid bacteria. Appl Environ Microbiol 2001;67(7):3086–91.

132. Shehata S, Richter WIF, Schuster M, et al. Adsorption of ochratoxin A, deoxynivalenol and zearalenone in vitro at different pH and adsorbents. Mycotoxin Res 2000;16(1):136–40.

133. De Mil T, Devreese M, Maes A, et al. Influence of mycotoxin binders on the oral bioavailability of tylosin, doxycycline, diclazuril, and salinomycin in fed broiler chickens. Poult Sci 2017;96(7):2137–44.

134. Piotrowska M. The adsorption of ochratoxin A by Lactobacillus species. Toxins 2014;6(9):2826–39.

135. Egner PA, Wang JB, Zhu YR, et al. Chlorophyllin intervention reduces aflatoxin–DNA adducts in individuals at high risk for liver cancer. Proc Natl Acad Sci 2001; 98(25):14601–6.

136. Muñoz R, Arena ME, Silva J, et al. Inhibition of mycotoxin-producing Aspergillus nomius VSC 23 by lactic acid bacteria and Saccharomyces cerevisiae. Braz J Microbiol 2010;41:1019–26.

137. Hassan YI, Bullerman LB. Antifungal activity of Lactobacillus paracasei ssp. tolerans isolated from a sourdough bread culture. Int J Food Microbiol 2008; 121(1):112–5.

138. Muhialdin BJ, Saari N, Meor Hussin AS. Review on the biological detoxification of mycotoxins using lactic acid bacteria to enhance the sustainability of foods supply. Molecules 2020;25(11):2655.

139. Shetty PH, Jespersen L. Saccharomyces cerevisiae and lactic acid bacteria as potential mycotoxin decontaminating agents. Trends Food Sci Technol 2006; 17(2):48–55.

140. Kim ST, Choi JH, Jeon HG, et al. Comparison between polymerase chain reaction and fungal culture for the detection of fungi in patients with chronic sinusitis and normal controls. Acta Otolaryngol 2005;125(1):72–5.
141. Braun H, Stammberger H, Buzina W, et al. Incidence and detection of fungi and eosinophilic granulocytes in chronic rhinosinusitis. Laryngorhinootologie 2003; 82(5):330–40.
142. Rabago D, Zgierska A. Saline nasal irrigation for upper respiratory conditions. Am Fam Physician 2009;80(10):1117–9.
143. Georgitis JW. Nasal hyperthermia and simple irrigation for perennial rhinitis: changes in inflammatory mediators. Chest 1994;106(5):1487–92.
144. CDC. "Mold". Available at: https://www.cdc.gov/mold/cleanup-guide.html, 2017

Social Determinants and Health Equity in Functional Medicine

Nazleen Bharmal, MD, PhD, MPP

KEYWORDS

- Functional medicine • Social determinants of health • Social connection
- Community health

KEY POINTS

- Social determinants of health (SDOH) and health-related social needs are important factors in patients' health journey.
- The functional medicine timeline and matrix are useful to map social determinants and social needs of patients and can help patients understand SDOH impact on different aspects of their health.
- Patient-centered trust and collaboration through community engagement are opportunities to adapt functional medicine practice to underserved communities and patients with increased risk of health disparities due to socio-demographics.

INTRODUCTION

Chronic diseases, or conditions that last 1 year or more and require ongoing medical attention and/or limit activities of daily living continue to the be the leading causes of death and disability in the United States. Heart disease, cancer, chronic lung disease, stroke, Alzheimer's disease, diabetes, chronic kidney disease, and obesity continue to be the leading drivers for the nation's health care costs.[1] Six in 10 adults in the United States have a chronic disease and 4 in 10 have 2 or more.[2] Traditional risk behaviors have included exposure to tobacco smoke, poor nutrition with diets low in fruits and vegetables and high in sodium and saturated fats, lack of physical activity, and excessive alcohol use.[2] In addition, the severity of mental health, substance use disorders, autoimmune, and infectious diseases, like COVID-19, may be worsened by chronic disease and/or exacerbate morbidity and mortality from chronic disease.

Population Health

The burden of chronic disease and illness is intertwined with population health. Population health is defined as the health outcomes for a group of individuals, including

Cleveland Clinic Community Care, 9500 Euclid Avenue, G10, Cleveland, OH 44195, USA
E-mail address: bharman2@ccf.org

Phys Med Rehabil Clin N Am 33 (2022) 665–678
https://doi.org/10.1016/j.pmr.2022.04.007

the distribution of such outcomes within the group.[3] It is a model for improving patient care quality and experiences while reducing costs for the health of the population with a focus on health outcomes or value versus services delivered. In essence, population health is focused on the prevention of disease or disease severity and helping people thrive as opposed to focusing on individuals when they are sick. As such, there is overlap with key tenets of functional medicine focused on lifestyle factors and health promotion, such as optimal stress management/reduction, sleep, physical activity, social connection.

Population health efforts in the United States are often broken down into 4 distinct factors with varying percentages of impact—health care (20%), physical environment (10%), health behaviors (30%), and social determinants (40%) **(Fig. 1)**.[4] Health behaviors include smoking, diet, exercise, alcohol intake; physical environment includes green space and access to clean air and water; and, social determinants include social and economic factors such as educational attainment, employment, and social support.

Social Determinants of Health

Social determinants of health (SDOH) are the conditions in which people are born, grow, live, work, and age.[5] These influencers of health are the wider set of forces and systems shaping the conditions of daily life. SDOH is impacted by economics, social policies, and politics and are often considered the root causes of health. Healthy People, which is a national effort that sets 10-year goals and measurable objectives to improve the health and well-being of people in the United States, breaks down SDOH into 5 domains: education access and quality, health care and quality, neighborhood and built environment, social and community context, and economic stability **(Fig. 2)**.[6]

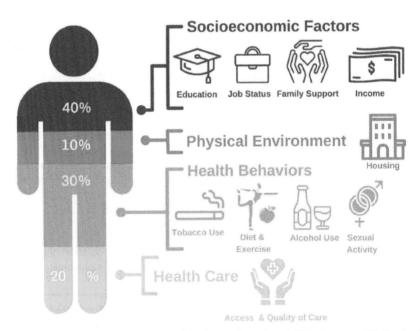

Fig. 1. Contributors to population health. (*Data from*: Hood CM, Gennuso KP, Swain GR, Catlin BB. County Health Rankings: Relationships Between Determinant Factors and Health Outcomes. *Am J Prev Med*. 2016;50(2):129-135.)

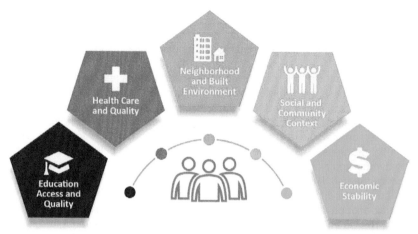

Fig. 2. Social determinants of health domains, healthy people 2030, office of disease prevention and health promotion, US Department of health and human services. (*From*: Office of Disease Prevention and Health Promotion. Healthy People 2030: Social Determinants of Health. U.S. Department of Health and Human Services. https://health.gov/healthypeople/objectives-and-data/social-determinants-health. Accessed January, 2022.)

Individual SDOH are important predictors of health outcomes and disparities in individual chronic disease risk. These individual factors, often referred to as individual *health-related social needs*, include an individual or family's socioeconomic status, food security, housing stability, social support, culture and language, access to health care, and residential environment. **Fig. 3** illustrates various health-related social needs and their areas of impact on health outcomes.[7]

Economic Stability	Neighborhood and Physical Environment	Education	Food	Community and Social Context	Health Care System
Employment	Housing	Literacy	Hunger	Social integration	Health coverage
Income	Transportation	Language	Access to healthy options	Support systems	Provider availability
Expenses	Safety	Early childhood education		Community engagement	Provider linguistic and cultural competency
Debt	Parks	Vocational training		Discrimination	
Medical bills	Playgrounds			Stress	
Support	Walkability	Higher education			Quality of care
	Zip code / geography				

Health Outcomes
Mortality, Morbidity, Life Expectancy, Health Care Expenditures, Health Status, Functional Limitations

Fig. 3. Social determinants of health and health-related social needs. (*From* Artiga S, Hinton E. Beyond health care: The role of social determinants in promoting health and health equity. Kaiser Family Foundation. https://www.kff.org/racial-equity-and-health-policy/issue-brief/beyond-health-care-the-role-of-social-determinants-in-promoting-health-and-health-equity/. Published 2018. Accessed January, 2022.)

Health Disparities and Health Equity

There is greater recognition of disparate health outcomes for cardiovascular disease, diabetes chronic kidney disease, neurologic conditions including dementia, lung disease, and COVID-19 for different populations based on SDOH.[8–12] Socioeconomic status, including education, income and occupation measures, food insecurity and healthy food access, social relationships and support, environmental factors such as air pollution, and social conditions such as chronic stress, racism, and discrimination are examples of SDOH that impact the development of chronic conditions such as obesity, cardiometabolic and cardiovascular diseases, and chronic kidney disease. Substantial progress has been made by researchers in data collection and stratification by demographic characteristics, in understanding the relationship between socioeconomic status and inequitable health care access and quality with health outcomes, and in the structural changes needed to achieve health equity.[13]

Vulnerable populations often have distinct experiences of health and illness. For example, the COVID-19 epidemic was felt differently if you were young or old with a chronic disease, paid by salary or paid by the hour, and/or if you were from a privileged or marginalized racial/ethnic group. Populations that often have a greater burden of poor health outcomes from chronic and acute illness, in part due to SDOH factors, include:

- Racial and ethnic minority groups, including indigenous populations
- Sexual and gender minority groups
- Low-income or lower socioeconomic status
- Limited English proficiency or low health literacy
- Residence in a disadvantaged, resource-challenged, and/or rural neighborhood
- Special populations, such as those who served in the military, were incarcerated and/or homeless, are newly settled refugees, and/or have developmental disorders or other disabilities

Health disparities cannot be reduced by targeting individual clinical conditions and the field is now focused on the exploration of structural factors, such as the role that structural racism plays in segregating society and limiting opportunities for health and well-being. An example of structural racism is redlining or discriminatory policies and practices that denied home loans to racial/ethnic minorities. As a result, geography of zip code can be more influential on your health than your genetic predisposition. **Fig. 4** illustrates a 20+ year difference in life expectancy between 2 neighborhoods in greater Cleveland, Ohio that is less than 2 miles apart.[14] In addition to disparity in life expectancy, individuals and families in these neighborhoods are experience differences in poverty, high school graduation rates, exposure to pollution or community violence, and prevalence of chronic disease.[14]

Structural factors are critical to achieve health equity and ensure that everyone has a fair and just opportunity to be healthy. The functional medicine model can help bring awareness to both patient and clinician of the structural and individual social determinants that impact the holistic health of an individual and can help guide steps for health improvement.

DISCUSSION

The appreciation of health disparities and social determinants that may be underlying chronic conditions is essential to the functional medicine approach when providing personalized care and developing patient-centered sustainable health plans. For example, nutrition-focused therapeutic interventions to combat lifestyle-focused

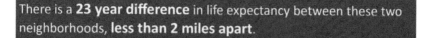

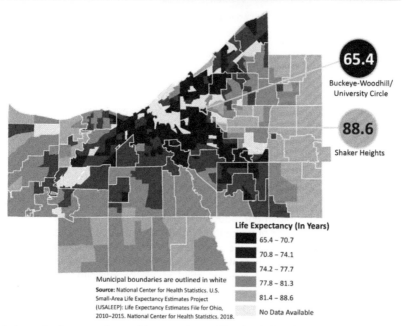

Fig. 4. Impact of geography on life expectancy, Cleveland, OH. (*From* Warren K, Ahern J. Correlations Exist Between Life Expectancy, Poverty and Race. In. *Correlations Exist Between Life Expectancy, Poverty, and Race.* Vol 2022. Cleveland, OH: The Center for Community Solutions; 2019.)

chronic disease may be impeded by patients who live in food-insecure households or in a food desert with limited access to affordable, nutritious foods.

Social Determinants of Health and the Functional Medicine Matrix

The functional medicine matrix provides us with an opportunity to understand how social determinants and individual health-related social needs may be root causes and contributors to current health and illness among patients (**Fig. 5**).[15] The matrix also allows us to map and recognize the intersectionality of SDOH on exposures and behaviors that influence antecedents, triggers, mediators (ATM), lifestyle factors, and clinical imbalances. Incorporating SDOH into clinical evaluations helps uncover the complex factors that lead to health disparities and provide more optimal patient-centered care.

Antecedents, Triggers, Mediators

- *Antecedents* are factors that predispose to illness. Population-level examples include slavery, forced migration, and other historical, intergenerational, and cultural trauma. Among individuals, SDOH antecedents are adverse childhood experiences, lack of access to medical care during childhood, and family migration experiences. An example of an antecedent impacting African Americans is redlining, or discriminatory policies and practices that denied home loans to Black Americans. This factor was so influential that if there were no redlining

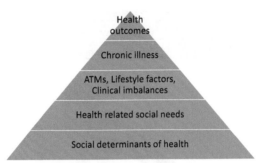

Fig. 5. Model of SDOH risks and outcomes. (Osinubi O, Satcher S, McCarron K, Robertson MW, Santos SL. Social Determinants of Health: COVID-19 Vulnerability and the Functional Medicine Model. https://www.ifm.org/news-insights/free-lecture-on-social-determinants-of-health-and-vulnerability/. Published 2021. Accessed January 15, 2022.)

practices that lead to residential racial segregation of Black Americans living in less desirable neighborhoods, then there would not be a black–white difference seen today in unemployment, education, and wealth.[16]

- *Triggers* are factors that provoke the symptoms and signs of illness. Events that cause trauma and inflict injury can include forced family separation, barriers to citizenship and voting, segregation, and incarceration. One can screen individuals for sexual or combat trauma, child abuse or intimate partner violence, identity-based trauma, discrimination and oppression experiences, and implicit bias in the health care setting. Implicit bias is defined as thoughts and feelings that exist outside of conscious awareness and subsequently can affect human understanding, actions, and decisions unknowingly.[17] Studies have found that implicit bias, while unintentional and often unrecognized, can affect how providers communicate with patients with people of color more likely to report lower satisfaction with health care provider interactions. Subtle biases may be expressed as approaching patients with a condescending tone, higher verbal dominance in communication, less interpersonal treatment which can lead patients to have a greater difficulty understanding or following recommendations; this in turn can then perpetuate biases held by the provider. Racial disparities in women's experience of trauma during birth in the United States are highly associated with provider interactions in which Black and Hispanic women are more likely to report provider mistreatment than White women. The perceived dismissals of women felt of legitimate concerns and symptoms, such as preeclampsia and hypertension, can help explain poor birth outcomes for Black women despite their level of income or education.[18]
- *Mediators* are factors, biochemical or psychosocial, that contribute to pathologic changes and dysfunctional responses. SDOH mediators or perpetrators that keep illness going include systemic racism and other forms of discrimination, income and education inequity, and lack of access to quality health care. Housing and transportation instability, stigma around mental health and substance use disorder, and geographic barriers to health are other examples. Repeated exposure to socioeconomic adversity, political marginalization, racism, and perpetual discrimination can harm health. Dr Geonimus who coined the term "weathering" hypothesized Black adults experience early health deterioration as a consequence of the cumulative impact of repeated experience with adversity and marginalization regardless of socioeconomic status or poverty. Linking allostatic

load biomarkers of stress (ie, cortisol levels, sympathetic nerve activity, cytokine production, waist-to-hip ratio, and glycated hemoglobin levels) to social measures (ie, socioeconomic status, occupation, birth outcome, and environmental risk), her team found allostatic load and biological age was much higher among Black populations in the United States compared with White adults, which likely contribute to poorer health outcomes.[19]

Lifestyle Factors

Lifestyle factors, such as sleep, exercise, nutrition, stress, and relationships are foundational to functional medicine and prevention and treatment of lifestyle-sensitive chronic disease. Social determinants often explain the variation in lifestyle behaviors that then leads to health disparities in disease.

Sleep and relaxation

Scientific research has found racial and economic disparities in sleep deficiency and people of color are more likely to have undiagnosed sleep disorders.[20] Occupational factors, such as shift work, long work hours, and multiple jobs contribute to this disparity.

Exercise and movement

Neighborhood factors such as safe, accessible sidewalks for physical activity and exposure to green space may be influenced by neighborhood disadvantage. A cross-sectional study of more than 44,000 adults reported that low neighborhood walkability predicted a 19% to 33% higher 10-year risk of cardiovascular events after adjustment for relevant covariates.[21] Neighborhood disadvantage has also been inversely related to duration and frequency of physical activity among African American adults.[22] Exercise and movement are also influenced by access to recreational spaces for people with all physical abilities, weight-based harassment and shaming, and limited time for exercise due to long work hours.

Nutrition

Patient's nutritional knowledge and dietary pattern may be influenced by living in a food desert, malnutrition, access to culturally appropriate nutritious foods, access to clean drinking water, and affordability of high-quality nutritional supplements. Supermarket presence, which is less prevalent in Black and Hispanic neighborhoods, may increase fruit and vegetable consumption. In a multi-site study of middle-aged and older adults, individuals who had proximity to supermarkets had a 17% lower prevalence of obesity, whereas the presence of convenience stores was linked to a 16% increased prevalence of obesity.[23] Early life nutritional disparities may be more prevalent among racial/ethnic patients as minority women continue to have lower breastfeeding rates than white women.[24] Low socioeconomic status and/or Black households are more likely to experience food insecurity, which is associated with increased inflammation.[23]

Stress

Stress for underserved and marginalized populations are experienced in discrimination, policing practices, acculturative stress, income disparities and inequity, lack of representation in the major sector of society, and being uninsured or underinsured. Coping with stress can be unhealthy behaviors to cope, such as excessive alcohol intake, smoking, substance use disorders, and binge eating. Childhood exposure to low socioeconomic status is associated with increased levels of adulthood inflammation.[25,26]

Relationships

Social connections are an important consideration for health, either in terms of social support or as a source of conflict or stress. Perceived discrimination or harassment based on socio-demographics (eg, sex identity, immigration status, national origin, race/ethnicity, religion, age, and disability) is a major influencer on relationships. Patient's socioeconomic status may influence support (or lack of) for eldercare and childcare. Loneliness or social isolation, which may be more prevalent in older adults, has been linked to increased immune compromise and mortality.[27]

Clinical Imbalances

SDOH factors impact the core clinical imbalances in the physical and function nodes of the matrix that lead to health inequities.

Assimilation

Assimilation refers to the digestion and absorption of nutrients in the gut, as well as the health, diversity, and balance of the microbes that inhabit the digestive tract. The gut microbiome, or the community of microbes that inhabit the human gastrointestinal tract, influences a person's nutrition, metabolism, and immune function. Alterations to the gut microbiome, possibly due to diet quality and/or environmental exposures, may lead to the dysregulation of immune, metabolic, and neuroendocrine processes involved in obesity, diabetes, atherosclerosis, asthma, allergies, depression, and anxiety.[28–30] Studies have shown that neighborhood factors are associated with the diversity of colonic microbiota with lower neighborhood socioeconomic status (eg, median household income, educational and employment characteristics, and median owner-occupied home value) associated with less diverse colonic microbiota in adults.[31,32]

Defense and repair

This node refers to chronic inflammation, how different parts of the body influence the immune system and the factors that lead to a breakdown in the normal role of the immune system. Race, education, income, and self-reported lifetime discrimination experiences are linked with inflammatory markers in midlife.[33] Personal experiences of racism and discrimination create chronic stress and are linked with inflammatory markers that result in negative health outcomes.[34]

Energy

Energy refers to the way that every cell in the body creates the fuel that it needs to carry out normal biological functions. Mitochondria are subcellular organelles that sustain life through energy transformation and intracellular signaling. Adverse childhood experiences and chronic stress have been linked to psychopathology in adulthood including major depression, depressive disorders, anxiety disorders, and substance use disorders through mitochondrial energy production capacity and mitochondrial morphology.[35] Behavioral, genetic, and dietary factors may also influence mitochondrial vulnerability to stress.[35]

Biotransformation and elimination

This node refers to the way for which the body handles products of metabolism, toxic elements, drugs, and other chemicals, and eliminates waste through the urine, stool, and sweat. Housing conditions, such as exposure to mold and lead, can lead to respiratory and neurodevelopmental abnormalities.[36] Exposure to air pollution or poor air quality, which is more prevalent in low socioeconomic neighborhoods due to their proximity to transportation- and industrial-based air pollution, is associated with respiratory conditions, cardiovascular disease risk, and early death.[37,38]

Transport
Transport involves the transport of nutrition, hormones, and enzymatic factors through blood vessels and lymphatics. Adverse childhood experiences impact several biological processes (eg, inflammatory, mitochondrial, immune) and are linked to many different diseases during adulthood, including adult heart disease, cancer, chronic lung or liver disease, diabetes, stroke, and mental illness.[39]

Communication
This node refers to hormones, neurotransmitters, and inflammatory mediators called cytokines. Perceived chronic discrimination is associated with heightened systemic inflammation, flattened diurnal cortisol slope, and higher blood pressure mediated through health behaviors and psychosocial factors.[40] One study found that among Black and Latina women, perceived stigma was associated with reduced immune function measured by higher cytokine IL-6, while in-group pride was associated improved endocrine function, measured by elevated DHEA (hormone dehydroepiandrosterone).[41]

Structural integrity
This node refers to the maintenance, repair, and replication of tissue and structure, often considered cellular integrity. Pain significantly impacts one's health and quality of life. Studies have consistently documented racial and ethnic disparities in the quality of care and under-treatment for acute and chronic pain.[42]

The mental, emotional, spiritual domain
This domain of the functional medicine matrix recognizes the mental-emotional-spiritual intersectionality to physical health. Clinical imbalances due to stress, internalized oppression, or moral injury may be mitigated through coping mechanisms, such as spiritual and religious practices and positive social relationships that may be rooted in race, culture, and shared trauma.

Summary - Social Determinants of Health Approaches in Functional Medicine

Understanding economic, social, and cultural barriers that may impede optimal health through a functional medicine model allows us to consider these factors in codeveloping treatment plans for illness. Approaches that enhance patient trust and access to care, including shared medical appointments (SMAs) and team-based care may support the health journey for patients who may be more vulnerable or live in underserved communities.

Patient-Centered Trust

A trusting and continuous relationship with a health care provider is associated with the utilization of preventive health services.[43] Trust can be eroded when clinicians do not recognize and accommodate a patient's health literacy, mistrust in the health care system due to past experiences (ie, Tuskegee syphilis experiment), cultural sensitivity, family history, and social determinants. Strengthening the patient–provider relationship may benefit from adhering to the key tenets of the functional medicine approach in clinical interactions, as well as systematic interventions. These include[44]

- Treat patients as the experts and being mindful of a patient's cultural background, primary language, traditional practices, and diet by screening for these factors[45]
- Use empathy, not arguments, for patient-oriented goals

- Attend to affordability and access barriers, including transparency about health care costs and flexible appointments in consideration of work schedules (eg, lack of paid time off)
- Adapt food plans to cultural awareness and sensitivity
- Create safe, welcoming environments by including patients in clinic or care design
- Commit to workplace diversity, especially physician diversity to match patient race and ethnicity, which has been shown to have higher scores on patient experience of their health care[46]
- Build relationships outside examination rooms and clinical settings

Shared Medical Appointments and Community Engagement

Clinical interventions can occur in community settings and can help build relationships outside the clinical walls. An example is SMAs, which offer an efficient and cost-effective approach to patient education and patient empowerment in the treatment of chronic diseases.[47] SMAs can improve clinical outcomes and patient satisfaction, as well as reduce costs among patients with obesity and diabetes.[48,49] The effectiveness of SMAs can be attributed to several factors[45,50,51]:

- Social connection and safety among peers with potentially similar lived experiences
- Time for education and time with providers (ie, health coach, physician, dietician)
- Collaborative patient–provider relationship whereby the provider functions as the leader and as a peer
- Participants' model each other after sharing thoughts and feelings

SMAs have been impactful for patients living in underserved communities and/or with working-class adults. Partnership with community organizations (eg, faith-based or social service organizations) or community members can allow SMAs to include multiple languages, the right level of health literacy for education and support, culturally appropriate food plans and affordable supplements, time for mindfulness and check-ins, and greater understanding of social determinants on lifestyle factors and clinical imbalances.

The Cleveland Clinic Center for Functional Medicine conducts 10-week community-based SMAs that consist of weekly, in-person group sessions with 4 sessions led by a clinical practitioner (PA-C) and health coach, and 6 sessions led by a registered dietitian. In the community-based SMA, providers deliver education and care in a shared environment plus a brief, individual medical assessment. Health coaches provide education related to exercise and movement, sleep, stress reduction, and tools to support lasting behavioral change. Dietitians focus on the use of food as medicine, and support participants in the implementation of a food plan that encourages the consumption of whole, unprocessed foods. The SMAs have taken place in a community-based health education center in a low-income neighborhood. In one SMA primarily focused on African American older adults from the neighborhood, we found improvements in blood pressure, weight, health status, daily fruit and vegetable intake, and sleep.[52] To address barriers to optimal health for underserved populations, this SMA included a cooking demonstration session, as well as in-kind laboratory testing, dietary supplementation, and weekly food delivery to households. In another SMA focused on working-class adults in the police department, we found a reduction in weight and improvements in blood pressure, stress, and nutritional health literacy among police officers who attended sessions.

Recognizing and addressing SDOH factors and committing to health equity can allow for a transformational relationship for vulnerable patients in health promotion.

CLINICS CARE POINTS

- Understanding economic, social, and cultural barriers that may impede optimal health through a functional medicine model allows us to consider these factors in co-developing treatment plans for illness.
- Approaches that enhance patient trust and access to care, including shared medical appointments and team-based care, may support the health journey for patients who may be more vulnerable or live in underserved communities.

DISCLOSURE

The author has nothing to disclose.

REFERENCES

1. Murphy S, Kochanek K, Xu J, et al. Mortality in the United States, 2020. In: Statistics NCfHNCHS data brief, 427. Hyattsville, MD: Center for Disease Control and Preevention; 2021.
2. National Center for Chronic Disease Prevention and Health Promotion. About chronic disease 2021. Available at. https://www.cdc.gov/chronicdisease/about/index.htm. Accessed January, 2022.
3. Kindig D, Stoddart G. What is population health? Am J Public Health 2003;93(3): 380–3.
4. Hood CM, Gennuso KP, Swain GR, et al. County health rankings: relationships between determinant factors and health outcomes. Am J Prev Med 2016;50(2): 129–35.
5. Marmot M, Friel S, Bell R, et al. Closing the gap in a generation: health equity through action on the social determinants of health. Lancet 2008;372(9650): 1661–9.
6. Office of Disease Prevention and Health Promotion. Healthy People 2030: Social Determinants of Health. U.S Department Health Human Services. Available at: https://health.gov/healthypeople/objectives-and-data/social-determinants-health. Accessed January 15, 2022.
7. Castrucci BC, Auerbach J. Meeting individual social needs falls short of addressing social determinants of health. Health Affairs 2019;2022.
8. Jilani MH, Javed Z, Yahya T, et al. Social determinants of health and cardiovascular disease: current state and future directions towards healthcare equity. Curr Atheroscler Rep 2021;23(9):55.
9. Grant T, Croce E, Matsui EC. Asthma and the social determinants of health. Ann Allergy Asthma Immunol 2022;128(1):5–11.
10. Quiñones J, Hammad Z. Social determinants of health and chronic kidney disease. Cureus 2020;12(9):e10266.
11. Rosendale N. Social determinants of health in neurology. Neurol Clin 2022;40(1): 231–47.
12. Walker RJ, Strom Williams J, Egede LE. Influence of race, ethnicity and social determinants of health on diabetes outcomes. Am J Med Sci 2016;351(4):366–73.

13. Lavizzo-Mourey RJ, Besser RE, Williams DR. Understanding and mitigating health inequities - past, current, and future directions. N Engl J Med 2021; 384(18):1681–4.

14. Warren K, Ahern J. Correlations exist between life expectancy, poverty and race. In: Correlations exist between life expectancy, poverty and race2022. Cleveland, OH: The Center for Community Solutions; 2019.

15. Omsinubi O, Satcher S, McCarron K, et al. Social determinants of health: COVID-19 vulnerability and the functional medicine model. 2021. Available at: https://www.ifm.org/news-insights/free-lecture-on-social-determinants-of-health-and-vulnerability/. Accessed January 15, 2022.

16. Williams DR, Collins C. Racial residential segregation: a fundamental cause of racial disparities in health. Public Health Rep 2001;116(5):404–16.

17. Hall WJ, Chapman MV, Lee KM, et al. Implicit racial/ethnic bias among health care professionals and its influence on health care outcomes: a systematic review. Am J Public Health 2015;105(12):e60–76.

18. Saluja B, Bryant Z. How implicit bias contributes to racial disparities in maternal morbidity and mortality in the United States. J Womens Health (Larchmt) 2021; 30(2):270–3.

19. Geronimus AT, Hicken M, Keene D, et al. "Weathering" and age patterns of allostatic load scores among blacks and whites in the United States. Am J Public Health 2006;96(5):826–33.

20. Egan KJ, Knutson KL, Pereira AC, et al. The role of race and ethnicity in sleep, circadian rhythms and cardiovascular health. Sleep Med Rev 2017;33:70–8.

21. Howell NA, Tu JV, Moineddin R, et al. Association between neighborhood walkability and predicted 10-year cardiovascular disease risk: The CANHEART (cardiovascular health in ambulatory care research team) cohort. J Am Heart Assoc 2019;8(21):e013146.

22. Barber S, Hickson DA, Wang X, et al. Neighborhood disadvantage, poor social conditions, and cardiovascular disease incidence among african american adults in the jackson heart study. Am J Public Health 2016;106(12):2219–26.

23. Morland K, Diez Roux AV, Wing S. Supermarkets, other food stores, and obesity: the atherosclerosis risk in communities study. Am J Prev Med 2006;30(4):333–9.

24. Jones KM, Power ML, Queenan JT, et al. Racial and ethnic disparities in breastfeeding. Breastfeed Med 2015;10(4):186–96.

25. Milaniak I, Jaffee SR. Childhood socioeconomic status and inflammation: a systematic review and meta-analysis. Brain Behav Immun 2019;78:161–76.

26. Liu RS, Aiello AE, Mensah FK, et al. Socioeconomic status in childhood and C reactive protein in adulthood: a systematic review and meta-analysis. J Epidemiol Community Health 2017;71(8):817–26.

27. Holt-Lunstad J, Steptoe A. Social isolation: An underappreciated determinant of physical health. Curr Opin Psychol 2021;43:232–7.

28. Chunxi L, Haiyue L, Yanxia L, et al. The gut microbiota and respiratory diseases: new evidence. J Immunol Res 2020;2020:2340670.

29. Foster JA, McVey Neufeld KA. Gut-brain axis: how the microbiome influences anxiety and depression. Trends Neurosci 2013;36(5):305–12.

30. Larsen N, Vogensen FK, van den Berg FW, et al. Gut microbiota in human adults with type 2 diabetes differs from non-diabetic adults. PLoS One 2010;5(2):e9085.

31. Amato KR, Arrieta MC, Azad MB, et al. The human gut microbiome and health inequities. Proc Natl Acad Sci U S A 2021;118(25).

32. Miller GE, Engen PA, Gillevet PM, et al. Lower neighborhood socioeconomic status associated with reduced diversity of the colonic microbiota in healthy adults. PLoS One 2016;11(2):e0148952.
33. Kershaw KN, Lewis TT, Diez Roux AV, et al. Self-reported experiences of discrimination and inflammation among men and women: The multi-ethnic study of atherosclerosis. Health Psychol 2016;35(4):343–50.
34. Harrell CJ, Burford TI, Cage BN, et al. Multiple pathways linking racism to health outcomes. Du Bois Rev 2011;8(1):143–57.
35. Picard M, McEwen BS. Psychological stress and mitochondria: a systematic review. Psychosom Med 2018;80(2):141–53.
36. Krieger J, Higgins DL. Housing and health: time again for public health action. Am J Public Health 2002;92(5):758–68.
37. Jilani MH, Simon-Friedt B, Yahya T, et al. Associations between particulate matter air pollution, presence and progression of subclinical coronary and carotid atherosclerosis: a systematic review. Atherosclerosis 2020;306:22–32.
38. Hajat A, Hsia C, O'Neill MS. Socioeconomic disparities and air pollution exposure: a global review. Curr Environ Health Rep 2015;2(4):440–50.
39. Soares S, Rocha V, Kelly-Irving M, et al. Adverse childhood events and health biomarkers: a systematic review. Front Public Health 2021;9.
40. Lockwood KG, Marsland AL, Matthews KA, et al. Perceived discrimination and cardiovascular health disparities: a multisystem review and health neuroscience perspective. Ann N Y Acad Sci 2018;1428(1):170–207.
41. Ratner KG, Halim ML, Amodio DM. Perceived stigmatization, ingroup pride, and immune and endocrine activity: evidence from a community sample of black and latina women. Social Psychol Personal Sci 2012;4(1):82–91.
42. Green CR, Anderson KO, Baker TA, et al. The unequal burden of pain: confronting racial and ethnic disparities in pain. Pain Med 2003;4(3):277–94.
43. Musa D, Schulz R, Harris R, et al. Trust in the health care system and the use of preventive health services by older black and white adults. Am J Public Health 2009;99(7):1293–9.
44. Hostetter M, Klein S. Understanding and ameliorating medical mistrust among black Americans. Commonwealth Fund. Transforming Care Web site. 2021. Available at: https://www.commonwealthfund.org/publications/newsletter-article/2021/jan/medical-mistrust-among-black-americans. Accessed January 15, 2022.
45. Supporting health in underserved populations. Institute for Functional Medicine. Available at. https://www.ifm.org/news-insights/supporting-health-underserved-populations/. Accessed January 15, 2022.
46. Takeshita J, Wang S, Loren AW, et al. Association of racial/ethnic and gender concordance between patients and physicians with patient experience ratings. JAMA Netw Open 2020;3(11):e2024583.
47. Egger G, Stevens J, Ganora C, et al. Programmed shared medical appointments: a novel procedure for chronic disease management. Aust J Gen Pract 2018; 47(1–2):70–5.
48. Trickett KH, Matiaco PM, Jones K, et al. Effectiveness of shared medical appointments targeting the triple aim among patients with overweight, obesity, or diabetes. J Am Osteopath Assoc 2016;116(12):780–7.
49. Beidelschies M, Alejandro-Rodriguez M, Guo N, et al. Patient outcomes and costs associated with functional medicine-based care in a shared versus individual setting for patients with chronic conditions: a retrospective cohort study. BMJ Open 2021;11(4):e048294.

50. Tsiamparlis-Wildeboer AHC, Feijen-De Jong EI, Scheele F. Factors influencing patient education in shared medical appointments: Integrative literature review. Patient Educ Couns 2020;103(9):1667–76.
51. Thompson-Lastad A. Group medical visits as participatory care in community health centers. Qual Health Res 2018;28(7):1065–76.
52. Bharmal N, Beidelschies M, Alejandro-Rodriguez M, et al. Feasibility of a nutrition and lifestyle focused shared medical appointment program in a resource-challenged community setting. BMC Public Health 2022;22(1):447.

Patient-Reported Outcomes and the Patient-Reported Outcome Measurement Information System of Functional Medicine Care and Research

Michelle Beidelschies, PhD[a,*], David Cella, PhD[b],
Irene Katzan, MD, MS[c], Christopher R. D'Adamo, PhD[d,e,f]

KEYWORDS

- Patient-centered care • Functional medicine • Patient-reported outcomes
- Global health

KEY POINTS

- Patient-reported outcomes (PROs) are integral to demonstrating value within the functional medicine model of care.
- Collection of PROs in clinical practice within the functional medicine model of care is feasible and provides useful data for clinicians, patients, and researchers.
- PROMIS Global is a general PROM well-suited for functional medicine care due to its brevity, public availability at no cost, relative ease of implementation, extensive research validation, and usefulness at the point of clinical care.

INTRODUCTION

"Health is a state of complete physical, mental and social well-being and not merely the absence of disease or infirmity."[1]

The World Health Organization defines health as "...a state of complete physical, mental and social well-being and not merely the absence of disease or infirmity."[1]

[a] Center for Functional Medicine, Cleveland Clinic Lerner College of Medicine, Cleveland Clinic, 9500 Carnegie Avenue, Q2-1 Glickman Tower, Cleveland, OH 44195, USA; [b] Department of Medical Social Sciences, Northwestern University Feinberg School of Medicine, 625 North Michigan Avenue, Chicago, IL 60611, USA; [c] Patient-Entered Data, Center for Outcomes Research & Evaluation, Neurological Institute, Cleveland Clinic, 9500 Carnegie Avenue, S8-859, Cleveland, OH 44195, USA; [d] Institute for Functional Medicine, 505 South 336th Street #600, Federal Way, WA 98003, USA; [e] Department of Family and Community Medicine, Center for Integrative Medicine, University of Maryland School of Medicine, 520 West Lombard Street, East Hall, Baltimore, MD 21201, USA; [f] Department of Epidemiology and Public Health, University of Maryland School of Medicine, 520 West Lombard Street, East Hall, Baltimore, MD 21201, USA
* Corresponding author.
E-mail address: beidelm2@ccf.org

Phys Med Rehabil Clin N Am 33 (2022) 679–697
https://doi.org/10.1016/j.pmr.2022.04.008

This definition embraces the biopsychosocial model of health care first introduced by Engel in 1977, which is critically centered on the delivery of patient-centered care and incorporates the social, psychological, and behavioral aspects of illness as well as its temporal nature.[2,3] It takes into consideration both the patient *and* the illness.[2] The biopsychosocial model was not intended to replace the conventional biomedical model of health care which uses a reductionist approach, attributing illness to a singular cause and considering other somatic disturbances as unrelated.[2,3] Instead, it aimed to *extend* the conventional biomedical model by providing a "more complete" account of health care and illness that goes beyond biological factors alone.[3]

Over a decade later, the functional medicine model of care was established to address the transition from a singular cause of disease to the management of more complex syndromes.[4] Seven defining characteristics of the model were established including being patient-centered versus disease-centered, using a systems biology approach, focusing on the dynamic balance of gene–environment interactions, personalizing care based on biochemical individuality, promoting organ reserve and sustained health, defining health as a positive vitality (not merely the absence of disease), and being function versus pathology focused.[4]

While this model aligns with the biopsychosocial model, it also contributes a framework, or "operating system," for the organization of clinical and patient-reported information to develop a personalized care strategy. Briefly, an extensive medical history identifies antecedents (genetic or acquired factors that predispose to illness), triggers (factors that provoke the symptoms of illness), and mediators (factors (biochemical or psychosocial) that contribute to pathologic changes and dysfunction) contributing to a patient's reported health status.[5,6] This information is then mapped across a timeline and within a matrix characterized by various somatic systems (eg, assimilation, biotransformation and elimination, defense and repair, and so forth) which takes into consideration mental, spiritual and emotional factors reported by the patient.[6]

At its inception, the awareness, accessibility, and application of the functional medicine model across and within health care organizations have not manifested as rapidly as its founders would have anticipated, but it is gaining traction. It, too, was intended to *extend*, not replace, the current health care model. However, an expansion of the evidence base evaluating functional medicine management strategies is warranted. Such evidence should include biological as well as patient-reported factors that may be keeping patients from achieving health and financially burdening the health care system. Together, this evidence is critical for establishing the value of functional medicine and its incorporation within the larger health care framework.

Therefore, this article provides practical insights for capturing patient-reported outcomes (PROs) in functional medicine clinical care and research. It will first introduce PROs and patient-reported outcome measures (PROMs) and briefly discuss their value within patient-centered care. The remainder of the article will discuss the utility of a specific PROM, Patient-Reported Outcome Measurement Information System (PROMIS) – Global Health ("PROMIS Global"), within functional medicine care, provide strategies for its implementation with clinical care and research, and discuss potential facilitators and barriers to its implementation.

PATIENT-REPORTED OUTCOMES

Patient-reported outcomes are defined as "any report of the status of a patient's (or person's) health condition, health behavior, or experience with health care that comes directly from the patient, without the interpretation of the patient's response by a clinician or anyone else."[7,8] First introduced in the 1970s, PROs were developed to capture self-representations of subjective well-being as part of the National Health and Nutrition Examination Surveys (NHANES).[9] Early studies examined how certain patient-reported socio-demographic, physical and mental factors explain variations in general well-being.[10] By the early 1990s, a perfect storm was developing in health care delivery. Patients were placing more attention on the value of health care services provided, and the idea of delivering patient-centered care (or enhancing the communication between patients and their providers) was emerging.[11,12] PROs were able to expand the original patient-centered care idealistic by incorporating the patient's experience of their own physical or mental well-being. Presently, PROs are a priority for achieving value-based care initiatives focused on providing high-quality patient care at a lower cost to improve population health.[13]

The National Quality Forum explains that "patients remain an untapped resource in assessing the quality of health care and of long-term support services."[8] The delivery of high-quality clinical care for a particular chronic condition is multi-dimensional, focusing not only on the attainment of an intended clinical outcome but also on the patient's reported experience of their condition as well as their experience of the intervention needed to achieve the intended clinical outcome. When combined with objective measures, patients' subjective experience of their condition provides further insight into the effectiveness of clinical intervention.

There are 5 domains reflected through PROs: Health-related quality of life, functional status (eg, daily activities), symptoms and symptom burden (eg, pain, bloating, and fatigue), health-related behaviors (eg, nutrition, smoking status, and exercise/movement) and experience with care (eg, Consumer Assessment of Healthcare Providers and Systems (CAHPS) surveys) (**Table 1**).[14] This article will focus on measuring the health-related quality of life domain as it reflects the physical, social, and emotional well-being associated with illness and its treatment,[15] all of which are particularly relevant to functional medicine as they can contribute to the inception and progression of chronic disease. Certainly, other domains are also relevant to functional medicine; however, they are beyond the scope of the current article.

PATIENT-REPORTED OUTCOME MEASURES

PROs are captured by PROMs, or "tools used to assess the PRO concept as perceived by the patient, obtained by directly asking the patient to self-report."[15] PROMs are standardized instruments that can measure and monitor the health of a population or the impact a specific management strategy has on a chronic condition. Historically, PROMs were an integral part of research,[16] but their utility within daily clinical care is expanding,[17–20] and information captured by PROMs is emerging as an indicator of health care quality and performance.[13] Validated PROMs are typically

Table 1
Five domains of patient-reported outcomes

PRO Domain	Description and Examples
1. Health-related quality of life	General physical and mental health
2. Functional status	Daily activities
3. Symptoms and symptom burden	Pain, bloating and fatigue
4. Health-related behaviors	Nutrition, smoking status, and exercise/movement
5. Experience with care	Consumer Assessment of Healthcare Providers and Systems (CAHPS) surveys

used in clinical care or research to ensure standardization among questions (or items) and response options; however, nonvalidated PROMs may also be used with the intent to validate the measure.

Selecting the appropriate PROM for a particular population or condition is of utmost importance. The National Quality Forum (NQF) developed 5 guiding principles to PROM selection for the monitoring and management of patients in clinical care and/ or research and include psychometric soundness, person-centeredness, meaningfulness, amenability to change, and ability to be implemented (**Table 2**).[15,21] Psychometric soundness speaks to the PROMs ability to measure the concept (or construct) in a particular population (eg, pain, stress, anxiety), to be translated across languages, to be interpreted, and ease with which it can be implemented in clinical care. Additionally, it speaks to the PROM's reliability and validity and its burden on the patient (eg, the number of questions and frequency of completion). Patient-centeredness is reflected in the PROMs ability to support the bidirectional flow of information between the patient and provider to the extent that both benefit. Meaningfulness is related to the interest of the patient, and how both the patient and provider use the information provided by a particular PROM. Amenability to change speaks to the PROMs ability to change based on targeted interventions implemented by the provider and patient. Lastly, the PROMs ability to be implemented speaks to how readily it is incorporated into clinical care. This encompasses its ability to be understood by the patient (eg, language literacy and health literacy), completed by the patient (eg, having the tools necessary to access the PROM [eg, phone, computer, and so forth]) and implemented in clinical care (eg, cost, acceptance, and so forth). While these are recognized as guiding principles for PROM selection, it is important to acknowledge that the

---

Table 2
Five guiding principles to PROM selection for the monitoring and management of patients in clinical care and/or research[15,21]

PROM Characteristic	Description
1. Psychometric Soundness	• Measures the concept of interest in a particular population • Reliable and valid • Translated across languages • Interpretable results • Recognized burden to the patient
2. Person-Centeredness	• Supports the bidirectional flow of information between the patient and provider (both benefiting) • Encourages shared decision-making
3. Meaningfulness	• Recognized as important to the patient and provider • Relates to how the patient and provider use the information
4. Amenability to Change	• Ability of PROM score to change based on targeted interventions recommended by the provider and implemented by the patient
5. Implementability	• Ability to be incorporated into clinical care from the perspective of the patient and provider

Data from Cella D HE, Jensen SE, Butt Z, Nowinski CJ, Rothrock N, Lohr KN. Patient-reported outcomes in performance measurement. RTI Press; 2015; and National Quality Forum. Patient-reported outcomes in performance measurement. 2012; https://www.qualityforum.org/publications/2012/12/patient-reported_outcomes_in_performance_measurement.aspx. Accessed November 29, 2021.

importance of each principle may depend on various factors including the type of care being delivered and/or the utility of the PROM within a specific model of care.

There are 2 specific types of PROMs–general or condition-specific. General PROMs can be used across various populations and a broad range of chronic conditions.[16] Such measures permit the overall evaluation of care evaluate general well-being and/or quality of life.[16,22] Examples of general PROMs include Patient-Reported Outcome Measurement Information System-Global 10 (PROMIS Global),[23] PROMIS-29,[24] 36-Item Short Form Survey (SF-36)[25] or the EuroQol-5 Dimension (EQ-5D).[26] Condition-specific PROMs evaluate the specific symptoms of a condition that manifest in body systems (eg, joints) such as pain or discomfort and limitations to mobility or function. Examples of condition-specific PROMs include the Knee Injury and Osteoarthritis Outcome Score (KOOS),[27] Inflammatory Bowel Disease Quality of Life Questionnaire (IBDQOL),[28] Asthma Quality of Life Questionnaire (AQLQ),[29] and the Functional Assessment of Cancer Therapy (FACT) measures.[30]

PROMIS Global and Functional Medicine Care

In 2004, the PROMIS initiative was formed under the NIH Roadmap for Medical Research Initiative to revolutionize the assessment of PROs in research and clinical care.[23] Since then, the PROMIS initiative has developed and evaluated more than 2000 items that assess symptoms, functional status, and health-related quality of life.[31]

Specific items as general indicators of health status were used to create the PROMIS Global scale.[32] PROMIS Global is a psychometrically validated dynamic system that measures self-reported health across multiple domains in patients with a wide range of diseases and demographic characteristics.[23] Because PROMIS Global does not reference a specific disease in its items, it permits comparisons across conditions.[33–35] Additionally, measurement of PROMIS Global provides a better understanding of a patient's well-being which can be tracked longitudinally. Lastly, it can support a therapeutic relationship between a provider and a patient by enhancing the provider's understanding of their patient's health and improving communication between them.

PROMIS Global includes 10 items that represent different domains of health including physical health, mental health, social health, pain, fatigue, and overall health-related quality of life to provide an overall measure of health status. Physical health is assessed by 4 items (Global03, Global06, Global07r, and Global08r) and mental health is assessed by 4 items (Global02, Global04, Global05, and Global10r) (**Table 3**). The items use various 5-point Likert scales and are used to produce 2 scores: Global Physical Health (GPH) and Global Mental Health (GMH). Two additional items are used to assess general health (Global01) and social activities (Global09r) as part of the survey; however, they are not used to score the survey. The raw item scores are transformed to summary T-Scores which are centered on the 2000 US Census with respect to age, sex, educational level, and race/ethnicity with a mean (SD) of 50 (10).[23] Higher scores indicate a better health-related quality of life and changes of 5 or more T-Score points suggest a meaningful or clinically important change.[36,37]

There are several reasons why PROMIS Global is a well-suited tool for establishing the evidence for the functional medicine model of care. First, it provides an accurate and reliable estimation of a patient's health status which includes their ability to function on various levels. As the name suggests, the functional medicine model of care is focused on improving a patient's *function* by mitigating the underlying contributors to the symptoms of chronic disease. In turn, patients experience improved physical, mental, and social functioning as well as the quality of life. Second, PROMIS Global

Table 3
PROMIS global v1.2 items

Variable Name	Global Health Domain	Item Context	Item Stem	Responses
Global01			In general, would you say your health is:…	5-Excellent 4-Very Good 3-Good 2-Fair 1-Poor
Global02	GMH		In general, would you say your quality of life is:…	5-Excellent 4-Very Good 3-Good 2-Fair 1-Poor
Global03	GPH		In general, how would you rate your physical health?..	5-Excellent 4-Very Good 3-Good 2-Fair 1-Poor
Global04	GMH		In general, how would you rate your mental health, including your mood and your ability to think?..	5-Excellent 4-Very Good 3-Good 2-Fair 1-Poor
Global05	GMH		In general, how would you rate your satisfaction with your social activities and relationships?..	5-Excellent 4-Very Good 3-Good 2-Fair 1-Poor
Global09r[a]			In general, please rate how well you carry out your usual social activities and roles. (This includes activities at home, at work and in your community, and responsibilities as a parent, child, spouse, employee, friend, and so forth)….	5-Excellent 4-Very Good 3-Good 2-Fair 1-Poor
Global06	GPH		To what extent are you able to carry out your everyday physical activities such as walking, climbing stairs, carrying groceries, or moving a chair?..	5-Completely 4-Mostly 3-Moderately 2-A Little 1-Not At All
Global10r[a,b]	GMH	In the past 7 d…	How often have you been bothered by emotional problems such as feeling anxious, depressed or irritable?..	5-Never 4-Rarely 3-Sometimes 2-Often 1-Always

(continued on next page)

Variable Name	Global Health Domain	Item Context	Item Stem	Responses
Global08r[a,b]	GPH	In the past 7 d...	How would you rate your fatigue on average?..	1-None 2-Mild 3-Moderate 4-Severe 5-Very Severe
Global07r[a]	GPH	In the past 7 d...	How would you rate your pain on average?..	0-No Pain 10-Worst Pain Imaginable

Table 3
(continued)

Abbreviations: GMH, global mental health; GPH, global physical health.
[a] Items in the original PROMIS Global v1.0/v1.1 were recoded to result in the current PROMIS Global v1.2.
[b] The response scores are reversed for these 2 items as they reflect negative health factors.
Adapted from Hays RD, Bjorner JB, Revicki DA, Spritzer KL, Cella D. Development of physical and mental health summary scores from the patient-reported outcomes measurement information system (PROMIS) global items. *Quality of Life Research.* 2009;18(7):873-880, with permission.

can assist in measuring treatment response[38,39] as it captures subjective domains not easily measured during clinical observation. When combined with objective outcomes commonly measured in clinical practice (eg, biometrics or biomarkers), these subjective domains become integral components in the delivery of functional medicine care as they foster the therapeutic relationship between the provider and patient. Third, PROMIS Global provides outcomes of care that are critical for achieving important value-based care initiatives including improving outcomes at a lower cost, improving health status, and reducing the incidence of chronic disease.[40] Utility scores can be estimated from the PROMIS Global summary scores through mapping the PROMIS Global items to the EQ-5D, allowing the use of PROMIS Global in cost-utility analyses.[41,42] Improving value-based care can, in turn, assist health care in achieving the Quadruple Aim: Improving population health outcomes, enhancing patient experience, reducing costs, and improving provider experience. Fourth, PROMIS Global is publicly available, without cost for use, and uses just 10 questions that take less than 5 minutes to complete. Lastly, PROMIS Global is a standardized measure that can be implemented within and across institutions which can have vast implications for clinical care and research needed for the advancement of functional medicine.

In 2019, a landmark study in *JAMA Network Open* demonstrated beneficial and sustainable associations of the functional medicine model of care with health-related quality of life as patients achieved significant greater improvements in PROMIS GPH at 6 and 12 months than patients receiving care at a family health center.[43] Additionally, 30% of functional medicine patients achieved a clinically meaningful improvement compared with 22% of family medicine patients.[43] Shortly thereafter, a study demonstrated that the functional medicine model of care significantly reduces pain and improves PROMIS GPH for patients with rheumatoid or psoriatic arthritis compared with standard rheumatological care.[44] More recently, shared medical appointments, or group visits, were shown to improve PROMIS GPH and GMH as well as important biological factors (eg, blood pressure and weight) beyond that which was achieved in individual appointment settings for those seeking functional medicine care.[45] Moreover, the SMA setting also permitted more time with the patient and was more cost-effective to deliver than individual appointments.[45]

While these 3 studies are important milestones for functional medicine, more studies are warranted to examine various aspects of the functional medicine model and evaluate strategies for the management of specific chronic conditions. Future studies should include various PRO domains including the aspects of health-related quality of life that are assessed by the individual PROMIS Global items. Therefore, it is important for those who deliver functional medicine-based care to appreciate how to incorporate PROMIS Global into clinical care as well as research.

INCORPORATING PROMIS GLOBAL INTO FUNCTIONAL MEDICINE CARE

Incorporating PROMIS Global into clinical care requires a strategy focused on education, implementation, and interpretation.

Considerations for Provider and Patient Education

One could argue that education (for both the provider and patient) is paramount to ensuring optimal data collection and accurate interpretation. Formal provider education, ideally by way of a clinical champion, should introduce PROMIS Global, discuss its value within the functional medicine model of care, explain how it is scored, and provide directions on how to access and use the scores. To support this type of education, the HealthMeasures website offers a prepared slide deck that can be delivered to a broad audience.[46] Providers can also review several landmark articles on PROMIS Global[23,32,36,37] as well as articles that have used PROMIS Global to evaluate functional medicine outcomes.[43–45]

Patient education regarding PROMIS Global can be delivered by various means and at various times throughout their care. Before their initial visit, patients can receive educational materials that introduce them to PROMIS Global, what it measures (ie, physical, mental, and social well-being), and how it relates to the functional medicine model of care. Expectations for how often they will be evaluated (ie, each visit), the length of the questionnaire (ie, 10 items), and amount of time to complete the questionnaire (ie, <5 minutes) can also be established (**Fig. 1**A). This type of education can be delivered as an educational document by way of email and/or language can be added to the practice's website. At the time of a patient's visit, the lobby or patient rooms can also offer reusable, laminated educational documents or provide this information on posters displayed in the clinic lobby. If a practice offers shared medical appointments (SMAs), this care model affords more educational time that can be used to deliver education on PROMIS Global to patients. Dedicated time within the SMA can also be used to complete the questionnaire (if in-person), or to remind patients to complete the online questionnaire (if virtual) (**Fig. 1**B).

Considerations for Implementation in Clinical Care

PROMIS Global can be implemented into clinical care in various ways and languages summarized herein. The HealthMeasures website provides comprehensive implementation guides.[47]

Formats and scoring

PROMIS Global is available in multiple formats including paper, computer, or an app. The paper form requires oversight by administrative or clinical staff to administer, ensure completion and answer any questions from the patient in real-time. The results from the paper form need to be transformed into T-Scores by hand using conversion tables available on the HealthMeasures website.[48] Results would then need to be scanned and securely saved, or transcribed into the electronic health record (EHR) used by the practice. Also, the paper form can only be used for in-person visits.

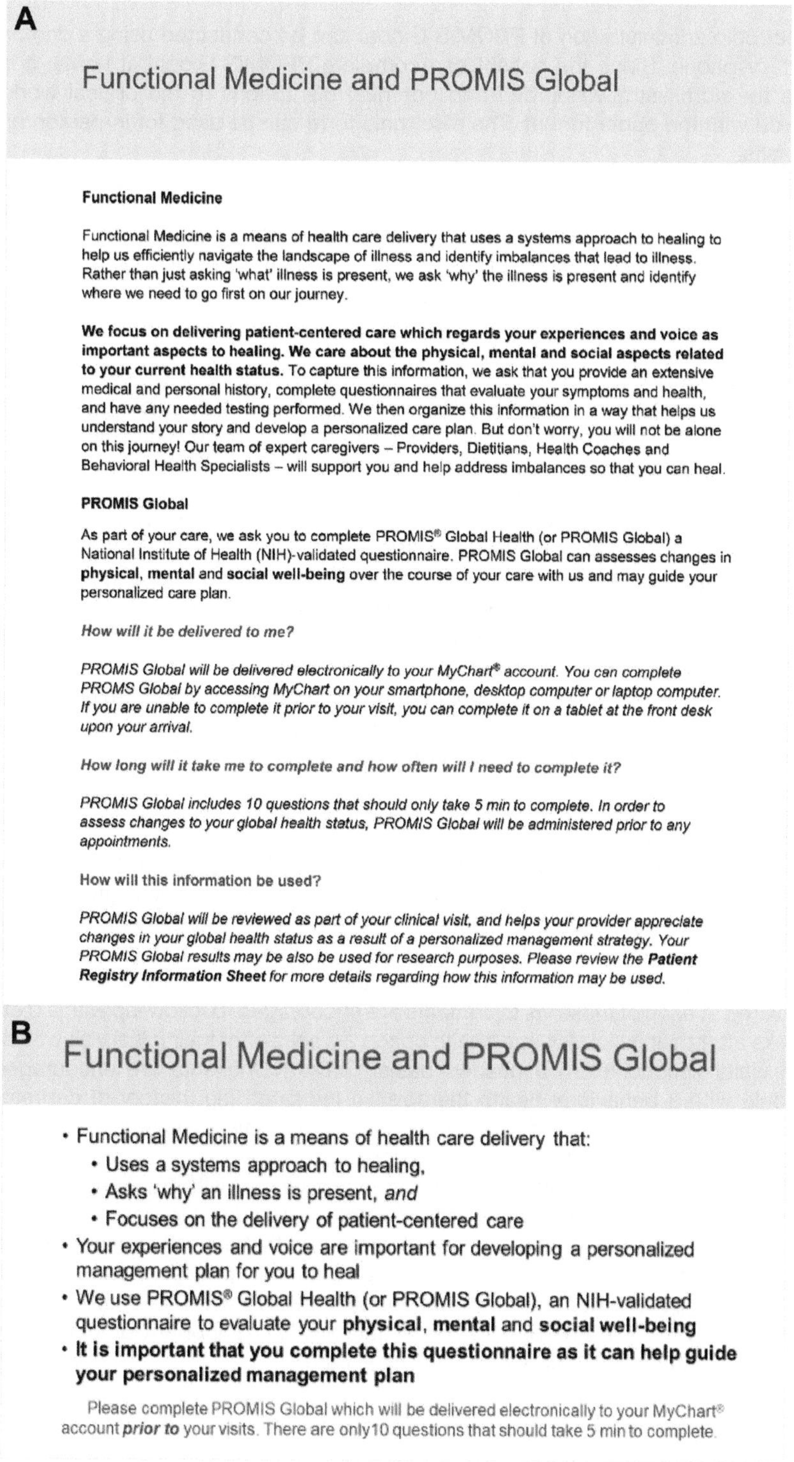

A

Functional Medicine and PROMIS Global

Functional Medicine

Functional Medicine is a means of health care delivery that uses a systems approach to healing to help us efficiently navigate the landscape of illness and identify imbalances that lead to illness. Rather than just asking 'what' illness is present, we ask 'why' the illness is present and identify where we need to go first on our journey.

We focus on delivering patient-centered care which regards your experiences and voice as important aspects to healing. We care about the physical, mental and social aspects related to your current health status. To capture this information, we ask that you provide an extensive medical and personal history, complete questionnaires that evaluate your symptoms and health, and have any needed testing performed. We then organize this information in a way that helps us understand your story and develop a personalized care plan. But don't worry, you will not be alone on this journey! Our team of expert caregivers – Providers, Dietitians, Health Coaches and Behavioral Health Specialists – will support you and help address imbalances so that you can heal.

PROMIS Global

As part of your care, we ask you to complete PROMIS® Global Health (or PROMIS Global) a National Institute of Health (NIH)-validated questionnaire. PROMIS Global can assesses changes in **physical, mental** and **social well-being** over the course of your care with us and may guide your personalized care plan.

How will it be delivered to me?

PROMIS Global will be delivered electronically to your MyChart® account. You can complete PROMS Global by accessing MyChart on your smartphone, desktop computer or laptop computer. If you are unable to complete it prior to your visit, you can complete it on a tablet at the front desk upon your arrival.

How long will it take me to complete and how often will I need to complete it?

PROMIS Global includes 10 questions that should only take 5 min to complete. In order to assess changes to your global health status, PROMIS Global will be administered prior to any appointments.

How will this information be used?

*PROMIS Global will be reviewed as part of your clinical visit, and helps your provider appreciate changes in your global health status as a result of a personalized management strategy. Your PROMIS Global results may be also be used for research purposes. Please review the **Patient Registry Information Sheet** for more details regarding how this information may be used.*

B

Functional Medicine and PROMIS Global

- Functional Medicine is a means of health care delivery that:
  - Uses a systems approach to healing,
  - Asks 'why' an illness is present, *and*
  - Focuses on the delivery of patient-centered care
- Your experiences and voice are important for developing a personalized management plan for you to heal
- We use PROMIS® Global Health (or PROMIS Global), an NIH-validated questionnaire to evaluate your **physical, mental** and **social well-being**
- **It is important that you complete this questionnaire as it can help guide your personalized management plan**

Please complete PROMIS Global which will be delivered electronically to your MyChart® account *prior to* your visits. There are only 10 questions that should take 5 min to complete.

Fig. 1. PROMIS Global patient education as (*A*) a handout and (*B*) a PowerPoint slide. MyChart® is a registered trademark of Epic Systems Corporation.

Electronic administration of PROMIS Global can be conducted using a computer, tablet, or phone. Since the patient can complete PROMIS Global at home, it minimizes the administrative burden and potential disruptions to the clinical workflow involved with the paper format. The electronic form can be used for in-person or virtual visits.

PROMIS Global is also available through the PROMIS iPad App or NIH Toolbox iPad App; however, the latter option requires extensive test administration training.[49] Once the data are collected by the app, it can be exported to transfer individual scores into the patient's electronic health record (EHR). PROMIS Global is available in both English and Spanish translations for all 3 types of the aforementioned means of administration.

Technical support

Several EHR systems have functionality allowing patients to complete questionnaires electronically.[50] In the Epic EHR (Epic Systems; Verona, Wisconsin) patient questionnaires are included in the electronic check-in process that patients can access through Epic's patient portal. In addition, invitations to complete questionnaires along with electronic links to the questionnaires can be sent to patients through the patient portal. If patients are unable to complete PROMIS GH before their visit through the patient portal, they can complete it using a tablet at the time of check-in for their visit. Patients can also complete the questionnaires on the examination room workstations using Epic's "captive mode," which locks the computer terminal to all other applications other than the patient's assigned questionnaires.

LivingMatrix, a cloud-based patient information management system used by subscribing to functional medicine practices (San Francisco, California), also offers the ability to collect PROMIS Global, but it may be necessary to manually transfer the results into the provider's EHR.

Timing of collection

Implementation also involves PROMIS Global being collected longitudinally within the functional medicine care continuum. This requires establishing meaningful time points for follow-up questionnaire completion following baseline assessment. At Cleveland Clinic Center for Functional Medicine, patients are instructed to follow-up with providers at 3, 6, 9, and 12 months following their initial visit and PROMIS Global is completed at each of these visits. Patients are encouraged to follow-up with a dietitian 4 weeks after their initial visit and health coach 2 weeks after their initial visit with additional visits scheduled on a needed basis. Similarly, patients are encouraged to schedule with a behavioral health therapist, if indicated (eg, history of depression, but not currently in care, or if they score high on the Patient Health Questionnaire-9 (PHQ-9), a measure of severity of depression).

Initially, PROMIS Global was only distributed at provider visits regardless of whether they were in-person or virtual; however, the Center expanded it to visits with any caregiver (provider, dietitian, health coach, behavioral health therapist) to ensure follow-up data were captured as scheduling follow-up visits with providers was challenging secondary to patient demand and appointment availability. This decision reduced potential gaps in follow-up PROMIS Global data and is an important factor to consider when implementing PROMIS Global in clinical care.

Considerations for Interpretation and Utilization in Clinical Care

Once PROMIS Global is implemented in the clinical care setting, it could be used to guide functional medicine-based management strategies. This would rely on appropriate interpretation of the PROMIS Global T-Scores and/or items. Higher PROMIS Global T-Scores indicate better function. Providers can discuss longitudinal improvements or declines in T-Scores with patients to help identify triggers or mediators in the patient's timeline that may have led to a change in health status and warrant adjustments in the management strategy.

Visualizing longitudinal changes in PROMIS Global T-Scores can support such provider–patient discussions. Providers can use visualizations to discuss how their treatment strategy has improved the patient's health status alongside biological factors (eg, blood glucose, blood pressure, weight, and so forth) or, conversely, discuss how other strategies may be warranted to move the needle, if you will (**Fig. 2**A). Recently, Cleveland Clinic began displaying PROMIS Global scores directly to patients immediately after they complete the scale. The display also indicates how the scores have changed since their last visit (**Fig. 2**B). Providing visualizations and interpretations of PROMIS Global to patients can foster bidirectional communication with the provider,[51,52] facilitate shared decision-making,[53] and support the delivery of patient-centered care.[54] When patients see that PROMs are used as the part of their care, they are more willing to complete them.[55] Therefore, incorporating PROMIS Global into the clinical care setting can enhance the ability to deliver patient-centered care which is integral to the functional medicine model.

Examination of longitudinal improvements or declines in individual item responses can provide more granularity with respect to the physical, mental or social factors contributing to the patient's self-reported health status. Targeted management strategies involving different treatment modalities or further symptom evaluation could potentially be implemented based on item responses (**Table 4**). For example, if a patient presents with a low item score for Global04 (Mental Health) and/or this item has not improved over time, then consider screening for depression using PHQ-9. If abnormal, a referral to behavioral health therapy may be indicated if the patient isn't already under the care of a mental health professional. If the patient is under the care of a medical health professional, a discussion regarding frequency or alternative, evidence-based therapies such as meditation may be warranted.

Incorporating PROMIS Global Into Functional Medicine Research

PROs are also integral to research initiatives focused on developing the evidence for and establishing the value of the functional medicine model of care. Incorporating PROMIS Global into research should consider the type of study being performed, objective of the study, frequency of data collection, and consistent interpretation and reporting.

Consider the type of study

When initiating research studies it is important to appreciate how the data will be obtained for analysis. Retrospective studies involve data being extracted from the EHR or another source into a useable format *after* patient encounters are complete. Therefore, this type of study relies heavily on the successful operational implementation of the measure and quality control (ie, the measure was fully completed by the patient, collected in a consistent and timely manner, and documented in a standard format). Cleveland Clinic Center for Functional Medicine developed an IRB-approved patient registry to collect demographic, biomarker, biometric, and PROs[43,45] with the intent of capturing outcomes such as PROMIS Global from the EHR to increase data access and improve research efficiency. Importantly, patients need to provide consent for this type of data collection which can facilitate performing deidentified retrospective analyses.

A

PROMIS Scale T-Scores - - HIGHER SCORES BETTER

PROMIS Global Health - (T-Scores - the mean of general population = 50. Five points is a clinically meaningful difference.)	3/3/2021	5/23/2021	9/12/21
Physical T-Score	42.3	44.9	48
Mental T-Score	48.3	50.8	50.8

Provider display of PROMIS Global scores automatically inserted into provider documentation templates within the EHR.

B

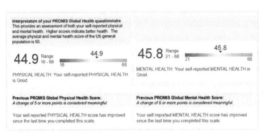

Domain	Range	Verbiage displayed to patients
Physical Health	16-34.99	Your self-reported PHYSICAL HEALTH score is Poor
	35-41.99	Your self-reported PHYSICAL HEALTH score is Fair
	42-49.99	Your self-reported PHYSICAL HEALTH score is Good
	50-57.99	Your self-reported PHYSICAL HEALTH score is Very Good
	58-68	Your self-reported PHYSICAL HEALTH score is Excellent
Mental Health	21-28.99	Your self-reported MENTAL HEALTH score is Poor
	29-39.99	Your self-reported MENTAL HEALTH score is Fair
	40-47.99	Your self-reported MENTAL HEALTH score is Good
	48-55.99	Your self-reported MENTAL HEALTH score is Very Good
	56-68	Your self-reported MENTAL HEALTH score is Excellent

Example of automated reporting provided directly to patients at the time of questionnaire completion through Epic's patient portal, MyChart® (a registered trademark of Epic Systems Corporation).

The bottom table is the verbiage displayed to patients according to their T-scores.

Fig. 2. Example (*A*) provider and (*B*) patient PROMIS Global reporting.

Prospective studies involve data being collected at predetermined time points and rely heavily on research coordinators, or other research personnel, to ensure PROMIS Global is distributed, collected, and documented. Prospective studies can collect PROMIS Global using paper or electronic format. Using the paper format requires an in-person visit, but ensures that the needed data are captured and also allows for quality control to occur at the time of collection (eg, confirming the patient answered all questions, understood the questions, and so forth). The use of the electronic questionnaire relies on timely completion by the patient which is not always feasible and quality control can, at times, be difficult to manage. However, electronic distribution can be implemented with minimal effort using a secure, online platform such as REDCap (Nashville, Tennessee) which has an expansive repository of

Table 4
Potential if/then scenarios for abnormal PROMIS global item responses

Item	If/Then Scenario...
Global04 – Mental health	If < 3, consider the following: • Screen for depression using PHQ-9. If abnormal, refer to behavioral health therapy • Referral to health coaching and consider meditation
Global05 – Satisfaction with social activities and relationships	If < 3, consider the following: • Referral to behavioral health therapy • Referral to a shared medical appointment, if available
Global06 – Ability to carry out physical activities	If < 3, consider the following: • Initiating TUG testing and, if indicated, referral to physical therapy and/or primary care physician
Global10r – Emotional problems	If < 4, consider the following: • Referral to behavioral health therapy
Global08r – Fatigue	If < 4, consider the following: • Reviewing LivingMatrix (eg, Tired on awakening) • Ordering a sleep apnea work-up • Implementing a detox food plan • Screen for depression using PHQ-9. If abnormal, refer to behavioral health therapy
Global07r – Pain	If pain, consider the following: • Referral for FSM • Referral for acupuncture • Implementing a detox food plan • Recommending Bromelain dietary supplementation

Abbreviations: Frequency Specific Microcurrent (FSM); Patient Health Questionnaire-9 (PHQ-9); Timed Up and Go (TUG).

programmed, validated questionnaires such as PROMIS Global. REDCap can be programmed to push out reminders to patients to complete questionnaires and quality control and completion rates can be easily monitored. Financial incentives by way of study stipends, discounted services, and so forth can also support patient engagement and participation.

Recently, the Enhancing Quality and Transparency of Health Research (EQUATOR) Network published the SPIRIT-PRO Extension to provide a consensus-based, PRO-specific research protocol guidance for information to be included within a clinical trial protocol when a PROM, such as PROMIS Global, is a primary or secondary outcome.[56,57] The intent of the SPIRIT-PRO Extension is to ensure studies are well-designed to collect high-quality data that can inform patient-centered care.

Consider the objective of the study
As research studies are being developed, it is important to appreciate how PROMIS Global aligns with the objective of the study. If examining the functional medicine model of care as a whole across patients with various chronic conditions, it is not ideal to select a biological factor as a primary outcome as this would vary among populations and conditions. Therefore, PROMIS Global would be an appropriate primary outcome to evaluate overall health status. Conversely, if the intent of the study is

the examine how an intervention can improve the diabetic status, change in hemoglobin A1c or insulin use would be more appropriate primary outcomes and PROMIS Global would then be a fitting secondary outcome.

Consider the frequency of data collection

The frequency of PROMIS Global data collection should also be considered when launching a research study. PROMIS is a dynamic measure that can change more frequently than other factors such as comorbidities.[58] Clinically meaningful changes have been reported as early as 3 months following intervention.[45] However, it is important to be cognizant of the frequency by which PROMIS Global is assessed especially in addition to other PROMs as the patient may experience questionnaire fatigue. Compounding this are the multi-modal nutrition and lifestyle-based interventions typically used by the functional medicine care model for the management of chronic conditions. Altogether, these can be cumbersome for patients and may reduce adherence and contribute to higher than normal withdrawal and loss of follow-up rates. Therefore, it is important to incorporate PROMs like PROMIS Global along the care continuum as needed with minimal burden to the patient.

Consider consistent reporting

Once PROMIS Global is collected it is important to be consistent with respect to reporting and interpretation. When reporting PROMIS Global, the T-Scores at baseline and follow-up can be used to determine if the population is "sicker" or "healthier" than the comparator population. Reporting the T-Score point change from baseline is important to appreciate if substantial improvements in global health have occurred as a result of a particular intervention. There are several studies that report on clinically meaningful T-Score point improvements for various PROMIS domains (eg, fatigue, anxiety, physical function, and so forth) as measured via different PROMIS forms.[48] Prior studies of functional medicine populations have used a T-Score change of 5 points or more points on the PROMIS Global 10-item questionnaire[43,45] to signify a clinically meaningful improvement.[37] T-Score point improvements or declines were also stratified in an effort to be fully transparent. Additionally, the amount of missing data was also reported and discussed in the limitations section. Missing data are a potential contributor to bias and reasons for this should be provided. Long-term, maintaining consistent PROMIS Global reporting across studies will aid in the comparison of studies that evaluate the functional medicine model of care, or aspects of its care, within and across practices or institutions. Such consistency can also serve as a guide for patients on the best treatment options for their care.[40]

Facilitators and Barriers to PROMIS Global Collection

There are several facilitators and barriers to PROMIS Global collection that are important to consider in clinical care or research settings. With respect to facilitators, PROMIS Global is an accurate, reliable, validated measure with standardized items and responses allowing for consistent evaluation within and among institutions. The questionnaire is a short-form version (only 10 items) that takes less than 5 minutes to complete. There is no cost to use the measure and it is open to anyone to download and use.

One of the most challenging barriers is failure to complete questionnaires, which can result in biased results. Patients who have not been adherent to the recommended nutrition and lifestyle-based interventions may be less likely to have improvements in PROMIS Global and may also be less likely to complete the questionnaire (also known as nonresponders). These patients may ultimately be excluded from a study whereby PROMIS Global is the primary outcome as they are missing pre/postdata leaving data for patients who have completed the questionnaire as asked (also known as responders). Therefore, the study may demonstrate a benefit simply because it is evaluating a subsample of responders. Other barriers to the collection include available practice resources (eg, personnel and financial), the potential for patient burden and loss to follow-up, and a belief among some providers that PROs are "soft" outcomes.

SUMMARY

An expansion of the evidence base evaluating the functional medicine model of care and its condition-specific management strategies is warranted. Such evidence should focus on biological factors as well as PROs to provide a "more complete" account of patient health. However, the successful incorporation of PROMIS Global into clinical care and research is imperative to expand on currently available evidence.

CLINICS CARE POINTS

- Validated general or condition-specific PROMs should be captured alongside biological factors as part of functional medicine care and research.
- Incorporating PROMIS Global into functional medicine care requires a strategy focused on education, implementation, and interpretation.
- PROMIS Global summary T-Scores and item responses can be implemented within clinical care to guide patient-centered, functional medicine management strategies.
- Providers should consider the format, timing of data collection, and visualization of longitudinal changes during PROMIS Global implementation in functional medicine clinical care.
- Providers should consider the type of study, objective of the study, frequency of data collection, and consistent reporting when performing research in functional medicine that incorporates PROMIS Global.

ACKNOWLEDGEMENTS

MB would like to thank The Institute for Functional Medicine for its educational and research support for the Center for Functional Medicine.

DISCLOSURE

M. Beidelschies reports personal fees from Cleveland HeartLab, Inc. outside the submitted work. In addition, she has a patent number 20110269150; issued. All other authors have nothing to disclose.

REFERENCES

1. World Health Organization. Constitution. 2021. Available at: https://www.who.int/about/governance/constitution. Accessed November 30, 2021.
2. Engel GL. The need for a new medical model: a challenge for biomedicine. Science 1977;196(4286):129–36.
3. Wade DT, Halligan PW. The biopsychosocial model of illness: a model whose time has come. Clin Rehabil 2017;31(8):995–1004.
4. Bland J. Defining function in the functional medicine model. Integr Med 2017; 16(1):22–5.
5. Galland L. Patient-centered care: Antecedents, triggers, and mediators. Altern Ther Health Med 2006;12(4):62–70.

6. Functional medicine: A clinical model to address chronic disease. The Institute for Functional Medicine. Updated October 11, 2021. https://functionalmedicine. widen.net/s/pkcvf2wzlj/ifm_functional_medicine_descriptive_paper.   Accessed May 11, 2022.

7. U.S. Department of Health and Human Services. Patient-reported outcome measures: use in medical product development to support labeling claims 2009. Available at: https://www.fda.gov/media/77832/download. Accessed November 29, 2021.

8. National Quality Forum. Patient-reported outcomes. 2021. Available at: https:// www.qualityforum.org/Patient-Reported_Outcomes.aspx. Accessed October 7, 2021.

9. U.S. Department of Health, Education, and Welfare. Proceedings of the Public Health Conference on Records and Statistics, meeting jointly with the National Conference on Mental Health Statistics: 14th National Meeting. Paper presented at: Public Health Conference on Records and Statistics; June 12–15, 1972, 1973; Washington, D.C.

10. Wan TT, Livieratos B. Interpreting a general index of subjective well-being. Milbank Mem Fund Q Health Soc 1978;56(4):531–56.

11. Cleary PD, Edgman-Levitan S, Roberts M, et al. Patients evaluate their hospital care: A national survey. Health Aff 1991;10(4):254–67.

12. Churruca K, Pomare C, Ellis LA, et al. Patient-reported outcome measures (PROMs): A review of generic and condition-specific measures and a discussion of trends and issues. Health Expect 2021;24(4):1015–24.

13. Centers for Medicare and Medicade Services. CMS measures management system blueprint. 2021. Available at: https://www.cms.gov/Medicare/Quality-Initiatives-Patient-Assessment-Instruments/MMS/Downloads/Blueprint.pdf. Accessed November 29, 2021.

14. National Quality Forum. Patient-reported outcomes: Best practices on selection and data collection. Natl Qual Forum 2020. Accessed November 29, 2021.

15. Cella DHE, Jensen SE, Butt Z, et al. Patient-reported outcomes in performance measurement. RTI Press; 2015.

16. Weldring T, Smith SM. Patient-Reported Outcomes (PROs) and Patient-Reported Outcome Measures (PROMs). Health Serv Insights 2013;6:61–8.

17. Walsh TL, Homa K, Hanscom B, et al. Screening for depressive symptoms in patients with chronic spinal pain using the SF-36 Health Survey. Spine Hournal 2006;6(3):316–20.

18. Ho B, Houck JR, Flemister AS, et al. Preoperative PROMIS scores predict postoperative success in foot and ankle patients. Foot Ankle Int 2016;37(9):911–8.

19. Mooney K, Berry DL, Whisenant M, et al. Improving cancer care through the patient experience: How to use patient-reported outcomes in clinical practice. Am Soc Clin Oncol Educ Book 2017;37:695–704.

20. LeBlanc TW, Abernethy AP. Patient-reported outcomes in cancer care: Hearing the patient voice at greater volume. Nat Rev Clin Oncol 2017;14(12):763–72.

21. National Quality Forum. Patient-reported outcomes in performance measurement 2012. Available at: https://www.qualityforum.org/publications/2012/12/patient-reported_outcomes_in_performance_measurement.aspx. Accessed November 29, 2021.

22. Kingsley C, Patel S. Patient-reported outcome measures and patient-reported experience measures. BJA Education 2017;17(4):137–44.

23. Cella D, Riley W, Stone A, et al. The Patient-Reported Outcomes Measurement Information System (PROMIS) developed and tested its first wave of adult self-reported health outcome item banks: 2005-2008. J Clin Epidemiol 2010;63(11):1179–94.

24. Cella D, Choi SW, Condon DM, et al. PROMIS® adult health profiles: Efficient short-form measures of seven health domains. Value Health 2019;22(5):537–44.

25. Ware JE Jr, Sherbourne CD. The MOS 36-item short-form health survey (SF-36). I. Conceptual framework and item selection. Med Care 1992;30(6):473–83.

26. Rabin R, de Charro F. EQ-5D: a measure of health status from the EuroQol Group. Ann Med 2001;33(5):337–43.

27. Roos EM, Roos HP, Lohmander LS, et al. Knee Injury and Osteoarthritis Outcome Score (KOOS)–Development of a self-administered outcome measure. J Orthop Sports Phys Ther 1998;28(2):88–96.

28. Love JR, Irvine EJ, Fedorak RN. Quality of life in inflammatory bowel disease. J Clin Gastroenterol 1992;14(1):15–9.

29. Juniper EF, O'Byrne PM, Guyatt GH, et al. Development and validation of a questionnaire to measure asthma control. Eur Respir J 1999;14(4):902–7.

30. Cella DF, Tulsky DS, Gray G, et al. The Functional Assessment of Cancer Therapy scale: Development and validation of the general measure. J Clin Oncol 1993;11(3):570–9.

31. HealthMeasures. Intro to PROMIS. 2021. Available at: https://www.healthmeasures.net/explore-measurement-systems/promis/intro-to-promis. Accessed October 10, 2021.

32. Hays RD, Bjorner JB, Revicki DA, et al. Development of physical and mental health summary scores from the patient-reported outcomes measurement information system (PROMIS) global items. Qual Life Res 2009;18(7):873–80.

33. Tinetti ME, McAvay GJ, Chang SS, et al. Contribution of multiple chronic conditions to universal health outcomes. J Am Geriatr Soc 2011;59(9):1686–91.

34. Tinetti ME, McAvay G, Chang SS, et al. Effect of chronic disease-related symptoms and impairments on universal health outcomes in older adults. J Am Geriatr Soc 2011;59(9):1618–27.

35. Working Group on Health Outcomes for Older Persons with Multiple Chronic Conditions. Universal health outcome measures for older persons with multiple chronic conditions. J Am Geriatr Soc 2012;60(12):2333–41.

36. Norman GR, Sloan JA, Wyrwich KW. Interpretation of changes in health-related quality of life: The remarkable universality of half a standard deviation. Med Care 2003;41(5):582–92.

37. Yost KJ, Eton DT, Garcia SF, et al. Minimally important differences were estimated for six Patient-Reported Outcomes Measurement Information System-Cancer scales in advanced-stage cancer patients. J Clin Epidemiol 2011;64(5):507–16.

38. Schalet BD, Hays RD, Jensen SE, et al. Validity of PROMIS physical function measured in diverse clinical samples. J Clin Epidemiol 2016;73:112–8.

39. Hays RD, Revicki DA, Feeny D, et al. Using Linear Equating to Map PROMIS® Global Health Items and the PROMIS-29 V2.0 Profile Measure to the Health Utilities Index Mark 3. PharmacoEconomics 2016;34(10):1015–22.

40. Kaplan RJL, Ko C, Pusic A, et al. Health care measurements that improve patient outcomes. NEJM Catalyst 2021;2(2):21.

41. Revicki DA, Kawata AK, Harnam N, et al. Predicting EuroQol (EQ-5D) scores from the patient-reported outcomes measurement information system (PROMIS)

global items and domain item banks in a United States sample. Qual Life Res 2009;18(6):783–91.

42. Thompson NR, Lapin BR, Katzan IL. Mapping PROMIS Global Health items to EuroQol (EQ-5D) utility scores using linear and equipercentile equating. PharmacoEconomics 2017;35(11):1167–76.

43. Beidelschies M, Alejandro-Rodriguez M, Ji X, et al. Association of the functional medicine model of care with patient-reported health-related quality of life outcomes. JAMA Netw Open 2019;2(10):e1914017.

44. Droz N, Hanaway P, Hyman M, et al. The impact of functional medicine on patient-reported outcomes in inflammatory arthritis: A retrospective study. PloS One 2020;15(10):e0240416.

45. Beidelschies M, Alejandro-Rodriguez M, Guo N, et al. Patient outcomes and costs associated with functional medicine-based care in a shared versus individual setting for patients with chronic conditions: A retrospective cohort study. BMJ Open 2021;11(4):e048294.

46. HealthMeasures. Slides introducing HealthMeasures. 2021. Available at: https://www.healthmeasures.net/resource-center/measurement-science/slides-introducing-healthmeasures. Accessed October 26, 2021.

47. HealthMeasures. Implement for Patient Care. 2021. Available at: https://www.healthmeasures.net/implement-healthmeasures/implement-for-patient-care. Accessed December 6, 2021.

48. HealthMeasures. PROMIS® scoring manuals: PROMIS Global Health short form scoring information. 2021. Available at: https://www.healthmeasures.net/images/PROMIS/manuals/Scoring_Manual_Only/PROMIS_Global_Health_Scoring_Manual.pdf.

49. HealthMeasures. NIH Toolbox® and PROMIS® iPad Apps. 2021. Available at: https://www.healthmeasures.net/implement-healthmeasures/administration-platforms/nih-toolbox-ipad-app. Accessed November 29, 2021.

50. Health IT Analytics. Cerner, epic to see improvements in EHR patient-reported outcomes 2016. Available at: https://healthitanalytics.com/news/cerner-epic-to-see-improvements-in-ehr-patient-reported-outcomes. Accessed December 27, 2021.

51. Freel JBJ, Hanmer J. Better physician ratings from discussing PROs with patients. Innovations in care delivery, 2021, 2018. Available at: https://catalyst.nejm.org/doi/full/10.1056/CAT.18.0150. Accessed November 29, 2021.

52. Detmar SB, Muller MJ, Schornagel JH, et al. Health-related quality of life assessments and patient-physician communication: A randomized controlled trial. JAMA 2002;288(23):3027–34.

53. Jayakumar P, Bozic KJ. Advanced decision-making using patient-reported outcome measures in total joint replacement. J Orthop Res 2020;38(7):1414–22.

54. Abernethy AP, Herndon JE 2nd, Wheeler JL, et al. Improving health care efficiency and quality using tablet personal computers to collect research quality, patient-reported data. Health Serv Res 2008;43(6):1975–91.

55. Gensheimer SG, Wu AW, Snyder CF. Oh, the Places We'll Go: Patient-reported outcomes and electronic health records. The Patient 2018;11(6):591–8.

56. Calvert M, Kyte D, Mercieca-Bebber R, et al. Guidelines for inclusion of patient-reported outcomes in clinical trial protocols: The SPIRIT-PRO Extension. JAMA 2018;319(5):483–94.

57. Calvert M, King M, Mercieca-Bebber R, et al. SPIRIT-PRO Extension explanation and elaboration: guidelines for inclusion of patient-reported outcomes in protocols of clinical trials. BMJ Open 2021;11(6):e045105.

58. Blumenthal KJ, Chang Y, Ferris TG, et al. Using a self-reported global health measure to identify patients at high risk for future healthcare utilization. J Gen Intern Med 2017;32(8):877–82.

Fasting and Fasting Mimicking Diets in Obesity and Cardiometabolic Disease Prevention and Treatment

Amrendra Mishra, PhD[a], Valter D. Longo, PhD[a,b,*]

KEYWORDS

- Obesity • Cadiometabolic health • Periodic fasting • Fasting mimicking diet
- Longevity

KEY POINTS

- The prevalence of obesity has been increasing for the past several decades.
- Obesity reduces both the healthspan and the lifespan.
- Fasting and fasting mimicking diet prevents obesity and increases lifespan in mouse models.
- Fasting mimicking diets are promising interventions for the treatment of obesity and related conditions including diabetes, hypertension, and high cholesterol.

INTRODUCTION: THE OBESITY PANDEMIC

The prevalence of obesity has been increasing consistently in the last 70 years generating a pandemic level. According to WHO estimates there were more than 1.9 billion overweight adults over the age of 18 or 39% of the world population and at least 650 million or 13% of the world population was clinically obese in 2016 (https://www.who.int/news-room/fact-sheets/detail/obesity-and-overweight). In the US, the prevalence of obesity has risen from 13.4% in 1960-1962 to 42.4% in 2017-2018.[1] Historically women have suffered from obesity more than men, but in recent years, in the United States the rate of obesity in men has increased faster than in women and hence according to 2017-2018 estimates obesity prevalence in men (43%) surpassed that in women (41.9%).[1] The increase in obesity is accompanied by an increase in diseases for which obesity is a risk factor, mainly diabetes, hypertension, cardiovascular disease, and metabolic syndrome but also cancer and neurodegenerative diseases.

[a] Longevity Institute and Davis School of Gerontology, University of Southern California, Los Angeles, CA 90089, USA; [b] IFOM, FIRC Institute of Molecular Oncology, Via Adamello, 16, Milano 20139, Italy
* Corresponding author.
E-mail address: vlongo@usc.edu

Phys Med Rehabil Clin N Am 33 (2022) 699–717
https://doi.org/10.1016/j.pmr.2022.04.009

The 2020 National Diabetes Statistics Report, estimates that 10.2% (26.8 million) of all US adults over the age of 18 has been diagnosed with diabetes and another 2.8% (7.3 million) have undiagnosed diabetes taking the total portion of diabetes to 13% (34.1 million) of all adults in the US in (US Department of Health and Human Services, 2020).,[2] a drastic rise from the 0.93% in 1958 (Centers for Disease Control and Prevention, 2017).[3]

Metabolic syndrome (MetS) is defined as a combination of conditions that are associated with increased risk of CVD, diabetes and all-cause mortality.[4],[5] The criteria comprise abdominal obesity in addition to any 2 of the following: elevated blood pressure, fasting hyperglycemia, elevated triglyceride and reduced high-density lipoprotein (HDL)-cholesterol or previously diagnosed type 2 diabetes.[5] The prevalence of the metabolic syndrome is 38.3% among all US adults for the year 2017-2018[6] up from 25.3% in the year 1988-1994.[7]

Similarly, 47.3% or more than 121 million adults in the United States of America suffered from hypertension according to National Health and Nutrition Examination Survey (NHANES) estimate for the years 2015 to 2018.[8] The total prevalence of CVD (including coronary heart disease, heart failure, stroke, and hypertension) for the year based on NHANES 2015 to 2018 data among US adults greater than 20 years of age is 49.2%, up from 34.2% in the year 2003.[8],[9]

In addition, midlife vascular disease, midlife hypertension, cardiovascular health and heart failure are associated with cognitive decline and neurodegenerative disease development in old age.[8],[10] There is also epidemiological data showing the relationship between diabetes and the development of dementia.[11] The prevalence of dementia subtypes in United States Medicare fee-for-service beneficiaries in the year 2011-2013 was 14.4%[12] but with the aging population in the United States and worldwide, the burden of dementia and associated neurodegenerative disease is expected to increase further in the future. In addition, obesity in itself has been implicated in reduced cognitive and motor function across the lifespan.[13],[14]

Adiposity is also implicated in the development of several tumors, possibly because it increases factors that can facilitate cancer cells' survival and growth including IGF-1, insulin, glucose and inflammatory markers.[15–17] Meta-Analyses of epidemiological studies have estimated the relative risk of cancers of the colon, gastric cardia, liver, gallbladder, pancreas and kidney to be 1.2 to 1.5 times for overweight and 1.5 to 1.8 times for obese individuals compared to normal weight individuals.[18] These epidemiological findings are also supported by animal studies wherein obesity is associated with a higher prevalence of multiple cancer types.[19] Based on these findings the International Agency for Research on Cancer (IARC) has concluded that the reduction in body fat can lower the risk of most cancers.[18]

In this review, we will focus on obesity and cardiometabolic diseases and how intermittent and periodic fasting interventions can prevent and treat them.

OBESITY, LIFESPAN, AND HEALTHSPAN

Obesity leads to a reduction in lifespan across various species including Drosophila, mice, rats, cats, dogs, monkeys and humans.[20–26] Among the high-income nations, the United States has one of the highest prevalences of overweight and obese individuals and one of the lowest life expectancies.[27] An estimation of the fraction of all-cause mortality attributable to obesity for the 16 high-income countries identified that the differences in the life expectancy can be partially attributed to a high prevalence of obesity in the United States, particularly in the age range of 50-59 (in the year 2006).[28] Another study analyzing human mortality data and individual level disability data to model and forecast future life expectancy for the year 2011-2040 among older adults in the United States concluded that the increase in lifespan due to reduced smoking among the US population will be partially offset by an increase in obesity, particularly among individuals born after 1955.[29]

Obesity increases the risk of several chronic and non-communicable diseases including type 2 diabetes, coronary heart disease, stroke, cancer, and asthma. Nyberg and colleagues performed a metanalysis of data from ten studies and 137,503 participants to identify loss of disease-free years attributable to obesity from age 40 years to 75 years in underweight (BMI $\leq$ 18.5 kg/m^2), overweight (BMI $\geq$ 25.0 kg/m^2 to $\leq$ 30.0 kg/m^2) and obese (BMI $\geq$ 30.0 kg/m^2 to $\leq$ 35.0 kg/m^2) and severely obese (BMI $\geq$ 35.0 kg/m^2) individuals when compared to normal-weight individuals (BMI $\geq$ 18.5 kg/m^2 to $\leq$ 25.0 kg/m^2).[30] The study estimated 29.3 (95% CI, 28.8 - 29.8) disease-free years among normal-weight men and 29.4 (28.7 - 30.0) disease-free years among normal-weight women. The loss of disease-free years was 1.8 (95% CI, 1.3 - 4.9), 1.1 (0.7 - 1.5), 3.9 (2.9 - 4.9), and 8.5 (7.1 - 9.8) years for underweight, overweight, obese, and severely obese men, respectively. Among women, the loss of disease-free years was 0.0 (−1.4 - 1.4), 1.1 (0.6 - 1.5), 2.7 (1.5 - 3.9), 7.3 (6.1 - 8.6) years for underweight, overweight, obese, and severely obese individuals. The loss of disease-free years increases with an increase in obesity in both sexes, among smokers and non-smokers, the physically active and inactive group, and across the socioeconomic stratum. Both obesity and severe obesity seems to cost more to men in terms of loss of disease-free years than to women.[30] A similar sex-dependent difference is also seen in overall life expectancy whereby in a study among Australian adults (age 20–69) where it was reported that men lose more years than women due to obesity and severe obesity.[31]

The data from the population-based Rotterdam study reported that obesity increases the risk of diabetes and CVD as well as the number of years spent with CVD and diabetes without impacting life expectancy.[32,33] However, data from the United States (the year 2000–2017) and Australia (the year 2006–2016) analysing death certificates for the overweight-and obesity-related causes of mortality including diabetes, chronic kidney disease, and hypertensive heart disease show a recent increase in incidence rate.[34] There was a larger increase in obesity-related mortality rate in younger cohorts, paralleling the higher lifetime obesity prevalence[34] indicating a direct impact of obesity on life expectancy.

Mice models are particularly important to study the effect of obesity because they mimic many of the comorbidities caused by obesity including, hyperglycaemia, insulin resistance, dyslipidaemia, poor glucose tolerance, and inflammation.[35] Obesity has been shown to cause the reduction in lifespan in both wild type C57Bl/6mice[26,36,37] as well as in genetic obesity models ob/ob mice and db/db mice[38–40] see **Box 1**.

In summary, adiposity and obesity are at the center of cardiometabolic but also neurodegenerative diseases leading to reduced disease-free years as well as lifespan, probably by generating insulin resistance, hyperglycemia and other changes which promote inflammation, oxidative damage, and multi-system dysfunction.

FASTING FOR LONGEVITY AND OBESITY TREATMENT

Early studies on substrate utilization during fasting in humans showed that more than 75% of calories come from fat.[42,43] Later, it was shown that during prolonged fasting the brain also utilizes β-hydroxybutyrate in addition to glucose as fuel.[44] β-Hydroxybutyrate also serves as stored energy in organisms across taxa. Bacteria, archaea and even protozoa use poly-β-hydroxybutyrate for energy storage.[45] The breakdown of

Box 1 Reduced longevity in commonly used mouse models of obesity	
Mice **Strain**	**Lifespan**
C57BL/6 SD[41]	
Male	878 days
Female	794 days
C57BL/6 HFD	
Male	779 days (HFD) vs 880 days (SD)[37]
Female	570 days (HFD) vs 836.5 days (SD)[26]
db/db[40]	
Male	349 days (SD)
Female	487 days (SD)
ob/ob	
Male	540 days (18 months) (SD)[39]
Female	552 (SD)[38]
Abbreviations: HFD, high fat diet; SD, standard diet.	

fats and generation of β-hydroxybutyrate and other ketone bodies during extended periods of fasting have allowed humans to survive seasonal food scarcity.[45] Notably, newborn humans are born obese[45,46] and the metabolism in the first few days is primarily ketogenic, since maternal colostrum contains high triglyceride and protein but little lactose.[47] If weight gain and obesity are evolved states necessary for survival during seasonal food scarcity, the currently prevailing "drug-based" method to treat and prevent diabetes and CVD should be preferably adopted when nutritional interventions implemented by a team of healthcare professionals fail to reverse the weight gain but also the health consequences of western or similar excess calorie diets. Notably, dietary interventions are often part of the therapies for the prevention and treatment of cardiometabolic disease but the lack of a sophisticated nutrition-centered treatment based on basic, clinical and epidemiologic studies together with the lack of a team able to understand, personalize and implement them in a drug-centered standard of care. Because fasting and severe calorie restriction has historically been at the center of the reversal of adiposity, different fasting methods could be combined with everyday nutritional recommendations to prevent and treat obesity and cardiometabolic diseases.

Notably, different types of fasting interventions, which avoid malnutrition, not only can prevent or reverse obesity but also can promote health-span and lifespan extension when compared to normal weight organisms on a standard and often relatively healthy diet.[25,48] These intermittent fasting interventions include Alternate Day Fasting (ADF), the 5:2 diet, and time-restricted feeding/eating (TRF for mice, TRE for humans), whereas periodic fasting includes prolonged water-only fasting and Fasting Mimicking Diets (FMDs) (reviewed in detail elsewhere (**Box 2, Fig. 1**)[48]

Time-Restricted Eating

Although absolute increase in calorie intake has been traditionally thought to be responsible for obesity, studies in the last decade have highlighted the role of circadian rhythm and night-time/extended feeding in obesity. Multiple studies using mouse models of diet-induced obesity have shown that the timing of food consumption affects obesity, and related disorders independently of calorie intake.[49–51] A study where mice were fed either an *ad libitum* HFD or an 8 hr TRF-HFD (food consumed daily within 8 hours), showed that TRF can protect mice from diet-induced obesity

Box 2	
Fasting interventions to promote health and lifespan	
Fasting Intervention	**Description**
Alternate Day Fasting	Zero-calorie every alternate day; 24 hr water-only fast followed by 24 h of the feeding period
Modified ADF	~25% calories every alternate days/fasting day
5:2 diet	2 days/week of complete fast or ~25% calories; can be either consecutive or non-consecutive days
Time-Restricted Eating	Food intake restricted to 6–12 hrs during the day; daily
Prolonged water only fast	4-5 days of water-only fasting once a month or less (humans) followed by a normal diet
Fasting mimicking diet	4–5 d of plant-based low caloric (30%–50% of normal), high fat, low protein and sugar diet; once a month in obese individuals, 2–4 times a year for normal-weight individuals depending on disease risk factors

even when eating the same number of calories as ad libitum HFD fed mice. These TRF mice were also protected from hyperinsulinemia, hepatic steatosis, and inflammation and showed improved motor coordination.[49] Furthermore, 8-9 hr TRF can also treat pre-existing diet-induced obesity and type II diabetes and reduce hypercholesteremia, triglyceride, hyperglycemia, hyperinsulinemia as well as adipose tissue inflammation in mice.[50]

In clinical studies among healthy overweight weight individuals (BMI $\geq$ 25.0 kg/m^2 to $\leq$ 30.0 kg/m^2), a 10hr-TRE was shown to cause a reduction in calorie intake and an average weight loss of 3.27 kg over a 16-week study period.[52] Among the obese individuals, an 8hr-TRE for a 12 weeks study period led to an average weight loss of 3 kg as well as a reduction in systolic blood pressure.[53] A more severe TRE of

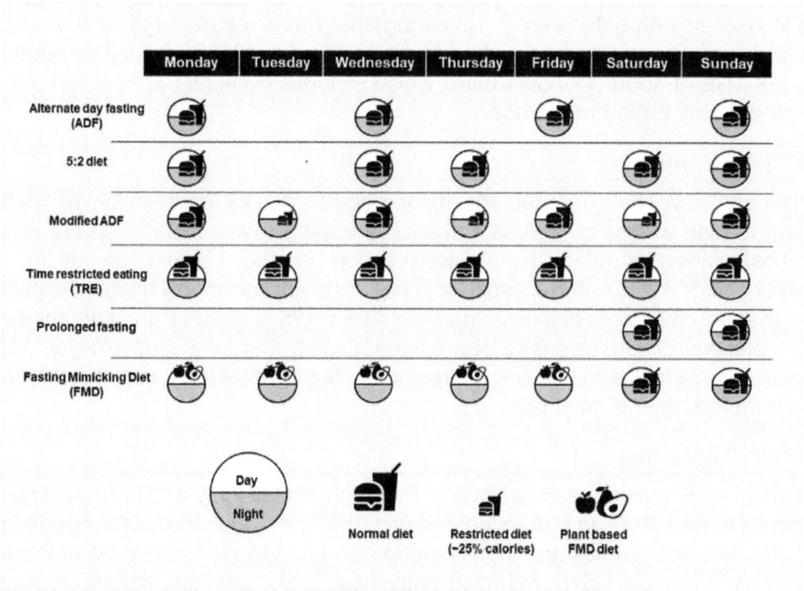

Fig. 1. A representative week on different dietary interventions used to promote health and longevity. Prolonged fasting and FMD are normally adopted once a month or less.

4 hr and 6 hr was compared by *Cienfuegos and colleagues*, for their effectiveness for weight loss among individuals with obesity.[54] During the 8-week study period, the participants lost 3.9% and 3.4% of the bodyweight on 4hr-TRE and 6hr-TRE, respectively. While both interventions produced similar reductions in insulin resistance and oxidative stress, participants also lost both fat mass as well as lean body mass[54] which is a concern for adults but especially the elderly.[55] Another study in individuals with metabolic syndrome reported a reduction in waist circumference, percent body fat, visceral fat, blood pressure, atherogenic lipids, and glycated hemoglobin upon 10hr-TRE for 12 weeks.[56]

In humans, numerous studies have correlated shift work with an increased risk of developing obesity.[57–61] Studies in mice have reported that nocturnal mice when fed only during the day (12 hr window) develop obesity, despite eating the same amount of calories as their counterparts that are fed only during the night (12 hr window).[62] A small clinical trial consisting of 11 overweight adults for 4 days to study the effects of early Time-Restricted Feeding (eTRF) (8 am-2 pm) vs normal schedule (8 am-8 pm) found that eTRF improves 24hr glucose, alters lipid metabolism, alters circadian clock gene expression, increases serum ketone, and increases levels of anti-ageing gene SIRT1 in humans in short term[63] eTRF also reduces appetite without affecting the total energy expenditure and increases fat oxidation.[64] In a study of obese men (mean BMI of 32.2 ± 4.4 kg/m^2) with prediabetes, eTRE for 5 weeks was found to increase insulin sensitivity, improve β-cell function, lower blood pressure and oxidative stress as well as reduce hunger but without any significant weight loss.[65] A recent metanalysis of 9 randomized clinical trials on eTRF concluded that it has significant beneficial effects on fasting blood glucose and insulin sensitivity (Homeostatic Model Assessment for Insulin Resistance [HOMA-IR])[66]

However, TRE is also associated with adverse effects, especially in epidemiologic studies. In fact, breakfast skipping has been consistently associated with increased cardiovascular and overall mortality[67–70] and fasting daily for more than 14 hours compared to less than 8 hours doubles the risk of hospitalization with gallstone disease in women with gallstones.[71] Taken together these results suggest that TRE of 14 hours or longer which involves breakfast skipping may be beneficial for short periods but TRE of about 12 hours daily, which includes breakfast appear to be more recommendable for long-term use.

Intermittent Fasting (IF)

IF regimens have been among the most popular dietary intervention for people wanting to lose weight as well as enthusiasts hoping to live longer and are among the most widely studied dietary intervention in the context of health and longevity.[25,72,73] Three different types of IF regimens are commonly used: ADF (fasting every alternate day; zero calories), modified ADF (~25% calories on alternate days), and 5:2 diet (low or zero calories 2 days a week, usually non-consecutive days).[61] TRF/TRE can also be included in the IF interventions, but here we have discussed it separately from the other IF methods.

Alternate-Day Fasting

Mice on an ADF regimen reach a lower body weight and display a 12% longer lifespan compared to their daily *ad libitum* fed counterparts,[74] although the longevity effects of ADF vary between studies and mouse models and can range from negative to major extensions.[75] In male C57BL/6J mice both mean and maximum lifespan increased when ADF was started at either 1.5 or 6 months of age, and only maximum lifespan increase when ADF started at 10 months of age.[75] In A/J mice mean and maximum lifespan- increased when ADF started at 1.5 months of age, remained unchanged when started at 6 months of age, and was reduced when started at 10 months of age.[75] Although the extent of its prolongevity effects differs with genotype, they seem to be more prominent when started at a young age and fade with age becoming negative after midlife.[75] In a diet-induced obesity model, ADF leads to significant weight loss irrespective of animals being fed a low fat or high-fat diet.[76]

Most human studies, that use a modified ADF regimen in which patients are provided a certain level of calories on the fasting days (reviewed in Ref 61) have reported improvement in bodyweight after 6 to 12 weeks.[77–86] In a small study to evaluate ADF as an alternative therapy for insulin-dependent type II diabetes, 3 out of three patients were able to discontinue insulin after days 5, 13, and 18 respectively. All patients showed improvement in BMI, waist circumference, and HbA1C. All patients lost more than 10% of their body weight in the 7 to 11 months period. The two patients who followed the diet for 11 months were able to get off all their diabetes medication and the 3rd one who followed the diet for 7 months, reduced the daily medications to one at the end of the study from four medications at the beginning.[87] In a study of 100 metabolically healthy obese individuals, modified ADF caused on average a 6% weight loss after 6 months of intervention, and the subjects maintained weight loss at 12 months after the start of the intervention.[88] ADF also led to an improvement in fat mass, blood pressure, heart rate, cholesterol, triglyceride, fasting glucose, fasting insulin, insulin resistance, and C-reactive protein[88] and the results were similar to that of daily calorie restriction at both 6 and 12 months.[88] However, HDL cholesterol levels were significantly increased among the participants in the ADF group at month 6, but not at month 12, relative to those in the daily calorie restriction group. Also, low-density lipoprotein (LDL) cholesterol level was significantly elevated by month 12 in the ADF group compared with that in the daily calorie restriction group.[88]

Stekovic and colleagues[89] reported that ADF was safe to be practiced by healthy non obese individuals for long term, and no adverse effects were reported after more than 6 months of use. ADF, which resulted in an average 37% reduction in calorie intake in the 4 weeks trial period, reduced fat mass, and improved fat to lean ratio and cardiovascular markers. Four-week ADF also increased the level of β-hydroxybutyrate and polyunsaturated fatty acids and reduced the levels of the proaging amino acid methionine (on fasting days). Long-term use of ADF (>6 months) led to reduction in both total and LDL- cholesterol, triglycerides and sICAM-1 (a marker of aging and atherosclerosis).[90] However, despite the weight loss achieved after 4 weeks of ADF (4.5%), no changes in insulin sensitivity (HOMA-IR) was observed between the control and ADF groups either at baseline or at the end of the intervention, although the HOMA-IR in both groups were already at a healthy level of around ~1.5 at baseline.[89,91–93]

5:2 Diet

The 5:2 diet is a popular form of intermittent fasting since calorie intake is restricted during only 2 days per week to either no calories or ~25% of normal intake. In a randomized clinical trial among 107 overweight or obese premenopausal women (mean BMI ± standard deviation [SD], 30.6 ±5.1 kg/m^2), a 25% energy restriction as achieved with a 5:2 diet was shown to be effective for weight loss, with an average weight loss of 6.4kg in the 6 months study period.[94] Participants also showed reductions in leptin, fasting insulin and insulin resistance, free androgen index, high-sensitivity C-reactive protein, total and LDL cholesterol, triglycerides, blood pressure, and an increase in sex hormone-binding globulin, and IGF binding proteins 1 and 2.[94] Another randomized clinical trial studying effects of the 5:2 diet among 137 obese individuals with type II diabetes for 12 months reported an average weight loss of 6.8 kg as well as a reduction in HbA1c, fasting glucose, serum cholesterol and triglycerides.[95]

In a larger recent randomized clinical trial studying the 5:2 diet and involving 300 individuals followed for 12 months, the results were moderate when compared to other regimens. The groups, which included the following: standard brief advice covering diet and physical activity (N = 100), 5:2 self-help instructions (N = 100), or 5:2 self-help instructions plus six once-weekly group support sessions (N = 100), produced similar weight loss results of 1.8 kg, 1.9 kg, and 2.3 kg, respectively.[96] An important finding, relevant to all the fasting regimens involving more than 12 hours of fasting and done every day to several times a week, was that adherence to the diet fell drastically with time. The adherence was initially high at 74% after 6 weeks but declined to 31% after 6 months and remained at 22% at the end of 12 month period.[96] This finding is of important consideration since long term adherence but also long-term side effects are of key importance to establish the efficacy, feasibility and potential clinical application of any dietary intervention.

Although no major side effects have been reported and IF is considered safe for most individuals, it should be used with caution for patients with type 2 diabetes using insulin/sulfonylureas due to the increased risk of hypoglycemia on fasting days.[97,98]

Therapeutic Fasting

Long periods of water only or similar types of fasting achieved by patients in specialized clinics, also known as therapeutic fasting, appear to have acute effects in reducing obesity, hypertension, metabolic syndrome and cardiovascular risk factors..[99–102] However, because these fasting periods require specialized clinics and/or physicians and in most cases are feasible/recommended only once a year or less, it remains to be determined whether and how they can be effective in disease prevention and treatment. In fact, the weight and lean body mass loss, hypoglycaemia, reduced blood pressure, and potential for micronutrient deficiencies associated with long periods of water-only fasting limit its use or make it very risky outside of these clinics.[103–105] Another concern is the effect of fasting periods lasting more than 1 week on metabolic rates since it was shown that obese and non-obese subjects maintained on a 800kcal/day modified fast diet for 4-14 weeks lost over 10% of body weight but displayed a reduction of 6-8 kcal of energy expenditure even when adjusted per kilogram of fat-free mass.[106] Similar long-term reductions in energy expenditures have been shown for calorie restriction studies in humans,[107] suggesting that these extreme and prolonged interventions may use the reduction in energy expenditure to favor a weight regain. For this reason, the long-term effects of weeks of therapeutic fasting on diseases and their risk factors remain to be determined.

Periodic Fasting

Periodic fasting is a term used for fasting periods lasting in most cases between 2 and 7 days and being adopted in most cases once every 2 weeks or less in rodents and once a month or less in humans.[48] It was developed to test the hypothesis that fasting periods lasting 2-7 days could generate changes able to slow down aging and reduce disease risk factors even when applied once a month or less. It can involve water-only fasting or low-calorie diets such as Fasting Mimicking Diets (FMD), which were developed to overcome the limitations of extended periodic water-only fasting and to harness the maximum benefits of it. FMD is a plant-based low calorie, low protein, and high dietary fat designed to mimic the effects of fasting while providing the essential nourishment and minimizing the side effects associated with water-only fasting.[108]

Most FMD interventions last between 4 and 7 days and are designed to provide between 10 to 50% of normal calorie intake in mice (commonly used version provide 50% on day 1 and 10% on day 2–4) or 30 to 50% (commonly used version provide 50% on day 1 and 30% on day 2–5) of normal calorie intake in humans, while providing high micronutrient nourishment.[48,108,109] A Bi-monthly FMD cycle in mice started at middle age lowered blood glucose, IGF1, and increased ketone bodies and IGFBP1, lowered visceral fat, reduced cancer incidence and skin lesions, rejuvenated the immune system, and retarded bone mineral density loss, leading to extended longevity.[108]

The increase in the rate of obesity has been paralleled by the increase in the incidence of autoimmune disorders, including rheumatoid arthritis, psoriasis and psoriatic arthritis, systemic lupus erythematosus, thyroid autoimmunity, multiple sclerosis (MS), inflammatory bowel disease (IBD), and type-1 diabetes (T1D).[110] Not surprisingly, FMD cycles were shown to be effective in the amelioration of MS symptoms by suppressing autoimmunity in a mouse model, as well to be a safe and promising treatment for patients with relapsing-remitting MS.[111] Periodic cycles of a 4-day FMD in mice were also shown to induce sequential Sox17, Pdx1 and Ngn3 expression driving the regeneration of insulin-producing pancreatic β cells, similar to that observed during pancreatic development, and restores both insulin secretion, and glucose homeostasis.[112] The regeneration of pancreatic β cells leads to the reversal of both type-1 diabetes and type-2 diabetes phenotype in mice. Similar β cell regeneration was also seen in the pancreatic islets derived from patients with type-1 diabetes following the FMD cycle.[112] In a dextran sodium sulfate (DSS)-induced colitis model commonly used to study IBD in mice, periodic cycles of 4-day FMD were shown to reduce IBD pathology and intestinal inflammation, and promote intestinal regeneration.[113] Notably, cycles of water-only fasting were not as effective as FMD cycles in reducing IBD-associated pathology/changes. The development of the inflammatory disease of the intestine and increased permeability of the intestine is accompanied by changes in the gut microbiota.[114] Periodic cycles of FMD in DSS induced mouse model of obesity led to beneficial changes in the gut microbiota of mice and increased the abundance of protective microbial families, such as Lactobacillaceae and Bifidobacteriaceae.[113]

In a mouse model of diet-induced obesity, periodic cycles of FMD once every 4 weeks, while eating a high fat and calorie diet (HFCD) for the rest of the month, was shown to counteract the negative effects of the unhealthy diet on lifespan, body weight, and several parameters of metabolic syndrome, diabetes, and cardiovascular ageing.[26] Periodic cycles of FMD prevented HFCD-dependent obesity by inhibiting the accumulation of visceral and subcutaneous fat without causing loss of lean body mass as well as prevented the development of hyperglycaemia, hypercholesterolaemia and hyperleptinemia and improved both impaired glucose and insulin tolerance. Mice undergoing periodic FMD also showed increased heart capillary density and reduced cardiomyocyte hypertrophy compared to mice on HFCD, a marker of cardiac health and youthfulness, and performed better when treated with cardiotoxin dobutamine.[26] The mice undergoing FMD cycles once every 4 weeks, although eating HFCD for the rest of the month, showed elevated serum ketone body levels even 4 days after the end of the FMD cycle as well as lack of compensatory feeding behaviour after the FMD cycle, suggesting a metabolic reprogramming towards preferential fat utilization resulting in overall reduction in calorie intake, compared with mice on continuous HFCD. Transcriptome sequencing of the adipose tissue revealed upregulation of mitochondrial biogenesis and metabolism in mice undergoing the periodic FMD cycles, while eating HFCD otherwise.[26] Notably, the effects of the FMD involve changes in inflammatory and stem cell markers during the fasting period but regenerative changes associated with the re-feeding period, indicating that the return to a normal calorie and protein diet is also important for regenerative and rejuvenating effects of periodic fasting.

Further, in a randomized controlled trial of 100 subjects to evaluate the potential of monthly 5-days of FMD to improve the markers/risk factors for aging, diabetes, cancer, and CVD, the diet cycles were shown to reduce bodyweight, BMI, total body fat and trunk fat, waist circumference, glucose, IGF-1, systolic and diastolic blood pressure, triglyceride, and c-reactive protein, and increase lean body mass. This study established FMD as a safe, effective, and feasible intervention for weight loss/obesity treatment and for reducing markers/risk factors for obesity and age-related diseases.[109]

In a randomized clinical trial to evaluate the efficacy of FMD as an adjunct to neo-adjuvant chemotherapy for HER2-negative breast cancer, patients in the FMD arm showed a radiologically complete or partial response more often than the control arm.[115] A 90–100% tumor-cell loss along with significantly reduced chemotherapy-induced DNA damage in T-lymphocytes was more likely to occur in patients using the FMD. Patients on the FMD had lowered blood glucose, insulin, IGF-1, and increased ketone bodies levels as compared to patients on the control diet.[115] In another study, in a mouse model of hormone-receptor-positive breast cancer, FMD enhanced the efficacy of tamoxifen and fulvestrant by lowering circulating IGF1, insulin and leptin and by inhibiting AKT–mTOR signalling via upregulation of EGR1 and PTEN.[116] The lowering of circulating IGF1, insulin, and leptin was also seen in patients undergoing FMD.[116] In conclusion, the safety and efficacy of FMD cycles have been tested in many clinical trials for the treatment of diseases including obesity, hypertension, diabetes, CVD, multiple sclerosis, and cancer.[108,109,111–113,115,116]

GENES AND DRUGS THAT MIMIC FASTING RESPONSES

Fasting and dietary restrictions promote health and longevity by modulating the levels of growth factors and hormones and the activity of evolutionarily conserved nutrient-sensing pathways.[25,48] These main nutrient-sensing pathways, namely those activated by GH, IGF-1, insulin and leptin and involving PI3K, mTORC, PKA and the down-regulation of downstream stress resistance transcription factors are modulated primarily by glucose and amino acids but are affected by adiposity and the resistance to their activities including insulin resistance.[48,117]

Rapamycin, a pharmacological inhibitor of mTORC1 signalling has been shown to prevent HFD-induced obesity as well as age-dependent obesity and to extend lifespan in mice.[118–120] Weekly rapamycin treatment in mice fed continuously an HFD lowered bodyweight, fatty liver score, adiposity, the level of serum leptin and insulin.[118] The age-dependent increase in mTORC signalling in hypothalamic POMC neurons contributes to age-dependent obesity and its inhibition by intracerebral rapamycin injection causes a reduction in food intake and bodyweight.[119] In a different study using a HFD-induced model of obesity, rapamycin was shown to inhibit obesity, reduce blood glucose, plasma triglyceride, and improve insulin sensitivity and glucose tolerance.[121] However, the effect of rapamycin on glucose tolerance is uncertain, with studies reporting that, while it reduces obesity, rapamycin causes mice to develop glucose intolerance upon long term treatment.[122,123]

Metformin is a widely used drug for the treatment of type 2 diabetes that effectively reduces blood glucose levels and improves insulin sensitivity in humans[124] and extends healthspan and lifespan in mice.[125] Multiple clinical trials have shown the effectiveness of metformin in reducing food intake as well as obesity, without causing hypoglycaemia in obese individuals.[126,127]

Laron syndrome is a genetic condition caused by a mutation in the growth hormone receptor (GHR) gene that leads to severe GHR and IGF-1 deficiencies. Individuals with GHR deficiency, despite being obese, rarely develop diabetes,[128] in agreement with the insulin-sensitizing effects of GHRD in mice and humans.[129,130] GHR deficient individuals have one-third of the serum insulin concentration than that of their relatives and are insulin sensitive with HOMA-IR of 0.34 for GHR deficient group but 0.96 for their relatives.[128] Although the mortality and cardiac and vascular disease effects of GHRD is not yet known, there are rare cases of mortality or morbidity owing to type 2 diabetes or cancer in GHRDs[128] underlining the important role played by GH/IGF-1 signalling in the development of insulin resistance, diabetes and cancer. Fasting appears to cause benefits in part by reducing GHR and IGF-1/insulin signalling but GHR mutant mice, although showing weight loss in response to IF (ADF), do not show any improvement in insulin sensitivity or survival.[131] It should be noted that GHR mutants have much higher insulin sensitivity and prolonged lifespan compared to their wild type counterparts.[131]

CONCLUSION AND FUTURE PERSPECTIVE

Preston and colleagues[132] quantified the role of rising BMI on mortality, proposing that it was responsible for 186,000 excess deaths in 2011.[132] However, the effect of adiposity on human health is much worse if we consider the increased incidence of diabetes, CVD, cancer and neurodegenerative diseases in the overweight and obese portion of the population. Projections for obesity prevalence in the US for the year 2030 predict an even worse situation with a 48.9% prevalence in adults nationwide and a minimum 35% prevalence in any state. Also, nearly one in four adults will be diagnosed with severe obesity (BMI $\geq$ 35.0 kg/m^2).[133]

Aside from the loss of health and lifespan at a personal level, obesity also presents an economic cost for society. The economic cost of obesity includes the direct healthcare cost and the productivity cost in terms of lost wages. Cawley and colleagues, estimated the cost of treating obesity-related illness among adults in the US to be $209.7 billion for the year 2008, representing 20.6% of the total US healthcare expenditure.[134] At an individual level, the estimated annual marginal effect of obesity (the difference between the medical expenditures of the non-obese and obese) was estimated to be $1152 for men ($1657 for non-obese and $2907 for obese men, respectively) and $3613 for women ($1928 for non-obese and $5363 for obese women, respectively).[134]

These projections point to the need of more sophisticated interventions to reduce adiposity that on one hand consider the physiological aspects of overfeeding but on the other hand identify and implement feasible, sustainable and effective dietary interventions. In addition to drugs, currently used treatment for severe obesity in the clinic, such as bariatric surgery, although effective in reducing adiposity and body weight quickly, are highly invasive and have limited effects effect on insulin sensitivity and risk factors for coronary heart disease[135] thus limiting its efficacy in maximizing healthspan. Instead, fasting methods including daily 12-hour TRE, periodic FMD, and everyday nutrition patterns such as the longevity diet[136] have been shown to result in long term beneficial effects on bodyweight, adiposity, fasting glucose, insulin sensitivity, serum level of cholesterol and triglycerides, blood pressure, and markers of cardiac health and aging, but to also be feasible and safe (**Fig. 2**). Thus, specific "fasting interventions" discussed in this article should begin to be considered by healthcare professionals for the prevention and treatments of a wide array of diseases.

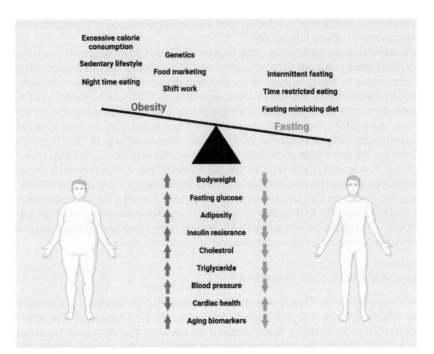

Fig. 2. Obesity is a systemic disease that is caused by multiple factors and leads to multiple adverse changes in the body at a systemic level. Fasting interventions are promising because they impact multiple pathways and prevent or reverse obesity as well as many of the disease risk factors to improve health and longevity.

DECLARATION OF INTERESTS

Funding was provided by the USC Edna Jones chair fund and NIH P01 AG055369-01 to V.D. Longo. V.D. Longo has equity interest in L-Nutra, which develops and sells medical food for the prevention and treatment of diseases.

REFERENCES

1. Fryar CD, Carroll MD, Afful J. Prevalence of overweight, obesity, and severe obesity among adults aged 20 and over: United States, 1960–1962 through 2017–2018. NCHS Health E-Stats; 2020.

2. US Department of Health and Human Services. National Diabetes Statistics Report, 2020. National diabetes Statistics Report, 2, 2020.

3. Centers for Disease Control and Prevention. Long-term Trends in diabetes. CDC's Division of Diabetes Translation; 2017.

4. Isomaa B, Almgren P, Tuomi T, et al. Cardiovascular Morbidity and Mortality Associated With the Metabolic Syndrome. Diabetes care 2001;24:683–9.

5. Alberti KGMM, Zimmet P, Shaw J. The metabolic syndrome - A new worldwide definition. Lancet 2005;366:1059–62.

6. Liang XP, Or CY, Tsoi MF, et al. Prevalence of metabolic syndrome in the United States National Health and Nutrition Examination Survey (nhanes) 2011–2018. Eur Heart J 2021;42:2011–8.

7. Moore JX, Chaudhary N, Akinyemiju T. Metabolic Syndrome Prevalence by Race/Ethnicity and Sex in the United States, National Health and Nutrition Examination Survey, 1988–2012. Preventing Chronic Dis 2017;14:160287.

8. Virani SS, Alonso A, Aparicio HJ, et al. Heart Disease and Stroke Statistics—2021 Update. Circulation 2021;143:E254–743.

9. Thom T, Haase N, Rosamond W, et al. Heart disease and stroke statistics - 2006 Update: A report from the American Heart Association Statistics Committee and Stroke Statistics Subcommittee. Circulation 2006. https://doi.org/10.1161/CIRCULATIONAHA.105.171600.

10. Gottesman RF, Schneider ALC, Zhou Y, et al. Association between midlife vascular risk factors and estimated brain amyloid deposition. JAMA - J Am Med Assoc 2017;317:1443–50.

11. Ninomiya T. Epidemiological Evidence of the Relationship Between Diabetes and Dementia. Adv Exp Med Biol 2019;1128:13–25.

12. Goodman RA, Lochner KA, Thambisetty M, et al. Prevalence of dementia subtypes in United States Medicare fee-for-service beneficiaries, 2011–2013. Alzheimer's Demen 2017;13:28–37.

13. Smith E, Hay P, Campbell L, et al. A review of the association between obesity and cognitive function across the lifespan: Implications for novel approaches to prevention and treatment. Obes Rev 2011;12:740–55.

14. Wang C, Chan JSY, Ren L, et al. Obesity Reduces Cognitive and Motor Functions across the Lifespan. Neural Plasticity 2016;2016:1–13.

15. Nam S, Lee E, Kim K, et al. Effect of obesity on total and free insulin-like growth factor (IGF)-1, and their relationship to IGF-binding protein (BP)-1, IGFBP-2, IGFBP-3, insulin, and growth hormone. Int J Obes 1997;21:355–9.

16. Shoelson SE, Herrero L, Naaz A. Obesity, Inflammation, and Insulin Resistance. Gastroenterology 2007;132:2169–80.

17. Salvadori G, Mirisola MG, Longo VD. Intermittent and periodic fasting, hormones, and cancer prevention. Cancers 2021;13:1–20.

18. Secretan BL, Scoccianti C, et al. Body Fatness and Cancer — Viewpoint of the IARC Working Group. New Engl J Med 2016;375:794–8.

19. Ray A, Cleary MP. Animal Models to Study the Interplay Between Cancer and Obesity. In: Kolonin MG, editor. Adipose tissue and cancer. New York: Springer New York; 2013. p. 99–119.

20. Mizuno T, Shu IW, Makimura H, et al. Obesity over the life course. Sci Aging knowledge Environ 2004;2004:1–8.

21. Piper MDW, Skorupa D, Partridge L. Diet, metabolism and lifespan in Drosophila. Exp Gerontol 2005;40:857–62.

22. Preston SH. Deadweight? — The Influence of Obesity on Longevity. New Engl J Med 2005;352:1135–7.

23. Alexander JG. The growing problem of obesity in dogs and cats. J Nutr 2006; 136:1940S–6S.

24. Skorupa DA, Dervisefendic A, Zwiener J, et al. Dietary composition specifies consumption, obesity, and lifespan in Drosophila melanogaster. Aging Cell 2008;7:478–90.

25. Fontana L, Partridge L, Longo VD. Extending healthy life span–from yeast to humans. Science (New York, NY) 2010;328:321–6.

26. Mishra A, Mirzaei H, Guidi N, et al. Fasting-mimicking diet prevents high-fat diet effect on cardiometabolic risk and lifespan. Nat Metab 2021;3:1342–56.

27. Ng M, Fleming T, Robinson M, et al. Global, regional, and national prevalence of overweight and obesity in children and adults during 1980–2013: a systematic analysis for the Global Burden of Disease Study 2013. Lancet 2014;384:766–81.

28. Preston SH, Stokes A. Contribution of obesity to international differences in life expectancy. Am J Public Health 2011;101:2137–43.

29. Cao B. Future healthy life expectancy among older adults in the US: A forecast based on cohort smoking and obesity history. Popul Health Metrics 2016; 14:1–14.

30. Nyberg ST, Batty GD, Pentti J, et al. Obesity and loss of disease-free years owing to major non-communicable diseases: a multicohort study. Lancet Public Health 2018;3:e490–7.

31. Lung T, Jan S, Tan EJ, et al. Impact of overweight, obesity and severe obesity on life expectancy of Australian adults. Int J Obes 2019;43:782–9.

32. Dhana K, Berghout MA, Peeters A, et al. Obesity in older adults and life expectancy with and without cardiovascular disease. Int J Obes 2016;40:1535–40.

33. Dhana K, Nano J, Ligthart S, et al. Obesity and Life Expectancy with and without Diabetes in Adults Aged 55 Years and Older in the Netherlands: A Prospective Cohort Study. PLoS Med 2016;13:1–13.

34. Adair T, Lopez AD. The role of overweight and obesity in adverse cardiovascular disease mortality trends: An analysis of multiple cause of death data from Australia and the USA. BMC Med 2020;18:1–11.

35. de Moura e Dias M, dos Reis SA, da Conceição LL, et al. Diet-induced obesity in animal models: points to consider and influence on metabolic markers. Diabetology Metab Syndr 2021;13. https://doi.org/10.1186/s13098-021-00647-2.

36. Ozanne SE, Hales CN. Catch-up growth and obesity in male mice. Nature 2004; 427:411–2.

37. Newman JC, Covarrubias AJ, Zhao M, et al. Ketogenic Diet Reduces Midlife Mortality and Improves Memory in Aging Mice. Cell Metab 2017;26:547–57, e8.

38. Harrison DE, Archer JR, Astle CM. Effects of food restriction on aging: Separation of food intake and adiposity. Proc Natl Acad Sci United States America 1984;81:1835–8.

39. Ren J, Dong F, Cai GJ, et al. Interaction between age and obesity on cardiomyocyte contractile function: Role of leptin and stress signaling. PLoS One 2010; 5:1–15.

40. Sataranatarajan K, Ikeno Y, Bokov A, et al. Rapamycin increases mortality in db/db mice, a mouse model of type 2 diabetes. Journals Gerontol - Ser A Biol Sci Med Sci 2016;71:850–7.

41. Kunstyr I, Leuenberger HW. Gerontological Data of C57BL/6J Mice. I. Sex Differences in Survival Curves1. J Gerontol 1975;30:157–62.

42. Benedict FG. A study of prolonged fasting. Carnegie Institution of Washington; 1915.

43. Cahill GF. Starvation in Man. New Engl J Med 1970;282:668–75.

44. Owen OE, Morgan AP, Kemp HG, et al. Brain metabolism during fasting. J Clin Invest 1967;46:1589–95.

45. Cahill GF. Fuel metabolism in starvation. Annu Rev Nutr 2006;26:1–22.

46. Cunnane SC, Crawford MA. Survival of the fattest: Fat babies were the key to evolution of the large human brain. Comp Biochem Physiol - A Mol Integr Physiol 2003;136:17–26.

47. Neville MC, Allen JC, Archer PC, et al. Studies in human lactation: milk volume and nutrient composition during weaning and lactogenesis. Am J Clin Nutr 1991;54:81–92.

48. Longo VD, Di Tano M, Mattson MP, et al. Intermittent and periodic fasting, longevity and disease. Nat Aging 2021;1:47–59.
49. Hatori M, Vollmers C, Zarrinpar A, et al. Time-restricted feeding without reducing caloric intake prevents metabolic diseases in mice fed a high-fat diet. Cell Metab 2012;15:848–60.
50. Chaix A, Zarrinpar A, Miu P, et al. Time-restricted feeding is a preventative and therapeutic intervention against diverse nutritional challenges. Cell Metab 2014; 20:991–1005.
51. Chaix A, et al. Time-Restricted Feeding Prevents Obesity and Metabolic Syndrome in Mice Lacking a Circadian Clock. Cell Metab 2019;29(2):303–19.e4.
52. Gill S, Panda S. A Smartphone App Reveals Erratic Diurnal Eating Patterns in Humans that Can Be Modulated for Health Benefits. Cell Metab 2015;22: 789–98.
53. Gabel K, Hoddy KK, Haggerty N, et al. Effects of 8-hour time restricted feeding on body weight and metabolic disease risk factors in obese adults: A pilot study. Nutr Healthy Aging 2018;4:345–53.
54. Cienfuegos S, Gabel K, Kalam F, et al. Effects of 4- and 6-h Time-Restricted Feeding on Weight and Cardiometabolic Health: A Randomized Controlled Trial in Adults with Obesity. Cell Metab 2020;32:366–78.e3.
55. Miller SL, Wolfe RR. The danger of weight loss in the elderly. J Nutr Health Aging 2008;12:487–91.
56. Wilkinson MJ, Manoogian ENC, Zadourian A, et al. Ten-Hour Time-Restricted Eating Reduces Weight, Blood Pressure, and Atherogenic Lipids in Patients with Metabolic Syndrome. Cell Metab 2020;31:92–104.e5.
57. Min Ju K, Kuk Hui S, Hyun Young P, et al. Association Between Shift Work and Obesity Among FemaleNnurses: Korean Nurses' Survey. BMC Public Health 2013;13:1–15.
58. Peplonska B, Bukowska A, Sobala W. Association of rotating night shift work with BMI and abdominal obesity among nurses and midwives. PLoS ONE 2015;10:1–13.
59. Liu Q, Shi J, Duan P, et al. Is shift work associated with a higher risk of overweight or obesity? A systematic review of observational studies with meta-analysis. Int J Epidemiol 2018;47:1956–71.
60. Sun M, Feng W, Wang F, et al. Meta-analysis on shift work and risks of specific obesity types. Obes Rev 2018;19:28–40.
61. Fanti M, Mishra A, Longo VD, et al. Time-Restricted Eating, Intermittent Fasting, and Fasting-Mimicking Diets in Weight Loss. Curr Obes Rep 2021;10:70–80.
62. Arble DM, Bass J, Laposky AD, et al. Circadian Timing of Food Intake Contributes to Weight Gain. Obesity 2009;17:2100–2.
63. Jamshed H, Beyl RA, Della Manna DL, et al. Early Time-Restricted Feeding Improves 24-Hour Glucose Levels and Affects Markers of the Circadian Clock, Aging, and Autophagy in Humans. Nutrients 2019. https://doi.org/10.3390/nu11061234.
64. Ravussin E, Beyl RA, Poggiogalle E, et al. Early Time-Restricted Feeding Reduces Appetite and Increases Fat Oxidation But Does Not Affect Energy Expenditure in Humans. Obesity 2019;27:1244–54.
65. Sutton EF, Beyl R, Early KS, et al. Early Time-Restricted Feeding Improves Insulin Sensitivity, Blood Pressure, and Oxidative Stress Even without Weight Loss in Men with Prediabetes. Cell Metab 2018;27:1212–21.e3.

66. de OM Pureza IR, Macena M de L, da Silva Junior AE, et al. Effect of early time-restricted feeding on the metabolic profile of adults with excess weight: A systematic review with meta-analysis. Clin Nutr 2021;40:1788–99.

67. Ofori-Asenso R, Owen AJ, Liew D. Skipping breakfast and the risk of cardiovascular disease and death: A systematic review of prospective cohort studies in primary prevention settings. J Cardiovasc Development Dis 2019;6:1–11.

68. Rong S, Snetselaar LG, Xu G, et al. Association of Skipping Breakfast With Cardiovascular and All-Cause Mortality. J Am Coll Cardiol 2019;73:2025–32.

69. Takagi H, Hari Y, Nakashima K, et al. Meta-Analysis of Relation of Skipping Breakfast With Heart Disease. Am J Cardiol 2019;124:978–86.

70. Chen H, Zhang B, Ge Y, et al. Association between skipping breakfast and risk of cardiovascular disease and all cause mortality: A meta-analysis. Clin Nutr 2020;39:2982–8.

71. Sichieri R, Everhart JE, Roth H. A prospective study of hospitalization with gallstone disease among women: role of dietary factors, fasting period, and dieting. Am J Public Health 1991;81:880–4.

72. Longo VD, Antebi A, Bartke A, et al. Interventions to slow aging in humans: are we ready? Aging Cell. Blackwell Publishing Ltd; 2015. p. 497–510. https://doi.org/10.1111/acel.12338.

73. Longo VD, Panda S. Fasting, Circadian Rhythms, and Time-Restricted Feeding in Healthy Lifespan. Cell Metab 2016;23:1048–59.

74. Xie K, Neff F, Markert A, et al. Every-other-day feeding extends lifespan but fails to delay many symptoms of aging in mice. Nat Commun 2017;8:155.

75. Goodrick CL, Ingram DK, Reynolds MA, et al. Effects of intermittent feeding upon body weight and lifespan in inbred mice: interaction of genotype and age. Mech Ageing Development 1990;55:69–87.

76. Gotthardt JD, Verpeut JL, Yeomans BL, et al. Intermittent Fasting Promotes Fat Loss With Lean Mass Retention, Increased Hypothalamic Norepinephrine Content, and Increased Neuropeptide Y Gene Expression in Diet-Induced Obese Male Mice. Endocrinology 2016;157:679–91.

77. Bhutani S, Klempel MC, Kroeger CM, et al. Alternate day fasting and endurance exercise combine to reduce body weight and favorably alter plasma lipids in obese humans. Obesity 2013;21:1370–9.

78. Eshghinia S, Mohammadzadeh F. The effects of modified alternate-day fasting diet on weight loss and CAD risk factors in overweight and obese women. J Diabetes Metab Disord 2013;12:4.

79. Klempel MC, Kroeger CM, Varady KA. Alternate day fasting increases LDL particle size independently of dietary fat content in obese humans. Eur J Clin Nutr 2013;67:783–5.

80. Hoddy KK, Kroeger CM, Trepanowski JF, et al. Meal timing during alternate day fasting: Impact on body weight and cardiovascular disease risk in obese adults. Obesity 2014;22:2524–31.

81. Hoddy KK, Kroeger CM, Trepanowski JF, et al. Safety of alternate day fasting and effect on disordered eating behaviors. Nutr J 2015;14:44.

82. Hoddy KK, Bhutani S, Phillips SA, et al. Effects of different degrees of insulin resistance on endothelial function in obese adults undergoing alternate day fasting. Nutr Healthy Aging 2016;4:63–71.

83. Catenacci VA, Pan Z, Ostendorf D, et al. A randomized pilot study comparing zero-calorie alternate-day fasting to daily caloric restriction in adults with obesity. Obesity 2016;24:1874–83.

84. Coutinho SR, Halset EH, Gåsbakk S, et al. Compensatory mechanisms activated with intermittent energy restriction: A randomized control trial. Clin Nutr 2018;37:815–23.
85. Cho A-R, Moon J-Y, Kim S, et al. Effects of alternate day fasting and exercise on cholesterol metabolism in overweight or obese adults: A pilot randomized controlled trial. Metab - Clin Exp 2019;93:52–60.
86. Hutchison AT, Liu B, Wood RE, et al. Effects of Intermittent Versus Continuous Energy Intakes on Insulin Sensitivity and Metabolic Risk in Women with Overweight. Obesity 2019;27:50–8.
87. Furmli S, Elmasry R, Ramos M, et al. Therapeutic use of intermittent fasting for people with type 2 diabetes as an alternative to insulin. BMJ Case Rep 2018; 2018. https://doi.org/10.1136/bcr-2017-221854. bcr-2017-221854.
88. Trepanowski JF, Kroeger CM, Barnosky A, et al. Effect of Alternate-Day Fasting on Weight Loss, Weight Maintenance, and Cardioprotection Among Metabolically Healthy Obese Adults: A Randomized Clinical Trial. JAMA Intern Med 2017;177:930–8.
89. Stekovic S, Hofer SJ, Tripolt N, et al. Alternate Day Fasting Improves Physiological and Molecular Markers of Aging in Healthy, Non-obese Humans. Cell Metab 2019;30:462–76.e5.
90. Morisaki N, Saito I, Tamura K, et al. New indices of ischemic heart disease and aging: Studies on the serum levels of soluble intercellular adhesion molecule-1 (ICAM-1) and soluble vascular cell adhesion molecule-1 (VCAM-1) in patients with hypercholesterolemia and ischemic heart disease. Atherosclerosis 1997; 131:43–8.
91. de A Salgado ALF, Carvalho L de, Oliveira AC, et al. Insulin resistance index (HOMA-IR) in the differentiation of patients with non-alcoholic fatty liver disease and healthy individuals. Arquivos de gastroenterologia 2010;47:165–9.
92. Gayoso-Diz P, Otero-González A, Rodriguez-Alvarez MX, et al. Insulin resistance (HOMA-IR) cut-off values and the metabolic syndrome in a general adult population: Effect of gender and age: EPIRCE cross-sectional study. BMC Endocr Disord 2013;13. https://doi.org/10.1186/1472-6823-13-47.
93. Shashaj B, Luciano R, Contoli B, et al. Reference ranges of HOMA-IR in normal-weight and obese young Caucasians. Acta Diabetol 2016;53:251–60.
94. Harvie MN, Pegington M, Mattson MP, et al. The effects of intermittent or continuous energy restriction on weight loss and metabolic disease risk markers: a randomized trial in young overweight women. Int J Obes 2011;35:714–27.
95. Carter S, Clifton PM, Keogh JB. Effect of Intermittent Compared With Continuous Energy Restricted Diet on Glycemic Control in Patients With Type 2 Diabetes: A Randomized Noninferiority Trial. JAMA Netw Open 2018;1:e180756.
96. Hajek P, Przulj D, Pesola F, et al. A randomised controlled trial of the 5:2 diet. PLoS ONE 2021;16. https://doi.org/10.1371/journal.pone.0258853.
97. Olansky L. Strategies for management of intermittent fasting in patients with diabetes. Cleve Clin J Med 2017;84(357):358.
98. Corley BT, Carroll RW, Hall RM, et al. Intermittent fasting in Type 2 diabetes mellitus and the risk of hypoglycaemia: a randomized controlled trial. Diabetic Med 2018;35:588–94.
99. Goldhamer AC, Lisle DJ, Sultana P, et al. Medically supervised water-only fasting in the treatment of borderline hypertension. J Altern Complement Med 2002; 8:643–50.
100. Goldhamer A, Lisle D, Parpia B, et al. Medically supervised water-only fasting in the treatment of hypertension. J Manipulative Physiol Ther 2001;24:335–9.

101. Horne BD, Muhlestein JB, Lappé DL, et al. Randomized cross-over trial of short-term water-only fasting: Metabolic and cardiovascular consequences. Nutr Metab Cardiovasc Dis 2013;23:1050–7.

102. Jiang Y, Yang X, Dong C, et al. Five-day water-only fasting decreased metabolic-syndrome risk factors and increased anti-aging biomarkers without toxicity in a clinical trial of normal-weight individuals. Clin Translational Med 2021; 11:1–7.

103. Hutcheon DA. Malnutrition-induced Wernicke's encephalopathy following a water-only fasting diet. Nutr Clin Pract 2015;30:92–9.

104. Finnell JS, Saul BC, Goldhamer AC, et al. Is fasting safe? A chart review of adverse events during medically supervised, water-only fasting. BMC Complement Altern Med 2018;18:1–9.

105. Ogłodek E, Pilis Prof W. Is Water-Only Fasting Safe? Glob Adv Health Med 2021; 10. https://doi.org/10.1177/21649561211031178.

106. Leibel RL, Rosenbaum M, Hirsch J. Changes in Energy Expenditure Resulting from Altered Body Weight. New Engl J Med 1995;332:621–8.

107. Bray G. EFFECT OF CALORIC RESTRICTION ON ENERGY EXPENDITURE IN OBESE PATIENTS. Lancet 1969;294:397–8.

108. Brandhorst S, Choi IY, Wei M, et al. A Periodic Diet that Mimics Fasting Promotes Multi-System Regeneration, Enhanced Cognitive Performance, and Healthspan. Cell Metab 2015;22:86–99.

109. Wei M, Brandhorst S, Shelehchi M, et al. Fasting-mimicking diet and markers/risk factors for aging, diabetes, cancer, and cardiovascular disease. Sci Translational Med 2017;9:eaai8700.

110. Versini M, Jeandel PY, Rosenthal E, et al. Obesity in autoimmune diseases: Not a passive bystander. Autoimmun Rev 2014;13:981–1000.

111. Choi IY, Piccio L, Childress P, et al. A Diet Mimicking Fasting Promotes Regeneration and Reduces Autoimmunity and Multiple Sclerosis Symptoms. Cell Rep 2016;15:2136–46.

112. Cheng C-W, Villani V, Buono R, et al. Fasting-Mimicking Diet Promotes Ngn3-Driven β-Cell Regeneration to Reverse Diabetes. Cell 2017;168:775–88.e12.

113. Rangan P, Choi I, Wei M, et al. Fasting-Mimicking Diet Modulates Microbiota and Promotes Intestinal Regeneration to Reduce Inflammatory Bowel Disease Pathology. Cell Rep 2019;26:2704–19.e6.

114. Cox AJ, West NP, Cripps AW. Obesity, inflammation, and the gut microbiota. Lancet Diabetes Endocrinol 2015;3:207–15.

115. de Groot S, Lugtenberg RT, Cohen D, et al. Fasting mimicking diet as an adjunct to neoadjuvant chemotherapy for breast cancer in the multicentre randomized phase 2 DIRECT trial. Nat Commun 2020;11:1–9.

116. Caffa I, Spagnolo V, Vernieri C, et al. Fasting-mimicking diet and hormone therapy induce breast cancer regression. Nature 2020;583:620–4.

117. Longo VD, Mattson MP. Fasting: Molecular mechanisms and clinical applications. Cell Metab 2014;19:181–92.

118. Chang GR, Chiu YS, Wu YY, et al. Rapamycin protects against high fat diet-induced obesity in C57BL/6J mice. J Pharmacol Sci 2009;109:496–503.

119. Yang SB, Tien AC, Boddupalli G, et al. Rapamycin ameliorates age-dependent obesity associated with increased mTOR signaling in hypothalamic POMC neurons. Neuron 2012;75:425–36.

120. Leontieva OV, Paszkiewicz GM, Blagosklonny MV. Weekly administration of rapamycin improves survival and biomarkers in obese male mice on high-fat diet. Aging Cell 2014;13:616–22.

121. den Hartigh LJ, Goodspeed L, Wang SA, et al. Chronic oral rapamycin decreases adiposity, hepatic triglycerides and insulin resistance in male mice fed a diet high in sucrose and saturated fat. Exp Physiol 2018;103:1469–80.
122. Chang GR, Wu YY, Chiu YS, et al. Long-term administration of rapamycin reduces adiposity, but impairs glucose tolerance in high-fat diet-fed KK/HIJ mice. Basic Clin Pharmacol Toxicol 2009;105:188–98.
123. Houde VP, Brûlé S, Festuccia WT, et al. Chronic rapamycin treatment causes glucose intolerance and hyperlipidemia by upregulating hepatic gluconeogenesis and impairing lipid deposition in adipose tissue. Diabetes 2010;59:1338–48.
124. Bailey CJ, Turner RC. Metformin. Wood AJJ, editor. New Engl J Med 1996;334:574–9.
125. Martin-Montalvo A, de Cabo R. Mitochondrial Metabolic Reprogramming Induced by Calorie Restriction. Antioxid Redox Signaling 2013;19:310–20.
126. Paolisso G, Amato L, Eccellente R, et al. Effect of metformin on food intake in obese subjects. Eur J Clin Invest 1998;28:441–6.
127. Ning HH, Le J, Wang Q, et al. The effects of metformin on simple obesity: a meta-analysis. Endocrine 2018;62:528–34.
128. Guevara-Aguirre J, Balasubramanian P, Guevara-Aguirre M, et al. Growth hormone receptor deficiency is associated with a major reduction in pro-aging signaling, cancer, and diabetes in humans. Sci Translational Med 2011;3:20–3.
129. Guevara-Aguirre J, Procel P, Guevara C, et al. Despite higher body fat content, Ecuadorian subjects with Laron syndrome have less insulin resistance and lower incidence of diabetes than their relatives. Growth Horm IGF Res 2016;28:76–8.
130. Junnila RK, Duran-Ortiz S, Suer O, et al. Disruption of the GH receptor gene in adult mice increases maximal lifespan in females. Endocrinology 2016;157:4502–13.
131. Arum O, Bonkowski MS, Rocha JS, et al. The growth hormone receptor gene-disrupted mouse fails to respond to an intermittent fasting diet. Aging Cell 2009;8:756–60.
132. Preston SH, Vierboom YC, Stokes A. The role of obesity in exceptionally slow US mortality improvement. Proc Natl Acad Sci United States America 2018;115:957–61.
133. Ward ZJ, Bleich SN, Cradock AL, et al. Projected U.S. State-Level Prevalence of Adult Obesity and Severe Obesity. New Engl J Med 2019;381:2440–50.
134. Cawley J, Meyerhoefer C. The medical care costs of obesity: An instrumental variables approach. J Health Econ 2012;31:219–30.
135. Klein S, Fontana L, Young VL, et al. Absence of an Effect of Liposuction on Insulin Action and Risk Factors for Coronary Heart Disease. New Engl J Med 2004;350:2549–57.
136. Brandhorst S, Longo VD. Dietary Restrictions and Nutrition in the Prevention and Treatment of Cardiovascular Disease. Circ Res 2019;124:952–65.

Environmental Medicine
Exploring the Pollutome for Solutions to Chronic Diseases

Anne Marie Fine, NMD, FAAEM*, Lyn Patrick, ND

KEYWORDS

- Environmental medicine • Endocrine-disrupting chemicals • Diabetes • Obesity
- Pollutome

KEY POINTS

- The Pollutome contributes to chronic diseases.
- Endocrine-disrupting chemicals induce pancreatic cell dysfunction and contribute to obesity.
- The emerging specialty of Environmental Medicine is necessary to address the global rise in noncommunicable diseases.

OVERVIEW OF ENVIRONMENTAL CONTAMINANTS

The global rise of noncommunicable diseases (NCD), particularly obesity and diabetes, neurologic diseases, reproductive health problems, and specific cancers has initiated a groundswell of research addressing the causative and contributing roles of environmental pollutants in NCD (**Tables 1 and 2**). There are currently 40,000 chemical compounds in use in the United States.[1] Five thousand of those are considered high production volume chemicals (HPVC)- defined as synthetic chemical compounds produced or imported in greater than 11,000 kg/y. Only half of the HPVC have any biomonitoring or safety data related to their toxicity.[2] HPVC are considered to be ubiquitous in the environment and the human population is estimated to have universal exposure.

The exposome, defined as the sum of all environmental exposures, is considered the source of causative agents for NCD as nongenetic contribution to these diseases increases steadily. The pollutome specifically refers to the chemical exposure aspect of the exposome. This aspect has traditionally been underestimated in its effect on human health. According to the Lancet Commission on pollution and health, pollution is the largest environmental cause of disease and premature death in the world today.[2]

Environmental Medicine Education International, LLC, PO Box 802, Mancos, CO 81328, USA
* Corresponding author.
E-mail address: Dr.annemariefine@gmail.com

Phys Med Rehabil Clin N Am 33 (2022) 719–732
https://doi.org/10.1016/j.pmr.2022.04.010
1047-9651/22/© 2022 Elsevier Inc. All rights reserved.

Table 1
Obesogens

Obesogens	NHANES Detection %	Mechanism of Action	PMID
BPA	95.7% (2013–2014)	PPAR-¡ Agonist	32796699
		Increased Adipocyte	27760374
		Proliferation	27760374
		and differentiation	31884733
		Increased lipid uptake	31256736
		Negatively associated with TSH levels, T4, and free T4	31256736
		Positively associated with TPO antibodies	
		Estrogen agonist and antagonist	
		Binds to aryl hydrocarbon receptor and affects toxin metabolism	
BPS (BPA substitute)	89.4 (2013–2014)	Interferes with thyroid hormone	29146198
		Decreased T3 and T4	25775505
		Estrogenic, estrogen receptor binding	25775505
		Antiandrogenic	25775505
		Targets the PGC1α and the ERRγ genes	34899613
BPF (BPA substitute)	66.5 (2013–2014)	Interferes with thyroid hormone	29146198
		Decreased T3, Increased T4	25775505
		Increased thyroid weight	25775505
		Estrogenic	25775505
		Decreased adiponectin and secretion	25775505
		Estrogenic, estrogen receptor binding	25775505
		Antiandrogenic	
Phthalate Metabolites	75%–100% various		
DEHP (MEHP)		PPAR-¡ agonist	22953781
		Adipogenesis PPAR-α agonist	34899613
DEP, DBP, DINP (MBP, MEP, MiNP, MBP)		Antiandrogens	17589594
DEHP (MBzP, MEHHP, Meohp, MEP)		Antiandrogens	17589594
DEP, DBP (MBP, MpzP, MEP)		Insulin resistance	17589594
PFAS (PFOA, PFOS)	98%	PPAR-α, PPAR-¡ agonists	33986457
DDE	99%	Mitochondrial damage increased firmicutes-to-bacteroidetes ratio in gut	30915030 32050320

Landrigan and colleagues[2] describe the pollutome-disease connection as a body of research that has 3 Zones. (**Fig. 1**). As modified from Landrigan and colleagues Zone 1 may be described as the group of identified toxicants for which the causative

Table 2
Diabetogens

Diabetogens	NHANES Detection	Mechanism of Action	PMID
BPA	95.7%	Insulin resistance, beta-cell dysfunction, disrupts glucose homeostasis, inflammation, oxidative stress	30400886
DDT/DDE	98%	estrogen receptor agonist and antiandrogen reduced gene expression in pancreatic beta cells for response to hyperglycemia	33557243 33794904 26186133
Phthalates		Block insulin receptor sites Impair glucose transporter 4 Induce epigenetic changes that disrupt blood sugar regulation and oxidation of glucose Interference with different cell-signaling pathways involved in weight and glucose homeostasis	24130215 27822670
PCBs		promotes large lipid droplet (LD) formation through fat-specific protein 27 (Fsp27) leads to the induction of insulin resistance can be reversed with resveratrol in animal models	27837308

relationship to disease has been clearly established: lead, arsenic, mercury, asbestos, hexavalent chromium, benzene, and so forth.

Zone 2 contains the body of knowledge for emerging effects whereby the relationship between toxicants and disease is not quantified, though evidence for causation is growing. This would include the effects of organochlorine and organophosphate pesticides, phthalates, bisphenols (BPA, BPF, BPS), polybrominated diphenyl ethers (PBDE flame retardants), polycyclic aromatic hydrocarbons (PAHs), PM 2.5 (air pollution particulate matter 2.5 microns in diameter or less), and polychlorinated biphenyls (PCBs). These toxicants have been connected to developmental damage to the nervous system, postnatal effects on the developing nervous system in children, and neurologic/mental health conditions in adults.[3–5] They have also been identified as carcinogens (PBDE, PCBs), and endocrine-disrupting toxicants.[6]

Zone 3 includes contaminants of concern that are only now emerging as neurotoxicants, immune toxicants, endocrine disruptors, and carcinogens. This would include per and polyfluorinated compounds (PFAS), neonicotinoid pesticides, glyphosate, nanoparticles, microplastics, and others not yet recognized as part of the human body burden. Many common chemical exposures are emerging that may have profound effects on insulin/glucose homeostasis and adipose dysregulation. An example is the contaminants found in human adipose tissue studies that have been shown to cause adipose tissue inflammation—a known mechanism for insulin resistance and obesity.[7] These chemicals: ethyl tetradecanoate, 2-phenyltetralin, and 4,4-diisopropylbiphenyl are found as common ingredients in personal care products and cleaning products. 4,4-Diisopropylbiphenyl—a plasticizer also used as a thermal transfer fluid in industry—can vaporize as an air pollutant but its release into the environment is not monitored or reported. Ethyl tetradecanoate (myristic acid ethyl ester) is used in perfumes, cosmetics, as a food additive flavoring agent listed as only "flavor," and for the manufacture of artificial fibers, paints, varnishes, and glue. 2-Phenyltetralin is commonly found in personal care products and conventional cleaning products.

Pellizari and colleagues also identified 36 environmental chemicals as priorities for biomonitoring in the National Institutes of Health's Environmental influences on Child

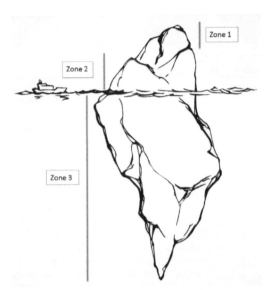

Fig. 1. The pollutome and current knowledge base related to toxicants and noncommunicable disease etiology.

Health Outcomes (ECHO) initiative.[1] Initially starting with 932 compounds, they identified a list based on risk for exposure, and identification as having endocrine, developmental, reproductive, and neurotoxic effects. Most of the listed chemicals would belong to Zone 3: alternative flame retardants, alternative plasticizers, alternative phenols: bisphenol B, bisphenol AF, organophosphorus-based flame retardants, perfluoroalkyl substances (PFAS), 11 organophosphate pesticides and finally, glyphosate. As health care providers, only one of these toxicants is currently available for testing in nonresearch practice settings (glyphosate).

ENDOCRINE DISRUPTORS

Endocrine-disrupting chemicals (EDCs) are chemicals that mimic, block, or interfere with hormones in the body's endocrine system. EDCs also have the ability to affect the immune and nervous systems. EDCs have been associated with a broad range of health issues, and affect the body at very low doses, in much the same way that hormones work at micromolecular levels, and often with nonmonotonic dose effects.

EDCs have rapidly gained recognition as troubling threats to public health. Certain organizations are spearheading the effort to accumulate the accelerating evidence for human health implications. They include the Endocrine Society, the International Federation of Gynecology and Obstetrics, and the American Academy of Pediatrics.[8] These organizations report both the impact of EDCs on fetal development, as well as the long latency between exposures in utero and disease, otherwise known as the Developmental Origins of Health and Disease or DOHaD.

The high cost of endocrine disruption has been documented in both the European Union and the United States. In the EU it is estimated that EDCs cost 157 billion Euros per year, or $209 billion USD. In the United States that figure is much higher at $340 billion USD per year or more than 2% of the nation's gross domestic product (GDP). The difference between the 2 nations was driven mainly by intelligence quotient (IQ) points lost and intellectual disability due to increased levels of exposure to polybrominated diphenyl ethers (11 million IQ points lost in the US with a cost of $266 billion vs 873,000 IQ points lost in the EU with a cost of $126 billion USD).[9]

These estimated costs document the urgent public threat caused by EDCs.

EDCs have been primarily demonstrated to cause diabetes and obesity, as well as contribute to deleterious effects on male and female reproductive health, alter the hypothalamic–pituitary–thyroid axis, and increase the risk of hormone-sensitive cancers.[8,10]

Type 2 diabetes is a silent, growing killer, with more than 450 million humans affected globally.[11] Around the world, the prevalence of obesity has nearly tripled between 1975 and 2015, with the death toll from obesity-related conditions reaching 1.6 million in 2015.[12] In 2012 the total estimated costs of diagnosed diabetes in the United States was $245 billion.[13]

Obesity added more than $342 billion to the US health care costs in 2013.[14] There is an urgent and unmet need to explore the underlying mechanisms for EDC exposure and how they predispose our population to obesity with its related comorbidities and increased risk for mortality.

This article will focus on 2 areas of human health that are directly related to endocrine disruptor exposure: obesity and type 2 diabetes.

OBESITY

The main toxicant contributors to obesity are BPA, phthalates, persistent organic pollutants (POPs), and DDT and its metabolite DDE.

BPA

EDCs such as Bisphenol A and its analogs BPS, BPF, and BPAF, phthalates, parabens, and PCBs have all been associated with the current epidemic of obesity and diabetes. Adipose tissue is an endocrine organ that is highly susceptible to perturbations by EDCs.[15]

Analyses have determined that activity, caloric intake, and genetics are insufficient to explain the magnitude and speed of the increase in the incidence of obesity. NHANES data compared BMI between US adults in 1988 and 2006 and found a 2.3 kg/m^2 increase in adult BMI in 2006 compared with 1988 even with the same amount of caloric intake (macronutrient specific) and energy spent.[16] Current evidence indicates that gene variants can only explain about 2.7% of the individual variation in BMI.[17]

Environmental chemicals, dubbed "obesogens," due to their promotion of adiposity, have been documented to contribute to these changes over the last 15 years. These chemicals impact metabolism through a variety of mechanisms such as microbiome disruption, effect on adipocytes, PPAR agonist activity, hormonal alterations of sex hormones or thyroid hormones, and promotion of insulin resistance.[10,18]

Bisphenol A or BPA is known as one of the top obesogens, a subset of EDCs that promote adiposity. Other obesogens include phthalates, tributyltin, pesticides, jet fuel, and dichlorodiphenyltrichloroethane (DDT).[6]

Over 600 peer-reviewed studies published since 2005 in scientific journals have examined the relationship between BPA (and its analogs) and obesity or diabetes. One recent meta-analysis concluded that *for every 1 ng/mL increase in urine BPA the risk for obesity was increased by 11%.*[19] The pooled OR of obesity for the highest versus lowest level of BPA exposure was 1.49.

BPA, BPS, and BPF were detected in 95.7%, 89.4%, and 66.5%, respectively, of randomly selected urine samples analyzed as part of NHANES 2013 to 2014.[20] As the awareness of the endocrine-disrupting effects of BPA have become known, the regrettable substitutions of BPS, BPF, and BPAF have entered chemical production. However, published research highlights similar endocrine-disrupting physiologic effects with these substitutions that are being marketed as "BPA-free."[21]

Bisphenol A is a monomer of polycarbonate plastics and one of the highest volume chemicals used in commerce. Polycarbonate is used in numerous consumer products that consumers are exposed to everyday, including food and water containers, baby bottles, lining of metal food and beverage cans, medical tubing, epoxy resins, and dental fillings.

BPA also demonstrates significant dermal exposure from thermal receipts, as free BPA applied to the outer layer of thermal receipt paper is present in very high (~20 mg BPA/g paper) quantities as a print developer.[22,23] In fact, BPA has been found to be even more absorbable transdermally following the use of hand sanitizer, on the order of the ranges provided in the 95th percentile according to the NHANES 2003/2004 data. At these values, epidemiologic evidence demonstrates a significant association with increased risk for developing cardiovascular disease and type 2 diabetes.[22]

PHTHALATES

Phthalates are plasticizers found in a variety of common consumer products; plastics, personal care products, food packaging, medical tubing, toys, house dust, and vinyl flooring. The high molecular weight phthalates such as di(2-ethylhexyl) phthalate (DEHP) are used primarily to make PVC plastic soft and flexible. Low molecular weight phthalates such as diethyl phthalate (DEP) are primarily used in personal care products. Phthalates are considered obesogens, diabetogens, and reproductive toxicants.[12,24]

In a cross-sectional study of postmenopausal women in the Women's Health Initiative, the sum total of DEHP metabolites in the 4th quartile versus the 1st quartile resulted in an odds ratio of 3.29 for obesity.[25] Other evidence arises from a large, population-based birth cohort whereby early and mid-pregnancy phthalate exposures were associated with higher weight gain 6 years postpartum, particularly among women who were overweight and obese before pregnancy.[26]

PERSISTENT ORGANIC POLLUTANTS

POPs are an identified group of toxicants known for their lipophilic nature and storage in adipose tissue. They are all organohalides (carbon chains bonded to chlorine, fluorine, and bromine) and as such do not degrade easily in or outside the body. They have long half-lives ranging from months to multiple decades in both adipose tissue and other organs, and as a result, they bioaccumulate over time in both humans and other animals, including fish.[6] The family of POPs includes organochlorine pesticides, PCBs, dioxins, difurans, the air pollutant PAH, brominated flame retardants, lindane and tributyltin—an organometal compound used on ships as a slimicide and also used in household items such as shower curtains. The family of perfluoronates (PFAS, commonly known as flame retardants, water-proofing, or nonstick chemicals) is considered POPs even though they are not stored in adipose tissue because of their persistence in the human body and long half-lives in the blood.[27]

The current list of identified POPs is not complete and new POPs are added as evidence of harm becomes available. The list is maintained by the Stockholm

Convention on Persistent Organic Pollutants, a global treaty enacted in 2004 as a part of the United Nations Environmental Programme.[28] This treaty seeks to have countries agree to reduce and eliminate the production and importation of POPs. As of December 2021, the United States is one of the very few countries that has not ratified nor enforced the treaty.

Specific individual POPs: DDE and PFOA, as well as groups of POPs (individual organochlorine pesticides and PCB congeners), have been linked in epidemiologic studies to increased risk for metabolic syndrome, type 2 diabetes, reproductive cancers, obesity, and nonalcoholic fatty liver disease.[29–32]

DICHLORO DIPHENYL TRICHLOROETHANE

DDT, a legacy pesticide banned in 1972, is currently found in most of the NHANES study population, as the metabolite p,p'-DDE.[33] DDT and DDE have been linked to increased risk for obesity in multiple studies. In a nested case-control study, Lee, and colleagues found that specific low levels of POPs at baseline could predict adiposity in a 20-year follow-up of controls who were diabetes-free.[18] The most consistent predictor of elevated BMI was serum levels of p,p'-DDE (a DDT metabolite that indicates historic exposure) which also predicted elevated triglycerides, higher HOMA-IR and lower HDL-cholesterol at year 20. The dose–response curve was a non-monotonic "U-shaped curve," which is not unusual for EDCs. Those in the 2nd and 3rd quartile of serum p,p'-DDE had a higher odds risk for increased BMI than those in the 4th quartile. In this population, serum PCBs (the higher chlorinated congeners PCB 146 and above) also predicted higher BMI, as well as higher triglycerides, higher HOMA-IR, and lower HDL-cholesterol at year 20.

Cirillo, and colleagues looked at generational effects of DDT in the Child Health and Development Studies cohort.[34] They assessed levels of serum DDT in the perinatal period of mothers (F0) and the relationship to risk for obesity and menarche in grand-daughters (F2). The F2 cohort that had normal weight grandmothers with elevated serum o,p'-DDT levels in the highest tertile were 2.6 times more likely to be obese than those with DDT levels in the 1st tertile. They were also 2.1 times more likely to have experienced early menarche.

In a meta-analysis of obesity and DDT levels, prenatal exposure to DDT has been shown to have either positive or no associations with obesity in overall populations of children followed out 20 to 50 years or in toddlers or school-aged children.[31] However, in that same meta-analysis, DDE showed consistent positive relationships with measurements of obesity.

In a small cohort of 100 obese and normal weight, diabetic and nondiabetic individuals in India, adipose tissue sampling of DDT revealed that obese individuals, regardless of their glycemic status had higher adipose concentrations of DDT that increased linearly with the degree of obesity.[35]

PER- AND POLYFLUOROALKYL SUBSTANCES

PFAS are a large chemical family of more than 4000 compounds used in a wide range of consumer products since the 1950s. Commonly known as nonstick, waterproofing, stain-proofing chemicals, the basic fluoride-carbon bond in PFAS is not vulnerable to degradation in biologic systems or in the environment. Therefore, PFAS have extremely long half-lives in the body from 1.5 to 21 years and have been detected in 98% of a representative sample of the US population.[36] They are identified by the Stockholm Convention as persistent organic compounds whose production should be reduced and eliminated. Public health concerns over drinking water contamination of PFAS in the United States and elsewhere have increasingly drawn public attention to these compounds. Continued exposure occurs through diet-the European Food Safety Authority (EFSA) estimated that "fish and other seafood" account for up to 86% of dietary PFAS exposure in adults.[37]

PFAS have been identified as obesogens in multiple studies. A meta-analysis of PFAS studies found positive associations between maternal PFOA (perfluoro-octanoic acid) concentrations but not PFOS or total PFAS and obesity indices in populations of preschoolers and school-aged children.[23]

In the POUNDS lost trial of 621 overweight and obese men and women, higher baseline levels of PFAS were significantly associated with a greater weight regain, primarily in women.[38] Women in the highest tertile of PFAS blood levels regained 1.7 to 2.2 kg more bodyweight than women in the lowest tertile. Higher levels of PFAS were also related to lower resting metabolic rate both during the weight loss period and the weight regain period.

DIABETES

The epidemic of diabetes is also largely influenced by the pollutome. While obesity has traditionally been thought of as the impetus for Type 2 diabetes, about 75% to 80% of obese people never develop Type 2 diabetes, data inferring that there are other environmental factors at play such as the endocrine disrupters listed above.[39] The diabetogens included in EDC-2 Scientific Statement: BPA, arsenic, phthalates, perfluorinates (PFOS), diethyl hexyl phthalate (DEHP), dioxin (TCDD), and the mixture of BPA, TCDD, PCB-153, and DEHP, are an incomplete list as more research has been published examining organochlorine and organophosphate pesticides as well as the drinking water contaminant arsenic. A more detailed review of recent literature than is possible in this article was published by one of the authors in 2020.[12]

BPA

BPA is a classic diabetogen. A diabetogen is an endocrine disruptor that is able to produce insulin resistance, or damage or disrupt pancreatic B-cells. BPA is also a well-known obesogen, but not all diabetogens are considered obesogens. This leads us to the concept of "metabolically obese despite normal weight" (MONW), an emerging group of individuals who have metabolic syndrome with insulin resistance and hypertriglyceridemia despite having a normal BMI.[6]

BPA in animal models produced hyperinsulinemia and insulin resistance that are associated with pancreatic B-cell disruption.[40] BPA is also an estrogen agonist and has been shown to impair glucose homeostasis, resulting in pancreatic beta-cell dysfunction, inflammation, oxidative stress, and insulin resistance. BPA binding to estrogen receptors at the physiologic range or below has the ability to disrupt the islets of Langerhans, which is responsible for glucose metabolism.[41] BPA binding to pancreatic beta-cells leads to insulin resistance.[6] In the meta-analysis described in this paragraph, BPA was found to be positively associated with Type-2 diabetes risk.[40]

While animal studies and cross-sectional human studies have demonstrated an association between BPA and insulin resistance, type 2 diabetes, and other metabolic diseases, the data are still emerging on human studies whereby BPA is administered to the individuals.

In the first study that directly administered BPA to individuals in a single oral dose, alterations in insulin/C-peptide secretion were found.[42] In this study they used the dose of 50 µg/kg body weight, which has been predicted by US regulators (Food and Drug Administration, Environmental Protection Agency) to be the maximum, safe daily oral BPA dose over the lifetime, a dose presumed safe.

PHTHALATES

Phthalates have been shown in animal research to block insulin receptor sites, impair glucose transporter 4, and induce epigenetic changes that disrupt blood sugar regulation and the oxidation of glucose for energy.[43] In addition, these effects begin *in utero* and the accumulation of phthalates continues through lactation. Due to their storage in fat, phthalate body burden continues throughout life.

Phthalates are also diabetogens. In the Nurses Health Study II (NHSII), the metabolites of DEHP were found to increase the risk of Type 2 diabetes.[44] In this study, the OR comparing the 4th quartile to the first, was nearly doubled.

Interestingly, analysis of joint associations between BPA and butyl phthalates in the NHSII showed that the effects of these 2 classes of compounds were multiplicative. As toxicants in our environment rarely, if ever, show up singly in our bodies, this is a useful research strategy for identifying true risk factor combinations and their magnitude in real-life populations.

PESTICIDES

Multiple studies have assessed risk for T2D based on pesticide exposure resulting in both increased risk for individual pesticides and pesticide groups.

Research published in 2006 showed that an identified group of POPs (organochlorine pesticides and PCBs) had an increased OR for T2D of 38.0 in a group of obese individuals based on a single measurement of a group of POPs (organochlorine pesticides and one PCB) as part of the NHANES database.[45] In 2015, another group published a nested case-control study following the young adults in the CARDIA cohort who had baseline measurements in 1987 to 1988.[29]

Follow-up from 2005 to 2006 showed that of all POPs tested (8 organochlorine pesticides, 22 PCBs congeners, and 1 polybrominated biphenyl (PBB)) risk for incident T2D was highest for the second sextile of trans-nonachlor, oxychlordane, mirex, highly chlorinated PCBs, and PBB 153—a finding that suggests low-dose effects. The adjusted OR in the second sextile versus the lowest sextile was 5.3 overall and 20.1 for body mass index $\geq$ 30 kg/m^2. This both implicates low-level exposure effects and increased risk for a diabetogenic toxicant effect in higher BMI individuals.

TREATMENT APPROACHES

For both BPA and its analogs, phthalates, and arsenic, the treatment approach follows the first rule of environmental medicine: Avoidance.[38] The half-lives of these substances are very short, and avoiding current exposures allows the substances to naturally be metabolized and excreted from the body. There is some evidence that both BPA and phthalates have some degree of storage in fat. In a small pilot study, both BPA and mono-ethylhexyl phthalic acid (MEHP) were found to be present in individuals who did not have detectable levels in serum and MEHP was found in the sweat at concentrations double that of the urine.[46,47] Many toxicants are sequestered in different body compartments such as bone, adipose tissue, and brain and thus do not show up on blood or urine testing. However, certain therapies such as sauna which induces sweating will increase the excretion of lipophilic toxicants into the sweat, which in the study just referenced, exceeded the amount excreted in the urine and serum.[48] This result showed that BPA and phthalates were able to be stored in fat, but could be voided via sweat.

For BPA avoidance, the focus should be on avoiding canned food and beverages, even the ones that claim to be BPA-free, plastic bottles and containers, and thermal receipts, which are coated in BPA. For avoiding thermal receipts, one strategy is to simply say "no receipt" to the cashier, as the BPA transdermal effects transpire in seconds.[49]

For avoiding phthalates, plastics must similarly be avoided. In addition, avoidance of all products that are fragranced including personal care products, laundry detergent, cleaning products can be recommended. The phthalates fall under the term "fragrance" on the label and will not be separately listed.

The main sources of intake of polychlorinated dibenzodioxins, dibenzofurans, and biphenyls in the body of an average US citizen have been shown to be represented by animal products (meat, fish, eggs, milk, and dairy products). In accordance with US national food traditions, the largest contribution to the accumulation in the human body of these toxicants from food is made by meat and dairy products.[32]

Treatment approaches for POPs whereby body burden has accumulated over long periods of time necessitate appropriate interventions; avoidance alone is inadequate.

There are few cohort studies addressing intervention for POP exposure, the majority coming from rice bran oil contamination with dioxins, difurans, and PCBs in Japanese and Taiwanese populations in 1968 and 1979 known as "Yusho" (oil disease) and "Yucheng" incidents.[50] Interventional pilot trials using rice bran fiber (10 g daily) and cholestyramine (4 g three times daily) significantly increased fecal elimination of difurans.[51] Oral chlorella pyrenoidosa at a dose of 2 g three times a day was shown to significantly decrease levels of dioxin and PCBs in breastmilk of women in the Yusho cohort. It was assumed this was due to increased fecal excretion of these toxicants, although that was not directly measured in the trial.[52]

SUMMARY

Standard medical interventions for type 2 diabetes and obesity concentrate on weight loss, caloric restriction, and increased exercise as well as medication improving glucose uptake and excretion, and appetite control. While these interventions may be helpful, they ignore the strong evidence for toxicant-induced endocrine disruption as controlling mechanisms in these diseases processes.

Adequate evaluation, laboratory testing, and both avoidance education and strategies for decreasing body burden may be necessary to stem the global epidemic of obesity and diabetes. Implementing environmental medicine-based education and strategies in medical approaches to endocrine disruptor-related conditions may be a crucial missing piece in current medical practice.

CLINICS CARE POINTS

- Educate your patients on the avoidance of BPA. No plastic water bottles, food containers, canned food or drink, don't touch thermal receipts, and eat mostly fresh food to avoid packaging.
- Educate your patients on avoidance of phthalates. This means avoiding plastics and especially polyvinyl chloride (PVC), and all scented personal care products including plug in air fresheners.

- Educate your patients on avoidance of Persistent Organic Pollutants (POPs)- -avoid farmed salmon and farmed fish due to their PCB and pesticide content. Avoid butter, organic and conventional due to high content of PCBs, and eat a plant-based, non-GMO organic diet due to its lower content of POPs.

DISCLOSURE

The authors have nothing to disclose related to this article

REFERENCES

1. Pellizzari ED, Woodruff TJ, Boyles RR, et al. Environmental influences on Child Health Outcomes). Identifying and Prioritizing Chemicals with Uncertain Burden of Exposure: Opportunities for Biomonitoring and Health-Related Research. Environ Health Perspect 2019;127(12):126001, 2019 Dec 18. Erratum in: Environ Health Perspect. 2020 Jan;128(1):19002. Erratum in: Environ Health Perspect. 2021 Apr;129(4):49001.
2. Landrigan PJ, Fuller R, Acosta NJR, et al. The Lancet Commission on pollution and health. Lancet 2018;391(10119):462–512. Erratum in: Lancet. 2018 Feb 3;391(10119):430. PMID: 29056410.
3. Grova N, Schroeder H, Olivier JL, et al. Epigenetic and Neurological Impairments Associated with Early Life Exposure to Persistent Organic Pollutants. Int J Genomics 2019;2019:2085496. https://doi.org/10.1155/2019/2085496.
4. Bellinger DC. Prenatal Exposures to Environmental Chemicals and Children's Neurodevelopment: An Update. Saf Health Work 2013;4(1):1–11.
5. Reuben A, Schaefer JD, Moffitt TE, et al. Association of Childhood Lead Exposure With Adult Personality Traits and Lifelong Mental Health. JAMA Psychiatry 2019; 76(4):418–25.
6. Gore AC, Chappell VA, Fenton SE, et al. EDC-2: The Endocrine Society's Second Scientific Statement on Endocrine-Disrupting Chemicals. Endocr Rev 2015;36(6): E1–150.
7. Rolle-Kampczyk U, Gebauer S, Haange SB, et al. Accumulation of distinct persistent organic pollutants is associated with adipose tissue inflammation. Sci Total Environ 2020;748:142458. https://doi.org/10.1016/j.scitotenv.2020.142458.
8. Kahn LG, Philippat C, Nakayama SF, et al. Endocrine-disrupting chemicals: implications for human health. Lancet Diabetes Endocrinol 2020;8(8):703–18.
9. Trasande L, Zoeller RT, Hass U, et al. Estimating burden and disease costs of exposure to endocrine-disrupting chemicals in the European union. J Clin Endocrinol Metab 2015;100(4):1245–55.
10. Gupta R, Kumar P, Fahmi N, et al. Endocrine disruption and obesity: A current review on environmental obesogens. Curr Res Green Sustainable Chem 2020;3: 100009. https://doi.org/10.1016/j.crgsc.2020.06.002.
11. Misra BB, Misra A. The chemical exposome of type 2 diabetes mellitus: Opportunities and challenges in the omics era. Diabetes Metab Syndr 2020;14(1): 23–38.
12. Patrick L. Diabetes and Toxicant Exposure. Integr Med (Encinitas) 2020;19(1): 16–23.
13. Cannon A, Handelsman Y, Heile M, et al. Burden of Illness in Type 2 Diabetes Mellitus. J Manag Care Spec Pharm 2018;24(9-a Suppl):S5–13.
14. Biener A, Cawley J, Meyerhoefer C. The High and Rising Costs of Obesity to the US Health Care System. J Gen Intern Med 2017;32(Suppl 1):6–8.

15. Janesick AS, Blumberg B. Obesogens: an emerging threat to public health. Am J Obstet Gynecol 2016;214(5):559–65.
16. Brown RE, Sharma AM, Ardern CI, et al. Secular differences in the association between caloric intake, macronutrient intake, and physical activity with obesity. Obes Res Clin Pract 2016;10(3):243–55.
17. Equsquiza R, Blumberg B. Environmental obesogens and their impact on susceptibility to obesity: new mechanisms and chemicals. Endocrinology 2020; 161(3).
18. Mohajer N, Du CY, Checkcinco C, et al. Obesogens: How They Are Identified and Molecular Mechanisms Underlying Their Action. Front Endocrinol (Lausanne) 2021;12:780888. https://doi.org/10.3389/fendo.2021.780888.
19. Wu W, Li M, Liu A, et al. Bisphenol A and the Risk of Obesity a Systematic Review With Meta-Analysis of the Epidemiological Evidence. Dose Response 2020;18(2). https://doi.org/10.1177/1559325820916949. 1559325820916949.
20. Lehmler HJ, Liu B, Gadogbe M, et al. Exposure to Bisphenol A, Bisphenol F, and Bisphenol S in U.S. Adults and Children: The National Health and Nutrition Examination Survey 2013-2014. ACS Omega 2018;3(6):6523–32.
21. Rochester JR, Bolden AL. Bisphenol S and F: A Systematic Review and Comparison of the Hormonal Activity of Bisphenol A Substitutes. Environ Health Perspect 2015;123(7):643–50.
22. Hormann AM, Vom Saal FS, Nagel SC, et al. Holding thermal receipt paper and eating food after using hand sanitizer results in high serum bioactive and urine total levels of bisphenol A (BPA). PLoS One 2014;9(10):e110509.
23. Bernier MR, Vandenberg LN. Handling of thermal paper: Implications for dermal exposure to bisphenol A and its alternatives. PLoS One 2017;12(6):e0178449.
24. Pizzorno J. Is the Diabetes Epidemic Primarily Due to Toxins? Integr Med (Encinitas) 2016;15(4):8–17.
25. Díaz Santana MV, Hankinson SE, Bigelow C, et al. Urinary concentrations of phthalate biomarkers and weight change among postmenopausal women: a prospective cohort study. Environ Health 2019;18(1):20.
26. Philips EM, Jaddoe VWV, Deierlein A, et al. Exposures to phthalates and bisphenols in pregnancy and postpartum weight gain in a population-based longitudinal birth cohort. Environ Int 2020;144:106002. https://doi.org/10.1016/j.envint.2020.106002.
27. Corsini E, Luebke RW, Germolec DR, et al. Perfluorinated compounds: emerging POPs with potential immunotoxicity. Toxicol Lett 2014;230(2):263–70.
28. Hung H, Katsoyiannis AA, Guardans R. Ten years of global monitoring under the Stockholm Convention on Persistent Organic Pollutants (POPs): Trends, sources and transport modelling. Environ Pollut 2016;217:1–3. https://doi.org/10.1016/j.envpol.2016.05.035.
29. Lee DH, Steffes MW, Sjödin A, et al. Low dose of some persistent organic pollutants predicts type 2 diabetes: a nested case-control study. Environ Health Perspect 2010;118(9):1235–42.
30. Lee DH, Steffes MW, Sjödin A, et al. Low dose organochlorine pesticides and polychlorinated biphenyls predict obesity, dyslipidemia, and insulin resistance among people free of diabetes. PLoSOne 2011;6(1):e15977.
31. Mohanto NC, Ito Y, Kato S, et al. Life-Time Environmental Chemical Exposure and Obesity: Review of Epidemiological Studies Using Human Biomonitoring Methods. Front Endocrinol (Lausanne) 2021;12:778737. https://doi.org/10.3389/fendo.2021.778737.

32. Deierlein AL, Rock S, Park S. Persistent Endocrine-Disrupting Chemicals and Fatty Liver Disease. Curr Environ Health Rep 2017;4(4):439–49.

33. Wattigney WA, Irvin-Barnwell E, Pavuk M, et al. Regional Variation in Human Exposure to Persistent Organic Pollutants in the United States, NHANES. J Environ Public Health 2015;2015:571839. https://doi.org/10.1155/2015/571839.

34. Cirillo PM, La Merrill MA, Krigbaum NY, et al. Grandmaternal Perinatal Serum DDT in Relation to Granddaughter Early Menarche and Adult Obesity: Three Generations in the Child Health and Development Studies Cohort. Cancer Epidemiol Biomarkers Prev 2021;30(8):1480–8.

35. Tawar N, Banerjee BD, Mishra BK, et al. Adipose Tissue Levels of DDT as Risk Factor for Obesity and Type 2 Diabetes Mellitus. Indian J Endocrinol Metab 2021;25(2):160–5.

36. Calafat AM, Wong LY, Kuklenyik Z, et al. Polyfluoroalkyl chemicals in the U.S. population: data from the National Health and Nutrition Examination Survey (NHANES) 2003-2004 and comparisons with NHANES 1999-2000. Environ Health Perspect 2007;115(11):1596–602.

37. Sunderland EM, Hu XC, Dassuncao C, et al. A review of the pathways of human exposure to poly- and perfluoroalkyl substances (PFASs) and present understanding of health effects. J Expo Sci Environ Epidemiol 2019;29(2):131–47.

38. Liu G, Dhana K, Furtado JD, et al. Perfluoroalkyl substances and changes in body weight and resting metabolic rate in response to weight-loss diets: A prospective study. Plos Med 2018;15(2):e1002502.

39. McLaughlin T, Abbasi F, Lamendola C, et al. Heterogeneity in the prevalence of risk factors for cardiovascular disease and type 2 diabetes mellitus in obese individuals: effect of differences in insulin sensitivity. Arch Intern Med 2007;167(7):642–8.

40. Alonso-Magdalena P, Ropero AB, Soriano S, et al. Bisphenol-A: a new diabetogenic factor? Hormones 2010;9:118–26.

41. Hwang S, Lim JE, Choi Y, et al. Bisphenol A exposure and type 2 diabetes mellitus risk: a meta-analysis. BMC Endocr Disord 2018;18(1):81.

42. Stahlhut RW, Myers JP, Taylor JA, et al. Experimental BPA Exposure and Glucose-Stimulated Insulin Response in Adult Men and Women. J Endocr Soc 2018;2(10):1173–87.

43. Crinnion W, Pizzorno J. Clinical environmental medicine. St. Louis, Missouri: Elsevier; 2019.

44. Sun Q, Cornelis MC, Townsend MK, et al. Association of urinary concentrations of bisphenol A and phthalate metabolites with risk of type 2 diabetes: a prospective investigation in the Nurses' Health Study (NHS) and NHSII cohorts. Environ Health Perspect 2014;122(6):616–23.

45. Lee DH, Lee IK, Song K, et al. A strong dose-response relation between serum concentrations of persistent organic pollutants and diabetes: results from the National Health and Examination Survey 1999-2002. Diabetes Care 2006;29(7):1638–44.

46. Genuis SJ, Beesoon S, Birkholz D, et al. Human excretion of bisphenol A: blood, urine, and sweat (BUS) study. J Environ Public Health 2012;2012:185731. https://doi.org/10.1155/2012/185731.

47. Genuis SJ, Beesoon S, Lobo RA, et al. Human elimination of phthalate compounds: blood, urine, and sweat (BUS) study. ScientificWorldJournal 2012;2012:615068. https://doi.org/10.1100/2012/615068.

48. Genuis S, Kelln K. Toxicant Exposure and Bioaccumulation: A Common and Potentially Reversible Cause of Cognitive Dysfunction and Dementia. Behav Neurol 2015. https://doi.org/10.1155/2015/620143.
49. vom Saal FS, Welshons WV. Evidence that bisphenol A (BPA) can be accurately measured without contamination in human serum and urine, and that BPA causes numerous hazards from multiple routes of exposure. Mol Cell Endocrinol 2014; 398(1–2):101–13.
50. Furue M, Ishii Y, Tsukimori K, Tsuji G. Aryl Hydrocarbon Receptor and Dioxin-Related Health Hazards— Lessons from Yusho. Int J Mol Sci 2021;22:708. https://doi.org/10.3390/ijms22020708.
51. Iida T, Nakagawa R, Hirakawa H, et al. Clinical trial of a combination of rice bran fiber and cholestyramine for promotion of fecal excretion of retained polychlorinated dibenzofuran and polychlorinated biphenyl in Yu-Cheng patients. Fukuoka Igaku Zasshi 1995;86(5):226–33.
52. Nakano S, Noguchi T, Takekoshi H, et al. Maternal-fetal distribution and transfer of dioxins in pregnant women in Japan, and attempts to reduce maternal transfer with Chlorella (Chlorella pyrenoidosa) supplements. Chemosphere 2005;61(9): 1244–55.

Functional Medicine Approaches to Neurodegeneration

Datis Kharrazian, PhD[a,b,c,*]

KEYWORDS

- Functional medicine • Neurodegeneration • Personalized medicine
- Lifestyle medicine

KEY POINTS

- Neurodegenerative diseases are progressive diseases that lead to the inability to work and function and induce significant costs to families and society.
- Drug interventions focused on protein aggregate end-products have been unsuccessful in reversing or slowing down the progression of the disease.
- Multivariate models that address upstream pathophysiological mechanisms show promise in reducing the progression of neurodegenerative diseases and potentially reversing symptoms.

INTRODUCTION AND BACKGROUND

Neurodegenerative diseases impact more than 6 million Americans, and current predictions estimate the rates of neurodegenerative diseases will double in the next 30 years.[1] These diseases are progressive with increasing loss of brain function throughout their course. Overtime, those suffering from neurodegenerative diseases will lose their ability to work and function efficiently in society.[2] Families and society are burdened with skyrocketing costs to provide care for those who are unable to perform activities of daily living.[3] There is an urgent need to develop treatment strategies to both reduce the incidence of neurodegenerative diseases and to delay the progression of the disease.

The pathophysiology of neurodegenerative diseases is complex and involves both genetic susceptibility (APOE, TREM2, APP/PS1/PS2, MAPT, C90RFZ2/GRN, SOD1) and various metabolic and lifestyle factors.[4] Attempts to treat neurodegenerative diseases as downstream proteinopathy diseases by designing drugs to reduce protein

[a] Department of Neurology, Harvard Medical School, Boston, MA 02155, USA; [b] Department of Neurology, Massachusetts General Hospital, Charlestown, MA 02155, USA; [c] Department of Preventive Medicine, Loma Linda University School of Medicine, Loma Linda, CA 92350, USA
* Department of Neurology, Harvard Medical School, Boston, MA 02155.
E-mail address: Datis_Kharrazian@hms.harvard.edu

Phys Med Rehabil Clin N Am 33 (2022) 733–743
https://doi.org/10.1016/j.pmr.2022.04.011
1047-9651/22/© 2022 Elsevier Inc. All rights reserved.

misfolding and aggregation have failed. These univariate models that attempted to treat the disease as a single biological end-product have been unsuccessful. More than 2000 clinical trials and billions of dollars have been spent unsuccessfully to treat neurodegenerative disease as a single end-product proteinopathy.[5]

It is becoming clear that the treatment of neurodegenerative disease involves managing upstream metabolic processes of the disease and that these multivariate upstream mechanisms may differ from one individual to another.[6] The development of personalized medicine models to treat these upstream multivariate processes has shown promise and provides proof of concept. A personalized 12-week multivariate treatment model called the "brain fitness program" was recently conducted. In this study, participants were given personalized counseling for diet, exercise, and goal-oriented behaviors as combined interventions. The results of these interventions found improved cognition and increased volume size of the hippocampus with pre and post-quantitative MRI.[7] Successful case study report series using an individualized multivariate functional medicine model have also been reported in the literature.[8] The functional medicine model develops personalized approaches to modulate upstream pathophysiological variables that, if left unchecked, could lead to downstream pathophysiological patterns promoting proteinopathies and neurodegenerative diseases.

According to the National Institutes of Health, upstream lifestyle factors that promote neurodegenerative diseases include lack of physical activity, unhealthy diet, toxin exposure, drug and alcohol abuse, and medical conditions such as obesity, hypertension, diabetes, chronic inflammatory conditions, certain infectious diseases, and certain medications.[9] The combination of these individualized multivariate mechanisms in combination with susceptible genes leads to neurodegenerative diseases. The development of a personalized approach to reduce and change the expression of these downstream multivariate risk factors is the hallmark of a functional medicine approach. The functional medicine model involves an individualized treatment plan that is unique to each patient and not generalized to the disease itself. In this article, a review of a functional medicine model to support individuals suffering from neurodegenerative disease will be presented.

EARLY DETECTION AND PREVENTIVE MANAGEMENT VERSUS LATE-STAGE DIAGNOSIS

A key feature of a functional medicine approach to neurodegenerative diseases involves early detection and a personalized treatment plan to prevent or delay the progression of the disease. Late-stage diagnosis leads to poor clinical prognosis in both functional medicine and conventional approaches to neurodegenerative disease management. Unfortunately, in the conventional health care system, the diagnosis of neurodegenerative diseases is not made until the late stages of the disease.[10] For example, the diagnosis and treatment of Alzheimer's disease are not provided until a patient has significant loss in 2 or more cognitive domains (executive function, complex attention, learning and memory, language, perpetual motor, or social cognition) and significant disability in performing activities of daily living. This typically occurs in Stage 5 of the 7 stages of Alzheimer's disease. In these late stages, significant irreversible amyloid and tau protein aggregation in the brain and signs of cortical atrophy make prognosis poor for any form of intervention.

One of the key differences in the clinical management of neurodegenerative diseases in a functional medicine model is to identify early loss of function associated with neurodegenerative disease and implement preventive strategies as soon as possible to avoid progression. A functional medicine model identifies potential dementia in Stages 2 to 3 of Alzheimer's disease, when the patient may have a subjective loss of cognitive function or mild cognitive impairments. Interventions in these early stages to reduce risk factors and improve cognitive function include dietary and lifestyle modifications, intermittent fasting, and nutraceuticals. These interventions reduce downstream risk factors to delay or prevent the progression of the disease and improve brain health and function. Functional medicine strategies offer no effective method to reverse brain atrophy or remove protein aggregates such as amyloid plaque or alpha-synuclein from the brain. Early intervention and treatment to reduce risk factors and to optimize general brain function is the hallmark of a functional medicine approach to neurodegenerative diseases. Therefore, the model has limitations in its ability to support neurodegenerative diseases.

PATHOPHYSIOLOGICAL VARIABLES OF NEURODEGENERATIVE DISEASES

The pathophysiology of neurodegenerative diseases includes mitochondria failure in neuron and neuroglia cellular bioenergetics, neuroinflammation, blood–brain barrier permeability, impaired neuron signaling, impaired mitophagy and autophagy, inefficient mitochondria biogenesis, excessive synaptic pruning, gut–brain axis dysfunction, loss of microglia synthesis of hormones, reduced brain-derived neurotrophic factor, inefficient cerebral circulation, oxidative stress, neuron insulin resistance, and impaired axonal branching.[11–16] These pathophysiological mechanisms ultimately lead to misfolding of proteins found in neurons. These misfolded proteins aggregate together to produce an inflammatory response and block healthy neurotransmission that leads to neuron death and brain atrophy.[17]

In a functional medicine approach to neurodegenerative disease, it is essential to identify and change the expression of these pathophysiological variables as uniquely expressed by each individual. Personalized approaches treat the patient rather than focus specifically on the disease itself. The clinical focus is on an individualized multivariate model to address physiologic factors that promote downstream neurodegenerative changes. In the subsequent paragraphs, a review of these pathophysiological variables and clinical approaches will be provided, starting with mitochondria dysfunction.

MITOCHONDRIA DYSFUNCTION AND NEURODEGENERATIVE DISEASES

Mitochondria impairment is a central feature of neurodegenerative disease.[18] Dysfunction in neuron ATP levels can lead to reduced neuron endurance, neurotransmission dysfunction, and increased breakdown leading to the production of misfolded proteins. Mitochondria dysfunction in neuroglia can lead to impaired protein-debris clearing and impaired autophagy, altered neuroinflammation modulation, and impaired neurotransmission modulation. As neurodegenerative diseases progress, they activate inflammatory and oxidative stress pathways that further uncouple and injure existing mitochondria, leading to a vicious feedforward cycle.[19]

Direct associations with brain mitochondria function and neurodegenerative changes exist.[20] Mitochondria homeostasis involves the ability to generate new mitochondria (mitochondria biogenesis), for mitochondria to combine together to meet energy demands (mitochondria fusion), to break apart mitochondria organelles (mitochondria fission), and to remove unhealthy mitochondria from the cellular space (mitophagy).[21]

A functional medicine model implements clinical strategies to optimize mitochondria function and homeostasis. Various lifestyle and physiologic mechanisms impact mitochondria homeostasis (**Fig. 1**). The development of mitochondria is

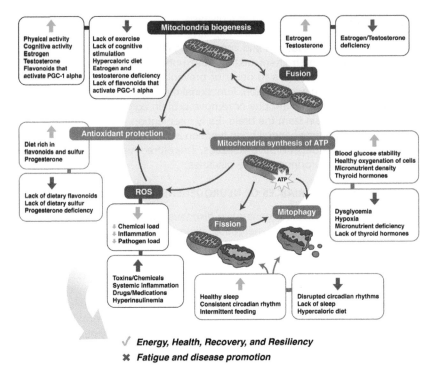

Fig. 1. Healthy and impaired bioenergetics.

essential for healthy brain function, neuroplasticity, and disease resistance.[22] Mitochondria biogenesis is activated by physical activity and cognitive activity.[23,24] In a functional medicine model, personalized approaches to support brain function include regular physical exercise and cognitive tasks such as jigsaw puzzles, crossword puzzles, chess, and sudoku. Hormones are also important for mitochondria biogenesis and neuroprotection. Specifically, estrogen and testosterone provide anabolic activity to support mitochondria biogenesis.[25] Many polyphenols found in fruits and vegetables have the ability to modulate the cellular expression of PGC-1 alpha and NrF2 to activate mitochondria biogenesis. These include flavonoids that are found in resveratrol, quercetin, curcumin, green tea, pomegranate, and many other colorful fruits and vegetables.[26] Several clinical trials and meta-analyses have shown that diets enriched in polyphenols may have protective effects against neurodegenerative diseases.[27] These protective flavonoid-rich diets and nutraceutical extracts are used in functional medicine to help reduce the expression of neurodegenerative diseases.

Mitochondria dysfunction and oxidative stress play a role in the pathophysiology of neurodegeneration. Increased oxidative stress damages mitochondria membranes and uncouples ATP production. This leads to energy-linked excitotoxic models of neuron injury that cause degenerative changes and altered neurotransmission.[28] Oxidative stress is promoted by exogenous factors such as environmental pollutants, heavy metals, UV radiation, and industrialized chemicals.[29] Functional medicine strategies to reduce chemical load includes reducing household xenobiotic exposures (pesticides, food additives, industrialized cosmetics, and so forth), using high-efficiency particulate air (HEPA) filters, nutraceuticals to support hepatic biotransformation, and polyphenolic nutraceuticals to combat oxidative stress. Natural compounds including alpha-lipoic acid, resveratrol, curcumin, n-acetylcysteine, and isolated polyphenols found in colorful fruits and vegetables have been shown to protect the mitochondria and exhibit neuroprotective properties.[30–32] Hormones play a significant role in supporting mitochondria bioenergetics and also exhibit neuroprotective properties.[33] Clinical evaluation of hormone status and potential hormone replacement therapy is a common feature of personalized approaches to neurodegenerative diseases in a functional medicine model.

Caloric intake has a tremendous impact on cellular bioenergetics and mitochondria function. A hypercaloric diet promotes neurodegenerative changes in animal models by reducing mitochondria biogenesis and increasing oxidative stress and mitochondria injury.[34] High caloric intake has been found to increase the relative risk of neurodegenerative disease development.[35] Conversely, caloric restriction has been found to attenuate proteinopathies such as beta-amyloid in animal models.[36] Clinical strategies to manage caloric intake and intermittent fasting strategies are commonly used in functional medicine approaches to neurodegenerative diseases. Intermittent fasting can promote autophagy and mitophagy, which are critical to remove protein aggregates that lead to neurodegenerative changes.[37] Recent research in animals found that intermittent fasting increases adult hippocampal neurogenesis.[38] Managing caloric intake and intermittent fasting strategies are used in a functional medicine model to address neurodegenerative diseases.

Mitochondria homeostasis and neurodegenerative disease risk are also significantly impacted by sleep and circadian rhythms. Disruption in circadian clocks has been found to impact neuroinflammation, redox status, synaptic homeostasis, proteostasis, neuronal metabolism, blood–brain barrier integrity, and glymphatic flow, all of which promote neurodegenerative pathophysiology.[39] Sleep disturbances and disrupted circadian rhythms have been implicated as risk factors for Alzheimer's disease, Parkinson's disease, and accelerated brain aging.[40] Targeting sleep and normal circadian function are therapeutic strategies in neurodegenerative diseases.[41] A functional medicine model uses strategies to improve sleep and optimize circadian rhythm consistency, such as sleep hygiene, melatonin, nutraceuticals, continuous airway pressure devices, light therapy, and other individualized approaches.

THE GUT–BRAIN CONNECTION

Developments in research on the gut–brain axis and the role the microbiome plays in neurodegenerative disorders are growing. Bidirectional communication between the microbiome and the brain via the vagus nerve, gut hormones, immunokines, lipopolysaccharides, and short-chain fatty acids exist.[42] Inflammation in the gut, dysbiosis, and intestinal permeability have been shown to upregulate microglia in the brain and promote neuroinflammatory changes associated with neurodegenerative pathophysiology.[43] Emerging evidence shows microbiome disruption may play a role in neurodegenerative diseases such as Alzheimer's and Parkinson's diseases.[44,45] Dietary and nutritional approaches to promote healthy microbiome function to protect against gut-induced mechanisms of protein aggregate accumulation have been reported in the literature as a potential therapeutic strategy.[46,47] Functional medicine approaches to chronic diseases always emphasize a healthy diet to optimize a healthy microbiome population and enhance intestinal impermeability. Dietary strategies to optimize healthy gut bacteria populations include the consumption of high fiber, prebiotics, probiotics, and nutraceuticals.

Box 1
Clinical strategies used in functional medicine approaches to neurodegeneration

Caloric modification

Intermittent fasting

Antiinflammatory diet to reduce neuroinflammation

Low-carbohydrate diet to manage insulin resistance

Diverse fiber diet to support microbiome diversity

Ketogenic diet to reduce glycemic metabolism

Physical exercise

Cognitive exercises (puzzles, word searches, Sudoku, chess)

Specific food restrictions based on dietary protein immune reactivity (IgG and or IgE)

Nutraceuticals to support microbiome health (prebiotics, probiotics, digestive enzymes)

Nutraceuticals to dampen neuroinflammation (omega 3, flavonoids, botanicals)

Nutraceuticals to support hepatic biotransformation and oxidative stress

Air filters to improve air quality

Reduction in household chemicals

Sleep hygiene interventions

Consistent feeding, exercise, and sleep schedules to establish circadian rhythms

Hormone replacement therapy

Management of acute and chronic infections

Conventional medications to address underlying risk factors

BLOOD GLUCOSE STABILITY

Stable blood sugar levels and proper insulin signaling are essential for healthy brain function. Hyperinsulinemia and insulin resistance in both peripheral and brain receptors have been implicated in the development of Alzheimer's disease and neurodegenerative diseases.[48] Insulin under normal conditions impacts cerebral bioenergetics, neurotransmitter synthesis and turnover, synaptic activity, and dendritic spine formations necessary for healthy brain function. In states of hyperinsulinemia due to excessive sugar and carbohydrate consumption, these functions are impaired, promoting unhealthy hyperphosphorylation of tau.[49] Functional medicine approaches to neurodegenerative disorders include a comprehensive evaluation for dysglycemia and clinical strategies with diet, lifestyle, medications, and target nutraceuticals to optimize glucose and insulin levels.[50]

MICROGLIA ACTIVATION AND NEUROINFLAMMATION

Neuroinflammation is a key feature of all neurodegenerative diseases and leads to neuronal injury and death. Systemic inflammatory triggers activate microglia in the brain, which promotes the development of protein aggregates in neurodegenerative diseases. Protein aggregates impair normal neuron signaling and activation leading to reduced neuronal metabolic activity, neuron atrophy, and neuron death.[51] Microglia-mediated inflammation is both a product of and a contributor to neurodegenerative disease. Protein aggregates developed from systemic inflammation trigger cellular mechanisms in a feedforward cycle to further activate microglia and increase neuroinflammation.[52] Increased microglia activation also leads to abnormal synaptic pruning. In normal conditions, microglia-mediated synaptic connections optimize synaptic efficiency. However, in pathologic conditions of heightened microglia activation, the microglia abnormally prune and damage essential circuits for healthy brain connectivity leading to further promotion of neurodegeneration.[53]

Clinical strategies to reduce the systemic inflammation that promotes microglia activation and to dampen neuroinflammation are essential functional medicine approaches. Mechanisms such as microbiome dysbiosis, intestinal permeability, blood–brain barrier permeability, chronic infection, dietary protein reactivities, environmental pollutant exposures, reduced antioxidant status, and hyperinsulinism are all variables that can activate microglia and perpetuate neuroinflammation.[54–61] A functional medicine model evaluates and manages each of these physiologic variables to reduce physiologic triggers that activate microglia inflammatory pathways. Additionally, this model may employ the use of protective and antiinflammatory targeted nutraceuticals, including omega-3 oils, flavonoids (resveratrol, quercetin, green tea, and so forth), and botanicals such as baicalin, huperzine, and Ginkgo biloba. Numerous human clinical trials and meta-analyses have shown these natural compounds are effective in reducing neuroinflammation and improving brain function.[62–66]

SUMMARY

A functional medicine approach to neurodegenerative diseases uses various personalized strategies to address upstream risk factors (**Box 1**). The clinical model is preventive and emphasizes the individual rather than the disease. The model has limited impact on late-stage disease. Early identification and personalized strategies to reduce risk and improve brain function and health are hallmark features of a functional medicine approach. Clinical strategies vary from one individual to another even if the neurodegenerative disease is the same. Furthermore, clinical strategies are dynamic and may change over the lifespan of the patient. Functional medicine approaches are not generalizable for the specific disease itself. Individual symptoms, clinical signs, risk factors, biomarkers, and imaging studies are used as a baseline and constantly reevaluated during the course of treatment. The emphasis of a functional medicine model is to address upstream pathophysiological variables that increase the risk for proteinopathies and to improve general health and brain function. The functional medicine model can be used preventively or in combination with current standards of care.

CLINICS CARE POINTS

- Early identification and strategies to reduce risk factors are essential in the management of neurodegenerative diseases.
- Clinical prognosis is poor in late-stage disease.
- Clinical factors that impact mitochondria homeostasis, gut–brain axis, neuroinflammation, and blood glucose/insulin are essential to modify.
- Functional medicine models can be used as preventive models or used in combination with current standards of care.

REFERENCES

1. Alzheimer's disease facts and figures [published online ahead of print, 2020 Mar 10]. Alzheimers Dement 2020. https://doi.org/10.1002/alz.12068.
2. Hou Y, Dan X, Babbar M, et al. Ageing as a risk factor for neurodegenerative disease. Nat Rev Neurol 2019;15(10):565–81.
3. Grabher BJ. Effects of Alzheimer Disease on Patients and Their Family. J Nucl Med Technol 2018;46(4):335–40.
4. Dugger BN, Dickson DW. Pathology of Neurodegenerative Diseases. Cold Spring Harb Perspect Biol 2017;9(7):a028035.
5. Liu PP, Xie Y, Meng XY, et al. History and progress of hypotheses and clinical trials for Alzheimer's disease. Signal Transduct Target Ther 2019;(4):37. https://doi.org/10.1038/s41392-019-0063-8.
6. Hampel H, Caraci F, Cuello AC, et al. A Path Toward Precision Medicine for Neuroinflammatory Mechanisms in Alzheimer's Disease. Front Immunol 2020;11:456. https://doi.org/10.3389/fimmu.2020.00456.
7. Fotuhi M, Lubinski B, Trullinger M, et al. A Personalized 12-week "Brain Fitness Program" for Improving Cognitive Function and Increasing the Volume of Hippocampus in Elderly with Mild Cognitive Impairment. J Prev Alzheimers Dis 2016; 3(3):133–7.
8. Bredesen DE. Reversal of cognitive decline: a novel therapeutic program. Aging (Albany NY) 2014;6(9):707–17.
9. Schneider J, Joen D, Gladman J, et al. The Alzheimer's disease-releated dementias summit. National Institute of Neurological Disorders and Stroke 2019.
10. Lane CA, Hardy J, Schott JM. Alzheimer's disease. Eur J Neurol 2018;25(1): 59–70.
11. Sweeney MD, Sagare AP, Zlokovic BV. Blood-brain barrier breakdown in Alzheimer disease and other neurodegenerative disorders. Nat Rev Neurol 2018; 14(3):133–50.
12. Phatnani H, Maniatis T. Astrocytes in neurodegenerative disease. Cold Spring Harb Perspect Biol 2015;7(6):a020628.
13. Xu L, He D, Bai Y. Microglia-Mediated Inflammation and Neurodegenerative Disease. Mol Neurobiol 2016;53(10):6709–15.
14. Golpich M, Amini E, Mohamed Z, et al. Mitochondrial Dysfunction and Biogenesis in Neurodegenerative diseases: Pathogenesis and Treatment. CNS Neurosci Ther 2017;23(1):5–22.
15. Ghaisas S, Maher J, Kanthasamy A. Gut microbiome in health and disease: Linking the microbiome-gut-brain axis and environmental factors in the pathogenesis of systemic and neurodegenerative diseases. Pharmacol Ther 2016;158:52–62.
16. Colucci-D'Amato L, Speranza L, Volpicelli F. Neurotrophic Factor BDNF, Physiological Functions and Therapeutic Potential in Depression, Neurodegeneration and Brain Cancer. Int J Mol Sci 2020;21(20):7777.
17. Ciccocioppo F, Bologna G, Ercolino E, et al. Neurodegenerative diseases as proteinopathies-driven immune disorders. Neural Regen Res 2020;15(5):850–6.
18. Lin MT, Beal MF. Mitochondrial dysfunction and oxidative stress in neurodegenerative diseases. Nature 2006;443(7113):787–95.
19. Wu Y, Chen M, Jiang J. Mitochondrial dysfunction in neurodegenerative diseases and drug targets via apoptotic signaling. Mitochondrion 2019;49:35–45. https://doi.org/10.1016/j.mito.2019.07.003.
20. Benaroya H. Brain energetics, mitochondria, and traumatic brain injury. Rev Neurosci 2020;31(4):363–90.

21. Akbari M, Kirkwood TBL, Bohr VA. Mitochondria in the signaling pathways that control longevity and health span. Ageing Res Rev 2019;54:100940. https://doi.org/10.1016/j.arr.2019.100940.

22. Raefsky SM, Mattson MP. Adaptive responses of neuronal mitochondria to bioenergetic challenges: Roles in neuroplasticity and disease resistance. Free Radic Biol Med 2017;102:203–16. https://doi.org/10.1016/j.freeradbiomed.2016.11.045.

23. Memme JM, Erlich AT, Phukan G, et al. Exercise and mitochondrial health. J Physiol 2021;599(3):803–17.

24. Valenzuela MJ, Matthews FE, Brayne C, et al. Multiple biological pathways link cognitive lifestyle to protection from dementia. Biol Psychiatry 2012;71(9):783–91.

25. Gaignard P, Liere P, Thérond P, et al. Role of Sex Hormones on Brain Mitochondrial Function, with Special Reference to Aging and Neurodegenerative Diseases. Front Aging Neurosci 2017;9:406. https://doi.org/10.3389/fnagi.2017.00406.

26. Chodari L, Dilsiz Aytemir M, Vahedi P, et al. Targeting Mitochondrial Biogenesis with Polyphenol Compounds. Oxid Med Cell Longev 2021;2021:4946711. https://doi.org/10.1155/2021/4946711.

27. Potì F, Santi D, Spaggiari G, et al. Polyphenol Health Effects on Cardiovascular and Neurodegenerative Disorders: A Review and Meta-Analysis. Int J Mol Sci 2019;20(2):351.

28. von Bernhardi R, Eugenín J. Alzheimer's disease: redox dysregulation as a common denominator for diverse pathogenic mechanisms. Antioxid Redox Signal 2012;16(9):974–1031.

29. Wadhwa R, Gupta R, Maurya PK. Oxidative Stress and Accelerated Aging in Neurodegenerative and Neuropsychiatric Disorder. Curr Pharm Des 2018;24(40):4711–25.

30. Ullah A, Munir S, Badshah SL, et al. Important Flavonoids and Their Role as a Therapeutic Agent. Molecules 2020;25(22):5243.

31. Jiang Q, Yin J, Chen J, et al. Mitochondria-Targeted Antioxidants: A Step towards Disease Treatment. Oxid Med Cell Longev 2020;2020:8837893. https://doi.org/10.1155/2020/8837893.

32. Pahrudin Arrozi A, Wan Ngah WZ, Mohd Yusof YA, et al. Antioxidant modulation in restoring mitochondrial function in neurodegeneration. Int J Neurosci 2017;127(3):218–35.

33. Siddiqui AN, Siddiqui N, Khan RA, et al. Neuroprotective Role of Steroidal Sex Hormones: An Overview. CNS Neurosci Ther 2016;22(5):342–50.

34. Pugazhenthi S, Qin L, Reddy PH. Common neurodegenerative pathways in obesity, diabetes, and Alzheimer's disease. Biochim Biophys Acta Mol Basis Dis 2017;1863(5):1037–45.

35. Pasinetti GM, Zhao Z, Qin W, et al. Caloric intake and Alzheimer's disease. Experimental approaches and therapeutic implications. Interdiscip Top Gerontol 2007;35:159–75. https://doi.org/10.1159/000096561.

36. Wang J, Ho L, Qin W, et al. Caloric restriction attenuates beta-amyloid neuropathology in a mouse model of Alzheimer's disease. FASEB J 2005;19(6):659–61.

37. Bagherniya M, Butler AE, Barreto GE, et al. The effect of fasting or calorie restriction on autophagy induction: A review of the literature. Ageing Res Rev 2018;47:183–97. https://doi.org/10.1016/j.arr.2018.08.004.

38. Baik SH, Rajeev V, Fann DY, et al. Intermittent fasting increases adult hippocampal neurogenesis. Brain Behav 2020;10(1):e01444.

39. Musiek ES, Holtzman DM. Mechanisms linking circadian clocks, sleep, and neurodegeneration. Science 2016;354(6315):1004–8.
40. Bonaconsa M, Colavito V, Pifferi F, et al. Cell clocks and neuronal networks: neuron ticking and synchronization in aging and aging-related neurodegenerative disease. Curr Alzheimer Res 2013;10(6):597–608.
41. Chang YC, Kim JY. Therapeutic implications of circadian clocks in neurodegenerative diseases. J Neurosci Res 2020;98(6):1095–113.
42. Dinan TG, Cryan JF. Gut instincts: microbiota as a key regulator of brain development, ageing and neurodegeneration. J Physiol 2017;595(2):489–503.
43. Rutsch A, Kantsjö JB, Ronchi F. The Gut-Brain Axis: How Microbiota and Host Inflammasome Influence Brain Physiology and Pathology. Front Immunol 2020;11: 604179. https://doi.org/10.3389/fimmu.2020.604179.
44. Goyal D, Ali SA, Singh RK. Emerging role of gut microbiota in modulation of neuroinflammation and neurodegeneration with emphasis on Alzheimer's disease. Prog Neuropsychopharmacol Biol Psychiatry 2021;106:110112. https://doi.org/ 10.1016/j.pnpbp.2020.110112.
45. Marogianni C, Sokratous M, Dardiotis E, et al. Neurodegeneration and Inflammation-An Interesting Interplay in Parkinson's Disease. Int J Mol Sci 2020;21(22):8421.
46. Uyar GÖ, Yildiran H. A nutritional approach to microbiota in Parkinson's disease. Biosci Microbiota Food Health 2019;38(4):115–27.
47. Wang Q, Luo Y, Ray Chaudhuri K, et al. The role of gut dysbiosis in Parkinson's disease: mechanistic insights and therapeutic options. Brain 2021;144(9): 2571–93.
48. Kellar D, Craft S. Brain insulin resistance in Alzheimer's disease and related disorders: mechanisms and therapeutic approaches. Lancet Neurol 2020;19(9): 758–66.
49. Neumann KF, Rojo L, Navarrete LP, et al. Insulin resistance and Alzheimer's disease: molecular links & clinical implications. Curr Alzheimer Res 2008;5(5): 438–47.
50. Liang Y, Xu X, Yin M, et al. Effects of berberine on blood glucose in patients with type 2 diabetes mellitus: a systematic literature review and a meta-analysis. Endocr J 2019;66(1):51–63.
51. Marsh AP. Molecular mechanisms of proteinopathies across neurodegenerative disease: a review. Neurol Res Pract 2019;1:35. https://doi.org/10.1186/s42466-019-0039-8.
52. Nichols MR, St-Pierre MK, Wendeln AC, et al. Inflammatory mechanisms in neurodegeneration. J Neurochem 2019;149(5):562–81.
53. Ho MS. Microglia in Parkinson's Disease. Adv Exp Med Biol 2019;1175:335–53.
54. Glass CK, Saijo K, Winner B, et al. Mechanisms underlying inflammation in neurodegeneration. Cell 2010;140(6):918–34.
55. Ray R, Juranek JK, Rai V. RAGE axis in neuroinflammation, neurodegeneration and its emerging role in the pathogenesis of amyotrophic lateral sclerosis. Neurosci Biobehav Rev 2016;62:48–55.
56. Stolp HB, Dziegielewska KM. Review: Role of developmental inflammation and blood-brain barrier dysfunction in neurodevelopmental and neurodegenerative diseases. Neuropathol Appl Neurobiol 2009;35(2):132–46.
57. Calderón-Garcidueñas L, Leray E, Heydarpour P, et al. Air pollution, a rising environmental risk factor for cognition, neuroinflammation and neurodegeneration: The clinical impact on children and beyond. Rev Neurol (Paris) 2016;172(1): 69–80.

58. McGrattan AM, McGuinness B, McKinley MC, et al. Diet and Inflammation in Cognitive Ageing and Alzheimer's Disease. Curr Nutr Rep 2019;8(2):53–65.

59. Więckowska-Gacek A, Mietelska-Porowska A, Wydrych M, et al. Western diet as a trigger of Alzheimer's disease: From metabolic syndrome and systemic inflammation to neuroinflammation and neurodegeneration. Ageing Res Rev 2021;70: 101397. https://doi.org/10.1016/j.arr.2021.101397.

60. Rakic S, Hung YMA, Smith M, et al. Systemic infection modifies the neuroinflammatory response in late stage Alzheimer's disease. Acta Neuropathol Commun 2018;6(1):88.

61. Pennisi M, Crupi R, Di Paola R, et al. Inflammasomes, hormesis, and antioxidants in neuroinflammation: Role of NRLP3 in Alzheimer disease. J Neurosci Res 2017; 95(7):1360–72.

62. Canhada S, Castro K, Perry IS, et al. Omega-3 fatty acids' supplementation in Alzheimer's disease: A systematic review. Nutr Neurosci 2018;21(8):529–38.

63. Calis Z, Mogulkoc R, Baltaci AK. The Roles of Flavonols/Flavonoids in Neurodegeneration and Neuroinflammation. Mini Rev Med Chem 2020;20(15):1475–88.

64. Guo LT, Wang SQ, Su J, et al. Baicalin ameliorates neuroinflammation-induced depressive-like behavior through inhibition of toll-like receptor 4 expression via the PI3K/AKT/FoxO1 pathway. J Neuroinflammation 2019;16(1):95.

65. Yang G, Wang Y, Tian J, et al. Huperzine A for Alzheimer's disease: a systematic review and meta-analysis of randomized clinical trials. PLoS One 2013;8(9): e74916.

66. Liao Z, Cheng L, Li X, et al. Meta-analysis of Ginkgo biloba Preparation for the Treatment of Alzheimer's Disease. Clin Neuropharmacol 2020;43(4):93–9.

Moving?

Make sure your subscription moves with you!

To notify us of your new address, find your **Clinics Account Number** (located on your mailing label above your name), and contact customer service at:

Email: journalscustomerservice-usa@elsevier.com

800-654-2452 (subscribers in the U.S. & Canada)
314-447-8871 (subscribers outside of the U.S. & Canada)

Fax number: 314-447-8029

Elsevier Health Sciences Division
Subscription Customer Service
3251 Riverport Lane
Maryland Heights, MO 63043

*To ensure uninterrupted delivery of your subscription, please notify us at least 4 weeks in advance of move.

Printed and bound by CPI Group (UK) Ltd, Croydon, CR0 4YY

03/10/2024

01040477-0020